Introduction to Plastic, Reconstructive and Microsurgery of Female Genitalia

Introduction to Plastic, Reconstructive and Microsurgery of Female Genitalia

Vishwa Prakash
MBBS, MS (Surgery), MCh (Plastic Surgery)
Ex Unit Head Plastic Surgery, Safdarjung Hospital and VMMC, New Delhi

Neeta Garg (Prakash)
MBBS, DGO
Ex Consultant, Flowerida Hospital
Agra

PEEPEE
PUBLISHERS and DISTRIBUTORS (P) LTD.

Introduction to Plastic, Reconstructive and Microsurgery of Female Genitalia

Published by
Pawaninder P. Vij
Peepee Publishers and Distributors (P) Ltd.
Head Office: 160, Shakti Vihar, Pitam Pura,
Delhi-110 034
Corporate Office: 7/31, Ansari Road, Daryaganj,
Post Box-7243, New Delhi-110002 (India)
Ph: 55195868, 9811156083
e-mail: peepee160@yahoo.co.in
e-mail: peepee160@rediffmail.com

First Edition: **2005**

ISBN: 81-88867-43-8

Printed at
Lordson, C-5/19, Rana Pratap Bagh, Delhi-110 007

Preface

This book would prove of immense benefit to the gynaecologists interested in plastic surgical procedures of female genitalia as well as the plastic surgeons interested in this field. Authors have tried to introduce the subject in easy way. Many a times the readers, both gynaecologists and as well plastic surgeons would come across the procedures, which they will think, Oh, it can also be done, or Oh, it can be done in this way. At places authors have described their techniques also which they have described after a long experience. Apart from authors' techniques all other procedures have been taken from standard Textbooks.

Vishwa Prakash
Neeta Garg (Prakash)

Contents

1

Anatomy of Female Genitalia

Female genitalia are divided into internal and external genitalia.

The internal genitalia are: The ovaries, uterine tubes, uterus and vagina.

The external genitalia are: mons, labia majora, labia minora, clitoris, bulb of the vestibule, greater vestibular glands and the vestibule itself.

Ovaries

- Paired structures.
- Situated one on each side of the uterus close to the lateral pelvic wall.
- These are attached to the posterior aspect of the broad uterine ligament of the uterus near its upper limit by a double fold of peritoneum—the mesovarium.
- Each ovary is 3 cm long, 1.5 cm wide and 1 cm thick, with a volume of about 6 cm.
- Ovarian fimbria of the uterine tube are attached to its upper tubal extremity.
- The uterine extremity is directed downwards towards the pelvic floor, and is attached to the lateral angle of the uterus by ovarian ligament.

Vessels

Ovary is supplied by ovarian artery and tubal branch of uterine artery.

- Ovarian arteries arise from aorta and at barium of lesser pelvic crosses the lower external iliac artery and vein to enter the true pelvic cavity.

- These then turn medially in the ovarian suspensory ligament and continue into the uterine broad ligament, below the uterine tune.
- At ovarian level the artery passes back in the mesovarium and divides into branches to the ovary.
- One of the branch passes to the side of uterus to units with uterine artery.
- Few other branches accompany the found ligament through the inguinal canal to the skin of the labia majora.
- Venous drainage is by pampiniform plexus which is drained by accompanying ovarian vein.

Uterine Tubes

Two uterine (fallopian tubes) lie on each side of the uterus in the upper margin of the broad ligament. Each tube is 10 cm long and opens medially into the uterine cavity and laterally into the peritoneal cavity near the ovary. It has four parts:

- Fimbriated end
- Ampulla
- Isthmus
- Intramural portion.

Fimbriated end: It is formed by a funnel like expansion of the uterus tube, which is called infundibulum. Many finger like processes emerge from infundibulum and are known as fimbriae. All fimbriae are lined by ciliated mucosa, which has longitudinal folds continuous with those in infundibulum. The deeply situated aperture within infundibulum is about 3 mm wide when relaxed.

Ampulla

It is expanded region of the tube. It has a thin wall and a tortuously folded luminal surface marked by 4-5 major longitudinal ridges, on which lie large number of secondary plicae, creating an extensive surface area. The widest luminal diameter is about 1 cm.

Isthmus

This part of the tube is rounded, muscular and firm and forms approximately its medial third. Its lumen is narrow and has from three to four major plicae.

Intramural Part

Lying within the wall of the uterus, it is about 1 cm long. It opens into the main cavity of the uterus near its upper end at the uterine cornu.

Microstructure of the Uterine Tube

The tube has:

- Internal mucosa,
- Intermediate muscular stratum, and
- External serosa.

Tubal mucosa is covered by folded simple ciliated and secretory epithelium.

Muscular layer is composed of external longitudinal and internal circular layers of smooth muscles.

Serosa is peritoneum with adjacent connective tissue, and is continuous with broad ligament.

Vessels

The vessels of the uterine tube arise from ovarian and uterine stems. Uterine artery usually supplies the medial two-thirds of the tube, and ovarian supplies lateral-third of the tube.

Uterus

The uterus is a hollow, thick-walled and muscular organ, situated in lesser pelvis between the urinary bladder and rectum. In adults nulliparous it is pear shaped, being about 7.5 cm long .5 cm wide and 2.5 cm thick. It is divided into body of uterus and cervix.

Uterine body narrows from the fundus down to internal os. Its anterior surface is covered by the peritoneum which is rejected on the bladder as the uterovesical fold. The posterior surface of the uterus is convex transversely. Its peritoneal covering continuous down to cervix and upper vagina and is reflected back to the rectum. The lateral margins of the body are convex, and on each side their peritoneum is reflected laterally to form the broad ligament, extending as a flat sheet to the pelvic wall.

The length of uterine cavity measures about 6 cm from the external os to the wall of the fundus.

Cervix is about 2.5 cm long in adult. It is divided into-supravaginal part of the cervix and vaginal part.

The supravaginal part of the cervix is separated in front from bladder by cellular connective tissue—The parametrium, which passes also to the sides of cervix and laterally between the two layers of the broad ligament. The uterine arteries flank the cervix in this tissue and ureters descend forward in it about 2 cm from the cervix.

The vaginal part of the cervix projects as a convex disc on to the anterior vaginal wall, forming grooves; known as vaginal fornices.

Vessels of the Uterus

The main arterial supply to the whole uterus is through the uterine branch of the internal iliac artery on each side. It anastomoses with the ovarian and vaginal arteries. The paired uterine arteries anastomose extensively with each other across the mid line. Each uterine artery gives numerous branches which immediately enter the uterine wall.

Vagina

The vagina is a fibromuscular tube lined by non-keratinized stratified epithelium. The inner surfaces of vaginal wall are ordinarily in contact with each other. Its anterior wall is 7.5 cm in length, the posterior 10 cm; its width, increases as it ascends. Its upper end surrounds the vaginal portion of the cervix uterine near the external os.

The lower vagina is surrounded by the skeletal muscle fibres of the bublospongiosus muscle.

The bulbospongiosus muscle covers the superficial parts of the vestibular bulbs and greater vestibular glands and passes forwards on each side of the vagina to attach to the corpora cavernous clitoridis. It is attached posteriorly to the perineal body, where its fibres decussate with those of sphincter ani externi and the contralateral transverse perinei. The action of the muscle is constriction of the vaginal orifice and expression of the secretions of the greater vestibular glands.

Vessels

Arterial supply is from vaginal, uterine, internal pudendal and middle rectal branches of the internal iliac arteries.

Mons Pubis

Rounded eminence situated anterior to the pubic symphysis, formed by a mass of the subcutaneous adipose connective tissue, covered by coarse hair limited above by horizontal boundary.

Labia Majora

There are two prominent, longitudinal, cutaneous folds extending back from the mons pubis to the perineum, from the lateral boundaries of the pudendal cleft, into which the vaginal and urethra opens.

The labia are thicker in front where they join to form the anterior commissure, posteriorly they don't join but merge into neighbouring skin forming posterior commissure, which overlies the perineal body, being posterior limit of the vulva.

Labia Minora

There are two small cutaneous folds, devoid of fat, between the labia majora, extend from the clitoris obliquely down, laterally and back for about 4 cm, flanking the vaginal orifice. In virgins their posterior ends may be joined by the cutaneous frenulum of the labia minora. Anteriorly each labium minus bifurcates, its upper layer passing above the clitoris to from with its fellow, a fold-prepuce. The lower layer passes below the clitoris to form with its fellow the frenulum clitoridis. Sometimes an extra labial fold (labium tertinum) is found on one or both sides between labia minora and majora.

Vestibule

The cavity lies between the labia minora and contains the vaginal and external urethral orifices and the openings of the two greater vestibular glands. Between the vaginal orifice and the frenulum of labia minora is a shallow vestibular fossa.

Clitoris

It is an erectile structure homologous with the penis, partially enclosed by the anterior, bifurcated ends of the labia minora. It has corpora cavernous and glans clitoridis.

Introitus

It is usually a sagittal slit, whose size varies inversely with that of hymen like vagina. It is capable of great distension during parturition and coitus.

Hymen Vaginae

It is a thin fold of mucosa membrane situated just within the vaginal orifice; the internal surfaces of the fold are normally folded to contact each other and the vaginal orifice appears as a cleft between them when it is ruptured, small found carunculae hymenales are left behind.

2

Anatomy and Physiology of Vagina

Vagina is the passageway between the vulva and uterine cervix referred as a potential space. In its resting state it is collapsed with anterior and posterior walls touching one another.

EMBRYOLOGY

The urethra and vagina have similar embryological origins. The epithelium of the female urethra is entirely derived from endoderm of the urogenital sinus, while the fibro-muscular layer is derived from surrounding splanchnic mesenchyme. The epithelium of the vagina is also derived from surrounding urogenital sinus endoderm.

Contact of the urovaginal primordium with the urogenital sinus induces formation of paired endodermal outgrowths, sinovaginal bulbs. These bulbs proliferate and fuse to form the vaginal plate. The vaginal plate elongates between the urogenital sinus and the caudal uterovaginal primordium and invades the latter upto the level of the future cervix. Central cells of the vaginal plate subsequently degenerate and form a vaginal lumen lined with the epithelium of sinus endoderm.

The fibromuscular layers of the vagina are derived from surrounding splanchnic mesenchyme.

ANATOMY

The vagina is a fibromuscular tubal structure bounded anteriorly by the bladder and urethra and posteriorly by the rectum. It extends from the vestibule to the cervix and is referred as a potential space because while in resting position, the anterior and posterior walls are in apposition to one another.

The vagina is lined by stratified squamous epithelium which thickens with hormonal stimulation. This thickened epithelium forms transverse folds or rugae. Underlying the epithelium is the lamina propria which contains a dense network of elastic fibres. Collagen fibres extend from the elastic fibres to the underlying muscular layers.

The muscular layer has been described as a bilayer of smooth muscles. Cranially, the muscle fibres merge into the myometrium. In the lower vagina, the smooth muscle is reinforced by striated muscle fibres which enclose caudal half of urethra and terminate in the lateral and posterior vaginal walls forming the urethrovaginal sphincter. The vagina's muscular layer is surrounded by the perivaginal portion of the endopelvic fascia.

Master and Johnson described that the unstimulated vagina has a length of 7-8 cm from forchette to the posterior fornix and transcervical width of 2 cm. With sexual arousal, the vagina is capable of significant enlargement. There is involuntary lengthening and distension of the inner two thirds of the vaginal barrel such that length increases by as much as 5 cm and the transcervical width increases by as much as 5.5 cm. The vagina's outer third distends minimally during early sexual arousal, but eventually becomes grossly engorged due to vasocongestion, reducing the outer luminal size and forming the orgasmic platform.

VAGINAL SUPPORT

The support to the vagina is formed by endopelvic fascia, the pelvic diaphragm, and the urogenital diaphragm.

The endopelvic fascia consists of the reflections of the superior fascia of the pelvic diaphragm on the urethra and bladder, the vagina and lower uterus, and the rectum. Fibrous connections between these reflections are from anteriorly, the pubovesicocervical fascia, and posteriorly the rectovaginal septum. The pubovesicocervical fascia extends from the symphysis pubis and from tendinous arch to insert onto the cervix at the level of internal os, therefore running the entire length of the anterior vaginal wall. The rectovaginal septum on the other hand, covers the middle two thirds of the posterior vaginal wall superiorly blending with the cardinal-uterosacral ligament and inferiorly with the perineal body. The upper 2-3 cm of the posterior vagina is covered on its outer surface by the peritoneum of the pouch of Douglas. The lower posterior vaginal wall and rectum diverge and are separated by the muscles of the perineal body.

Further support of the vagina, along with the urethra, bladder and rectum is provided by the pelvic diaphragm and urogenital diaphragm.

Pelvic diaphragm is composed of levator ani, the coccygeus, the obturator internus and piriformis muscles while the urogenital diaphragm lies external and inferior to levator ani and composed of the striated muscles (Fig. 2.1).

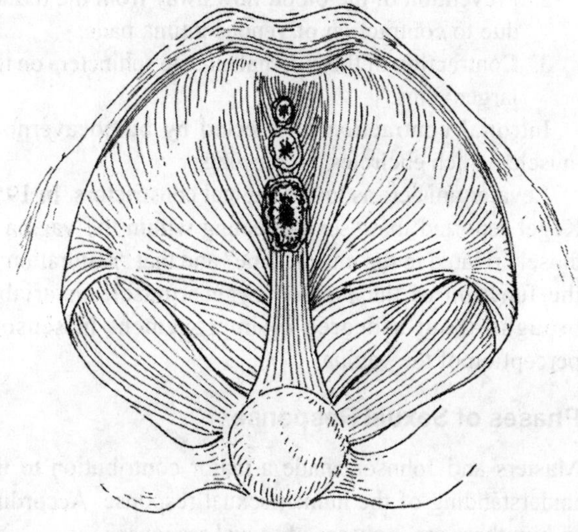

Fig. 2.1: The pelvic diaphragm, composed of the levator ani, the coccygeus, the obturator internus, and piriformis muscles. The levator ani, consisting of the medial pubococcygeus and the lateral iliococcygeus, are divided in the midline by the interlevator cleft through which pass the urethra, vagina and rectum

SEXUAL PHYSIOLOGY

Vaginal Pressure Areas

Masters and Johnson asserted that the vagina provides the "primary means of heterosexual expression of the human female". It undergoes marked physical changes in response to psychogenic and somatogenic erotic stimuli. It can also impart as well as mediate perception of intensely pleasurable erotic sensation during coitus by virtue of its pressure areas.

The outer third of the vagina constricts and generates increased pressure both voluntarily and involuntarily during arousal and orgasmic response. The constriction occurs by

- Introital and lower vaginal muscle contractions.
- Vasocongestion of erectile genital tissues.
- Vasocongestion is caused by
  1. Relaxation of the arterial intima pads allowing increased blood flow into the cavernous bodies.
  2. Prevention of the blood flow away from the tissues due to contraction of venous intima pads.
  3. Contraction of the external muscle sphincters on the larger veins.

Introital contraction is effected by bulbocavernous muscle, which encircles the introitus.

Levator ani acts as lower vaginal constrictors. In 1952 Kegel reported that "sexual feeling within the vagina is closely related to the muscle tone" and that "restoration of the function of the pubococcygeus muscle invariably brought about a degree of improvement in sensory perception of the vagina.

Phases of Sexual Response

Masters and Johnson made a major contribution to the understanding of the human sexual response. According to him there are 3 phases of sexual response.

1. *Excitation and plateau phase:* In this phase, there is arousal in response to psychogenic or somatogenic stimuli. This is manifested by
   - in the vagina by lubrication
   - lengthening of the inner two thirds of the vagina and widening and the expansion of the transcervical diameter
   - vasocongestion and swelling of the outer third of the vagina, to the extent that the central lumen is markedly reduced.

2. *Orgasmic phase:* During this phase
   - Inner two thirds of the vagina remain expanded
   - Outer third goes a series of regular involuntary contractions. These orgasmic contractions involve all muscles of the urogenital diaphragm as well as levator ani
   - Vaginal and anal orgasmic contractions occur simultaneously with the anal contractions having greater amplitude than vaginal contractions. It is due to the fact that fibres of iliococcygeus muscles interdigitate with external anal sphincter.
3. *Resolution phase:* During this phase
   - vasocongestion regresses
   - the diameter of the outer lumen increases
   - the expansion of inner two thirds decreases.

VAGINAL VERSUS CLITORAL ORGASM

Freud postulated that there are two types of female oragsms—vaginal and clitoral. However Masters and Johnson asserted that clitoris is the centre of female sensual focus and all orgasmic responses result either from direct or indirect clitoral stimulation. The relative lack of vaginal sensory innervation favours Masters and Johnson theory. Krantz did the microscopic studies of the vaginal nerve supply and revealed no mediators of touch or pressure within the vaginal walls. In contrast, clitoris contains both Meissner corpuscles and Merkel tactile discs. Kinsey found that vaginal walls are quite insensitive to touch while clitoral stimulation evoked intense and immediate erotic response.

Another proposed source of vaginal erotic sensitivity which sparked considerable controversy is the Grafenberg Spot (G-Spot). This erotically sensitive area palpable through the anterior vaginal wall has been suggested to be composed of periurethral glandular tissue homologous to the male prostate. Width digital or penile tactile stimulation through the anterior vaginal wall, this area, which was reported to range in diameter from 2-4 cm swells and is possibly the source of an ejaculatory release from the female urethra at the time of orgasm.

Few authors found that vagina is erotically sensitive through out the whole length of the anterior vaginal wall. In spite of the vaginal erotic sensitivity, the incidence of coital anorgasmia is quite high Alzat emphasizes the pressure exerted at an angle to the vaginal wall is necessary to most efficiently evoke erotic response. Coitus performed in missionary positional allows the penis to move parallel to the axis of the vagina, failing to adequately provide direct pressure to the anterior vaginal wall. Indeed, coitally orgasmic women have reported the most optimal coital positions to be the female superior and rear entry positions.

3

The Pubococcygeus Muscle

In women with pelvic relaxation there is usually associated damage to the pubococcygeus muscle. Examination reveals that this muscle is lax, atrophied, and of poor tone. Symptoms include urinary stress incontinence, genital prolapse, sexual problems, and rectal stasis.

Pelvic relaxation syndrome is a lifelong neuromuscular disorder that can be prevented or reversed by early recognition and treatment of pathological pubococcygeus muscle dysfunction.

Anatomy and Function of Pubococcygeus Muscle

Pubococcygeus muscle occupies the central location and has its origin in the arch of the os pubis and its insertion not only into the tip of coccyx but also into the intrinsic musculature of urethra, the vagina, and the rectum.

The muscle consists of heterogeneous population of large diameter, slow twitch (type 1) and fast twitch (type 2) muscle fibres. The predominance of the slow twitch, type 1 fibers suggests that the major role of the pubococcygeus muscle is to provide static visceral support. However, the significant number of fast twitch, type 2 fibres found in pubococcygeus indicate that this muscle also helps in maintenance of urethral, vaginal and rectal tone and assists in active closure of these structures.

The pubococcygeus muscle neuromuscular dysfunction can be prevented or reversed through muscle education and exercise.

ASSESSMENT OF THE FUNCTION

Inspection

In women with advanced relaxation:

- Perineum bulges downward
- The vaginal introitus opens
- Mucosa of vagina is exposed
- Anus appears everted.

On per speculum examination presence of cystocele, rectocele, and or prolapse can be determined by asking the patient to bear down.

Patient is asked to draw up, and the amount of upward movement of the perineum shows the function of the muscle.

Palpation

Vaginal palpation is done with index finger. A well developed pubococcygeus muscle is manifested by firm tone throughout the entire length of the vagina. In genital relaxation on the other hand, the vaginal walls offer little resistance and feel thin and loose as if detached from the surrounding structures (Fig. 3.1).

The muscle can be palpated on the lateral vaginal wall when the index finger is introduced to a depth of 3-5 cm

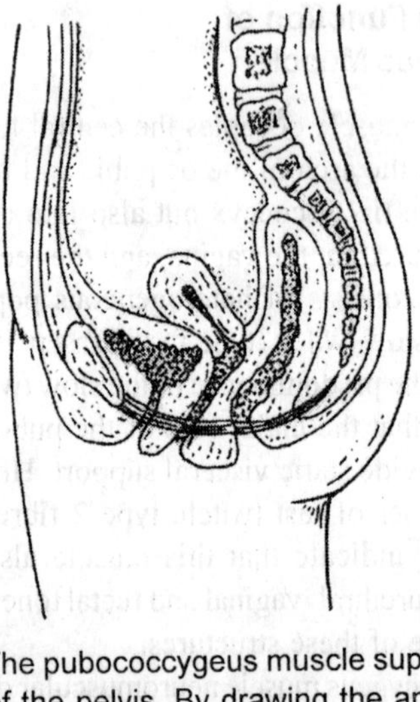

Fig. 3.1: The pubococcygeus muscle supports and raises the floor of the pelvis. By drawing the anus, vagina, and urethra toward the pubis, these structures are constricted and their sphincteric functions are enhanced

beyond the vaginal introitus. The muscle can be further demonstrated by asking the patient to contract it. This is done by asking the patient to pretend that they have to stop the urinary flow or contract the rectal sphincters.

Vaginal Pressure Manometry

Vaginal pressure manometry and physiotherapy of the pelvic floor muscles as treatment of urinary stress incontinence and pelvic relaxation syndrome was popularized by Dr. Arnold Kegel.

The perineometer is a pneumatic device designed to help the clinician assess pubococcygeus muscle strength, help women establish awareness of pubococcygeus function, and therapeutically exercise and strengthen this muscle. It consists of vaginal pressure sensor connected to a manometer calibrated from zero to 100 mmHg (Fig. 3.2).

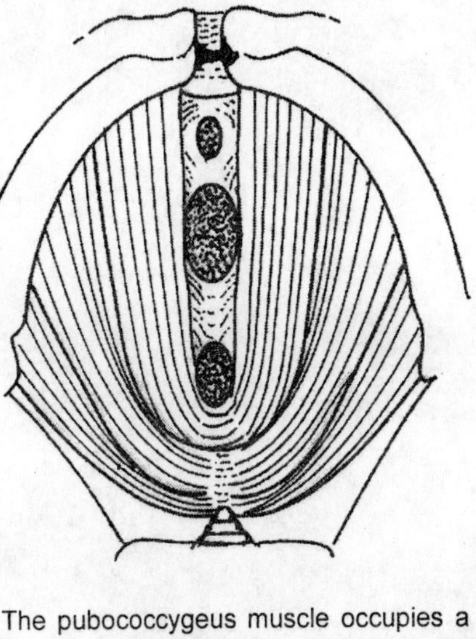

Fig. 3.2: The pubococcygeus muscle occupies a key position within the supporting musculofascial diaphragms that comprise the pelvic floor. Its origin is from the inner surface of the superior ramus of the pubis and the spine of the ischium and also from the connecting fascia (arcus tendinous ligament) which runs along the lateral wall. Its posterior fibers insert into the coccyx; the anterior fibers insert in the midline behind and in front of the anus, vagina, and urethra. A = urethra; B= vagina; C=anus; D = pubococcygeus muscle; E=iliococcygeus muscle; F=ischiococcygeus muscle

When the pressure sensor is introduced into the vagina and pelvic muscles are in a relaxed state, a static pressure reading between 15-20 mmHg indicates a normal pubococcygeus muscle resistance and normal vaginal tone. A static pressure reading of 10 mmHg or lower usually indicates poor muscle resistance and decreased vaginal tone.

Contraction of an intact, well developed pubococcygeus muscle can generate a pressure change of 20 mmHg or more above the initial static pressure.

The perineometer can also be used for starting the exercise of the pubococcygeus muscle.

4

Reconstructive Surgery of Vulva

ABNORMALITIES OF HYMEN

Imperforate Hymen

In this condition vaginal orifice is not patent but covered by hymen having no opening.

It is usually congenital condition but sometimes, though rarely, gonococcal vulvovaginitis of children may also lead to adhesions.

Clinical Features

Patient usually presents with:

- Delay in menses
- Pain in abdomen at monthly intervals
- Lump in abdomen
- On vaginal examination the imperforate hymen bulges externally and the retained dark colored blood can be seen through thin almost translucent septum.

Hematocolpos

It is the condition in which blood is collected in vagina as it can't escape outside. When condition is not relieved blood may be retained in uterus giving a lump like appearance, when it is called hematometra.

Diagnosis

1. Clinical
2. Ultrasound of abdomen.

Treatment

1. Under anaesthesia septum is excised and few sutures are placed.

2. Blood is evacuated from vagina.
3. Cervix should be examined, if it is closed, nothing further is required. If cervix is open a course of antibiotic is given, and patient kept under observation for disappearance of abdominal tumour.

Author's Modification

Author recommends that complete excision of hymen should not be done. It should be divided in central half and flaps so created are folded upon remaining hymen, after abrasion.

Advantage

As intact hymen is important sign of virginity, it should not be excised in toto. Preservation of hymen retains virginity.

Chronic Epithelial Dystrophy of the Vulva

These are:
- Simple atrophic vulvitis (kraurosis)
- Lichen scleroses
- Leukoplakia.

Kraurosis

It is a progressive sclerosing atrophy of the skin of the vulva. The clinical features are:
- Gradual narrowing of vaginal introitus.
- Labia minora, clitoris and frenulum together with the vestibule and urinary meatus are involved. These area become dry and shining. Color may vary from a waxy white or yellow to red.
- In late stages the vaginal orifice is so much narrowed that coitus becomes impossible.
- Disease is common in patients of menopausal or post menopausal age though it may occur in quite young women.

Treatment

- Bland local application such as zinc oxide ointment.
- Oestrogen cream can be used.
- If problem is disabling, plastic surgery may be done.

PLASTIC SURGERY

As affected skin lacks elastic tissue in dermis, it is to be excised in toto. After excision the area is to be resurfaced with flap. There are various flaps which can be used. Details are given in chapter for vaginal reconstruction.

Why flap cover and not skin graft or simple dressings

Flap cover is required because it has normal dermis with normal elastic tissue, which will not contract. Grafting or healing with second intention would result in severe contracture and recurrence of condition.

Lichen Sclerosis

Lichen sclerosis is an atrophic form of scleroderma.

- Starts as small flat very white papule, which fuse with similar other lesions.
- Spreads to perineal region and into genito-crural folds, thigh and buttock.
- As in kraurosis, labia minora, clitoris and sometimes introitus is involved resulting in dyspareunia.

Treatment

- Usual treatment is local application of steroids.
- If condition is very disabling excision of involved area and resurfacing with flap is advised.

Leukoplakia Vulvae

It is a condition in which the skin is thickened and indurated and patches of white skin are scattered irregularly over the vulva.

- Usually involves the labia majora, and sometimes labia minora.
- Rarely it extends beyond the perineum.
- The vestibule and the vaginal orifice are not involved.
- Symptoms are local discomfort, pruritus and discharge.

Treatment

Local excision and skin grafting.

Pruritus Vulvae

Pruritus vulvae is defined as irritation or pruritus of vulva. There are various causes of pruritus vulvae, which can be found in any textbook of gynecology.

Plastic Surgery in Pruritus Vulvae

Prolonged scratching for any reason produces lichenification of vulvae. Here comes the role of plastic surgery. After the primary cause has been removed, simple vulvectomy followed by flap cover is the treatment of choice.

Carcinoma of Vulva

Carcinoma of vulva is usually squamous cell carcinoma which spreads by lymphatics. Treatment is by radical vulvectomy with node dissection.

Role of Plastic Surgery

After vulvectomy area is resurfaced with skin graft. If vessels are exposed during node dissection one of many available flaps can be used like extended deep inferior epigastric artery flap from contralateral side.

Hidradenitis Suppurativa

In this condition apocrine sweat glands are infected and multiple pus discharging sinuses appear over vulva and mons pubis.

Treatment

Treatment of this condition is thorough removal of all sinuses along with skin. Resulting raw area is skin grafted.

Vulvodynia and Vestibulitis

Chronic vulvar pain was first described in the late 1800s as hyperesthesia by Skins. In 1984 the International society for the study of vulvar diseases published a standard definition for vulvodynia as chronic vulvar discomfort characterized by the patient's complaints of burning, stinging, irritation or rawness.

Friedrich defined a subset vestibulitis as:

- Severe pain on vestibular touch
- Introital dyspareunia
- Vestibular erythema of various degrees.

Treatment

1. Medical
    - Tricyclic antidepressants

Amitriptyline
10 mg/day
which can be increased to 100 mg/day.

2. Surgical
Surgical treatment is carried out if medical treatment fails.
Aim is to remove all sensitive vestibular tissue and resurfacing with flap.
Woodruff advised partial vestibulotomy (modified perineoplasty), where all the sensitive areas of the vestibule to a depth of 2 mm, as well as hymen is removed. He advised advancement of vaginal mucosa to cover the excised area.
Many other surgeons advocate excision of localized area of pain such as the posterior, lateral or anterior vestibule without advancement of the vagina (Figs 4.1 to 4.3).

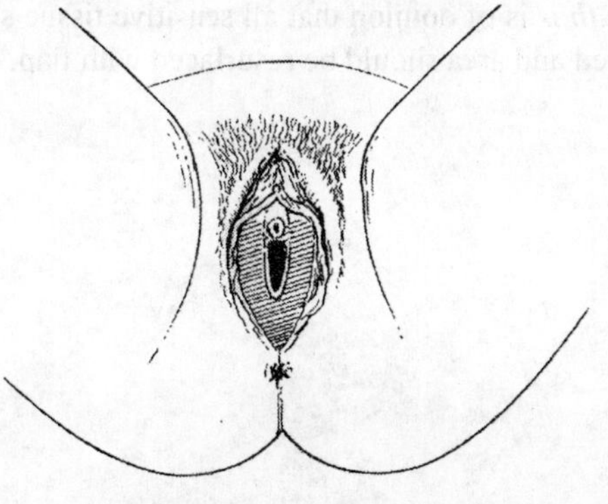

Fig. 4.1: Woodruff's perineoplasty—shaded area to be excised

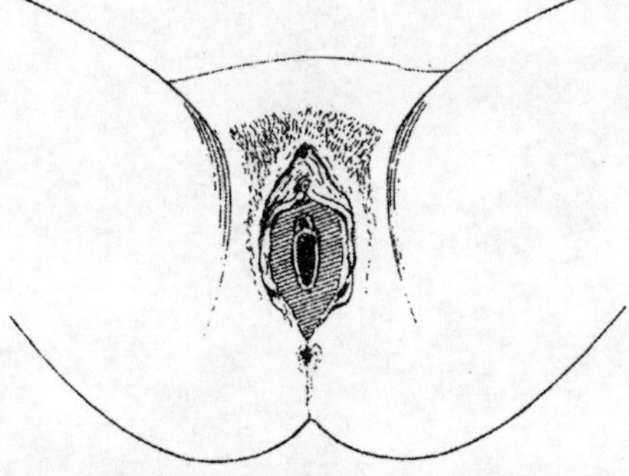

Fig. 4.2: Total vestibulectomy—shaded area to be excised

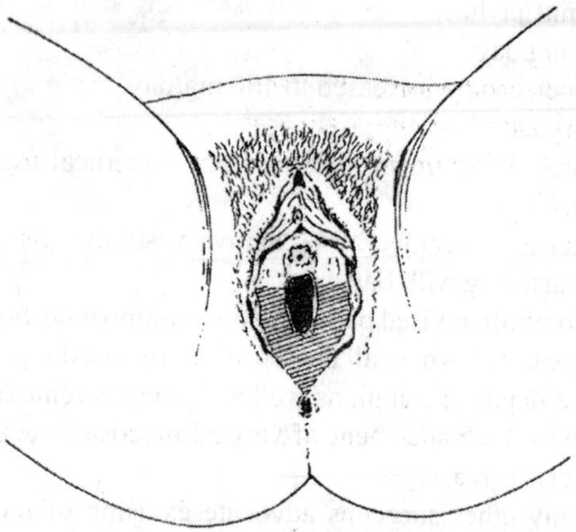

Fig. 4.3: Vestibulaplasty—shaded area to be excised

Author is of opinion that all sensitive tissue should be excised and area should be resurfaced with flap.

5

Reconstructive Surgery of Vagina

DYSPAREUNIA

Dyspareunia is defined as pain with intercourse. According to DSM IV, diagnostic criteria for dyspareunia are:

- Recurrent or persistent genital pain associated with sexual intercourse in either a male or a female.
- The disturbance causes marked distress or interpersonal difficulty.
- Not caused exclusively by vaginismus or lack of lubrication.

Clinically dyspareunia is divided into:

Superficial or Entry: Pain associated with attempted penetration, usually as a result of irritation or anatomical factors.

Vaginal: Pain related to lubrication/friction problems, often due to atrophy or medication; arousal disorders are included in this category.

Deep: Pain related to thrusting, often related to pelvic disease, anatomic distortion or relaxation.

Physical Examination

a. External genitalia
   - Assess muscle tone—Vaginismus
   - Skin color/texture—Vulvar dystrophy
   - Q tip test vestibule —Vestibulitis
   - Examine posterior forchette and hymenal ring—Episiotomy scars and strictures.

b. Manual examination
   - Palpate rectovaginal surface—Rectal disease
   - Palpate levator ani—Levator ani myalgia and vaginismus

- Palpate bladder/urethra—Urethritis
- Cervical motion tenderness—Infection
- Assess vaginal depth—Postoperative changes and stricture formation
- Palpate uterus/adnexa
  - Retroversion
  - Endometritis
  - Masses

c. Speculum examination
Vaginal discharge—Vaginitis
Vaginal mucosa—Atrophy

Management

Here we would limit to plastic surgery of conditions causing dyspareunia. Few operations have been described in individual chapters.

1. Urethral Meatus Surgery

In 1959 O' Donnel described a condition in which inadequate rupture of the hymenal ring caused lower urinary tract inflammation and dyspareunia. It is because with sexual intercourse eversion of urethral meatus occurs due to hymenal attachment.

Surgery

- Hymen is excised (Fig 5.1and 5.2).
- Bulbo cavernous pads are transposed to the area beneath the urethra (Martius procedure).

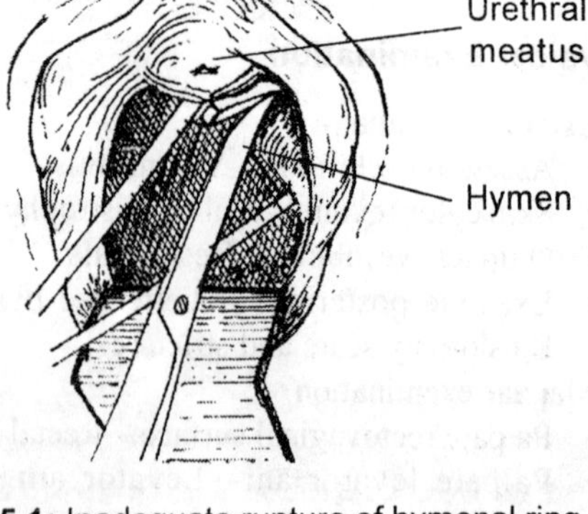

Fig. 5.1: Inadequate rupture of hymenal ring

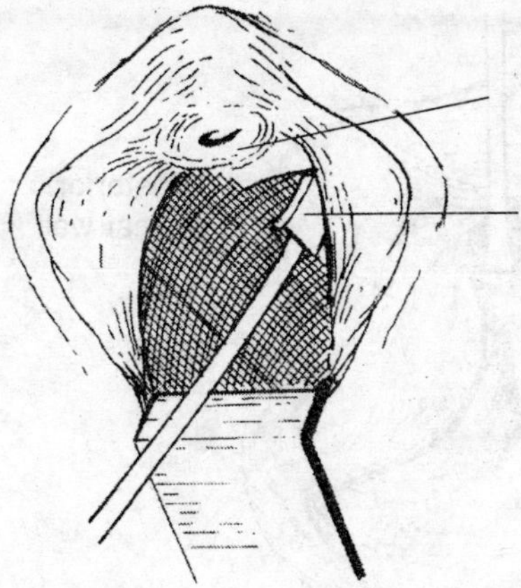

Fig. 5.2: Removal of hymenal piece

2. Introital Contracture

There are two types:
- Contracture due to chronic vulvar dystrophy.
- Contracture following perineorrhaphy.

Correction of Contracture following Perineorrhaphy

In these patient alongwith skin contracture, musculature of perineal body is also involved, which is fibrosed and adhered medially. The only treatment of this condition is plastic surgery of the perineum—Perineoplasty.

Perineoplasty

- Patient in placed in lithotomy position.
- Skin incision is made horizontally along the line of the posterior commissure.
- Skin flaps are elevated by undermining and freeing.
- With finger in the rectum, external anal splinter is identified and protected and the large amount of fibrous tissue removed.
- It results in perineal musculature to go laterally.
- Now closure is made transversely (Figs 5.3 to 5.6).

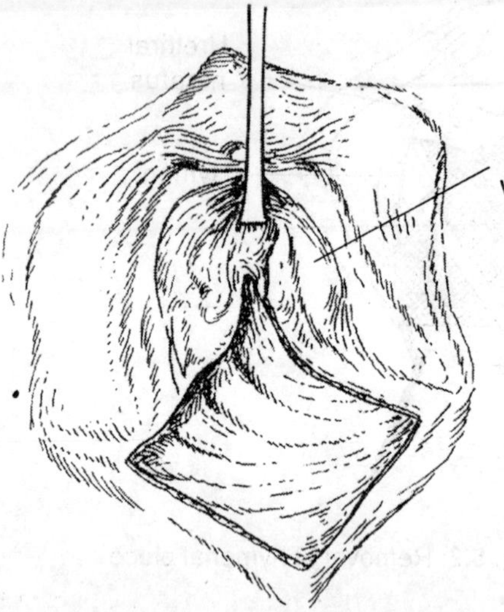

Fig. 5.3: Perineoplasty: Skin incision

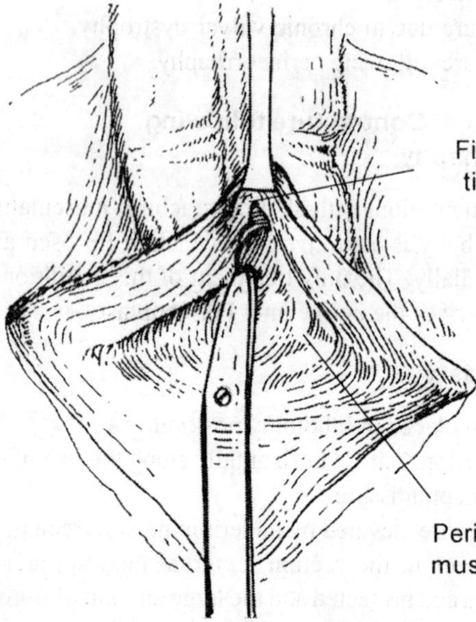

Fig. 5.4: Perineoplasty: Excision of fibrous tissue

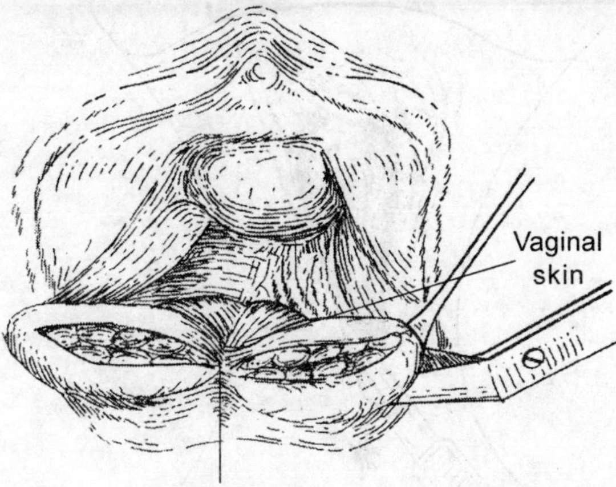

Fig. 5.5: Perineoplasty: Closure transversely

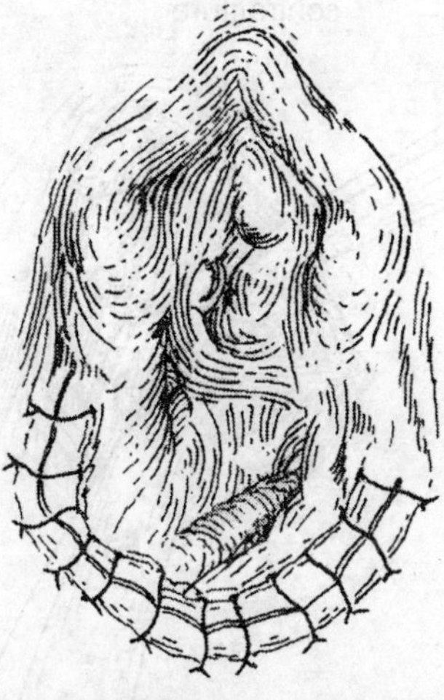

Fig. 5.6: Perineoplasty: Final closure by bringing down vaginal mucosa

Correction of Contracture Secondary to Dystrophy

The main difference between both contractures is that in dystrophy flap cover is required (Figs 5.7 to 5.11).

- Patient is placed in lithotomy position.
- Posterior vaginal wall is split in posterior longitudinal axis and undermined until introitus and lumen are of adequate size.

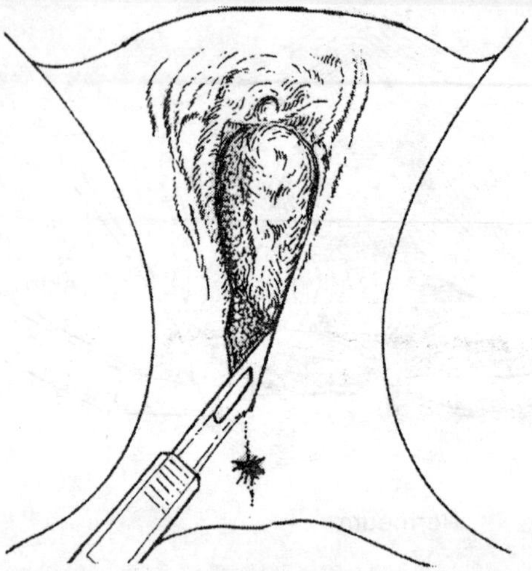

Fig. 5.7: Contracture secondary to dystrophy: Incision in contracture

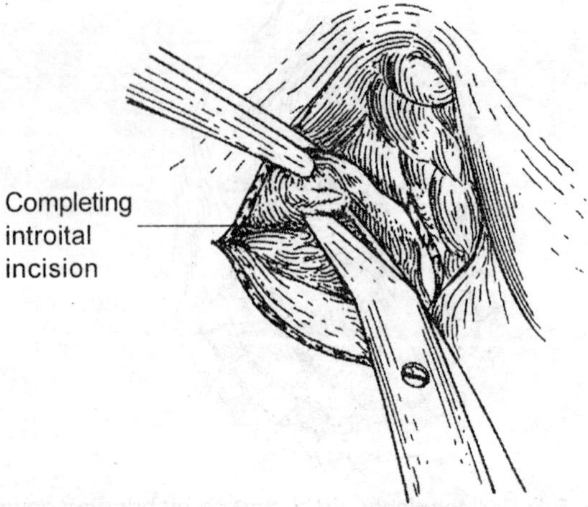

Fig. 5.8: Contracture secondary to dystrophy: Excision of fibrous tissue

- Then flap is used to resurface the defect.
- Various flaps can be used as described in vaginal agenesis.

Vaginal Laxity

Vaginal relaxation or laxity is important problem because it reduces the pleasure of sex. Every patient presenting with

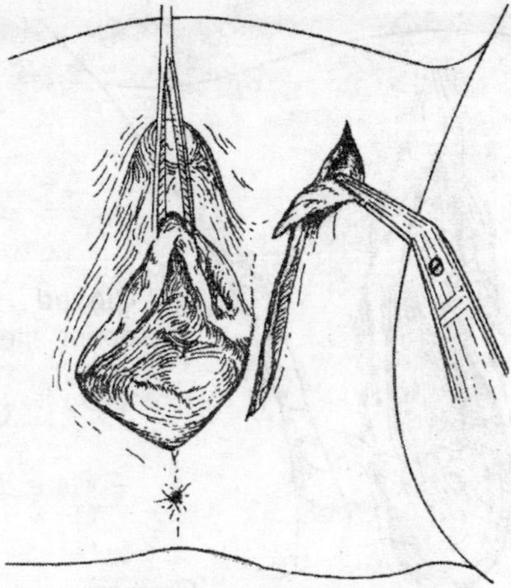

Fig. 5.9: Contracture secondary to dystrophy: Raising the labial flap

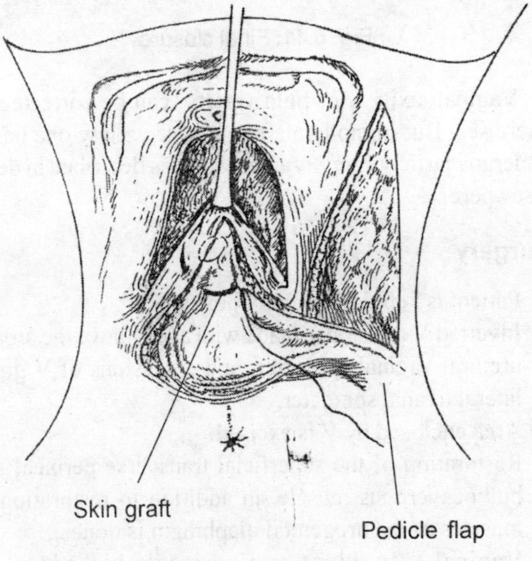

Fig. 5.10: Contracture secondary to dystrophy: Flap transposed over the defect

vaginal laxity should be carefully evaluated for different defects. Usual defects are:

- Excess vaginal mucosa with chronic perineal tears.
- Loss of muscular activity.

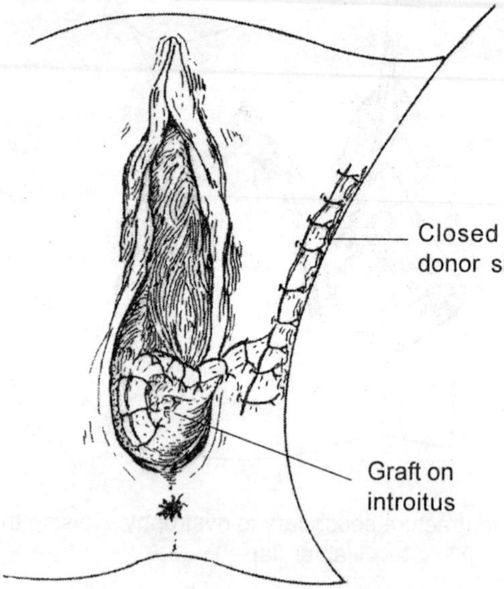

Fig. 5.11: Final closure

Vaginal laxity if of mild variety can be corrected by exercises. But in moderate and severe variety one has to undergo plastic surgery. Vaginal laxity is described in detail elsewhere.

Surgery

- Patient is kept in lithotomy position.
- Inverted V incision is made with apex above the area of urethral vaginal sphincter, and extensions of V going lateral to anal sphincter.
- Area enclosed by V is excised.
- Restoration of the superficial transverse perineal and bulbocavernous muscle, in addition to restoration of muscles of the urogenital diaphragm is done.
- Vaginal skin edges and perineal skin edges are approximated.

Vaginal Agenesis

Vaginal agenesis is described as a condition in which vagina is not formed. It is an indication of vaginal reconstruction. Different procedures are described for vaginal reconstruction in the literature. Vaginal reconstruction has two parts.

1. Creation of space between bladder and rectum.
2. Resurfacing the space.

Creation of Space

It is almost standard procedure:

- Patient is placed in lithotomy position.
- Foley's catheter is passed.
- Incision is made at the site of vaginal orifice usually marked by a hymenal dimple.
- By blunt dissection space is created between bladder and rectum.
- If there is tightness laterally few cuts should be made in the fascia laterally.
- Bleeders are coagulated under direct vision.

Resurfacing the Space

Following methods are used to resurface the space.

- Mc Indoe's split thick skin graft (Figs 5.12 to 5.14).
- Horton's full thickness skin graft.
- Rectus abdominis myocutaneous flap.
- Pudendal thigh flap.
- Transfer of sigmoid colon.
- Prefabricated peritoneal radial fascial flap (Authors).
- Resurfacing with SIS (Authors).

Mc Indoe's Procedure

In this procedure split skin graft is taken from the flexor surface of the thigh.

Though in text books of Gynaecology it is described that skin graft should be taken from the flexor surface of the thighs, authors don't agree. Plastic surgeons never advice to take the graft from the thighs of a female. They always advice to take the graft from the buttocks. Reasons are:

- It is well hidden in every society.
- Donor area problems, if occur, are not much problematical in buttocks as compared to medial thigh.
    1. Graft is harvested.
    2. It is wrapped over mould with raw surface outside.
    3. Standard mould is made of plastic material and is hollow. It measures 10 by 4.5 cm.

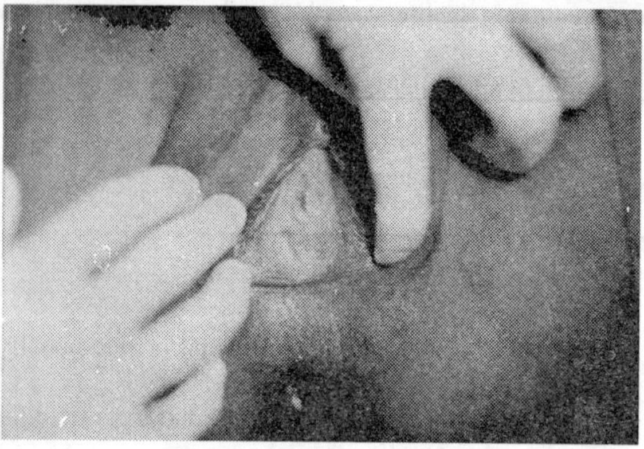

Fig. 5.12: Vaginal agenesis

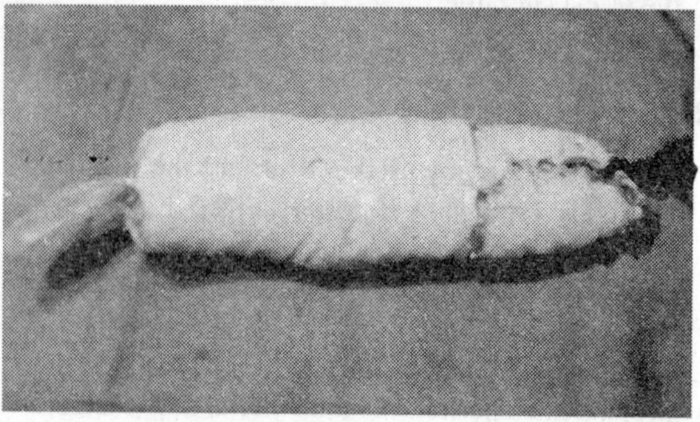

Fig. 5.13: Split thick graft taken from thigh and wrapped over mould

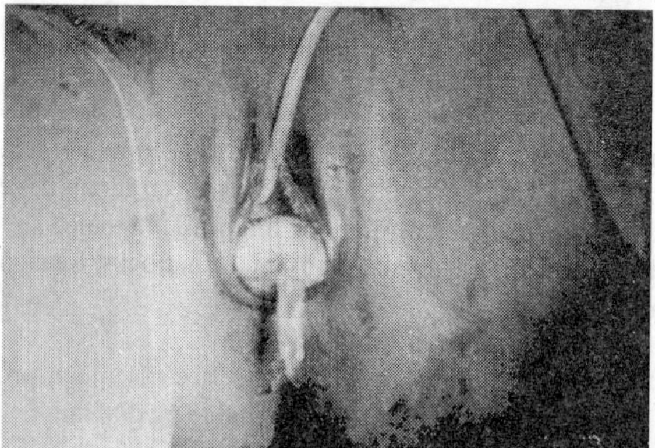

Fig. 5.14: Mould with graft placed in space created between anal and bladder canal

4. Alternatively polythene sponge mould is placed inside Ferguson's speculum over which graft is placed.
5. Graft-carrying speculum or mould is now inserted gently into the prepared new vaginal cavity.
6. Speculum is next gently withdrawn, so that sponge mould is left inside the graft, against which, by its elastic compression, it exerts a gentle and uniformly equal pressure in all directions.
7. The labias are closed over the distal end of the sponge.
8. The sponge mould is removed on the 14th day and cavity is inspected for failure of take or presence of granulation tissue. (This programme is described in textbook of Gynecologies. But authors don't agree. They are of opinion that dressing should be inspected after 7 days and if there is failure of takeof graft immediate regrafting should be done).
9. An acrylic mould is now placed inside the cavity and retained there by stitching the labia over the mould after splitting them upto urethra, where mould is left in the cavity for 2-3 months.
10. After removal of mould she should have regular dilatation for six months. Split thick skin graft is harvested from thigh and wrapped over a mould with raw surface outside.

Disadvantages

The main disadvantage of this procedure is severe contraction of graft, which is very difficult to correct.

Prefabricated Peritoneo Radial Fascial Flap (V. Prakash et al)

- Author has taken peritoneum and placed over radial fascia.
- After three weeks whole peritoneoradial flap is raised based on radial artery (Fig. 5.15).
- The whole flap is transferred using microsurgical principle.

Fasciocutaneous Flaps

Different fasciocutaneous flaps have also been described but main problem is their bulk. *Author* has used ultra thin

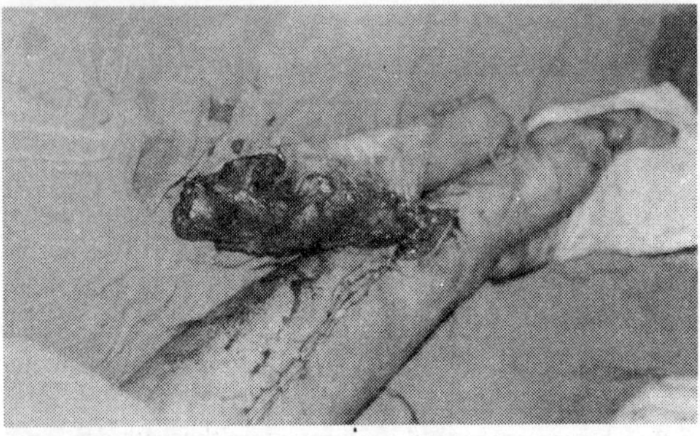

Fig. 5.15: Prefabricated peritoneal radial fascial vagina over forearm

fasciocutaneous flap and found good result in vaginal reconstruction.

Pudendal Thigh Flap

Pudendal thigh flap is useful flap for not only resurfacing the created vaginal space but also various other problems of vulva/vagina/perineum where flap covered is required.

Blood Supply

The pudendal thigh flap is an axial and sensate fasciocutaneous flap based on the terminal branches of the superficial perineal artery.

The perineal artery is a continuation, below the urogenital diaphragm, of the internal pudendal artery, which is a major branch of the hypogastric or internal iliac artery.

The perineal artery, after giving off the transverse perineal artery, continues as the posterior scrotal artery (in females as corresponding artery).

Flap Elevation

- Incision begins at tip of flap.
- Deepened through skin and subcutaneous tissue down to the deep fascia on two sides, except for the posterior margin of the flap.
- Flap is elevated including deep fascia and epimysium over proximal part of adductor muscles.

(Author does not agree that epimysium should be included in flap as it is not going to increase the blood supply of flap).

- Tunnel is created by elevating the labia off the public rami, and each flap is passed through so that both come to lie together in the mid line without tension.
- The ventral and dorsal margins are sutured together to form a tubular structure, which is then turned in to form the new vagina.

Author is of opinion that flap is very bulky and difficult to use in patients of congenital absence of vagina. However it is good for carcinoma patients. So he has used the flap using the principle of ultra thinning (super thin flaps).

Resurfacing the Space with SIS (V Prakash et al)

Author has used small intestine submucosa for lining the space created for vagina and found it the best procedure. The advantage of the procedure are:

- Thin flap.
- Spontaneous resurfacing with mesothelial cells.
- Pliable and smooth lining.

Vaginismus

Vaginismus is defined as hyperaesthesia which leads to spasm of sphincter vaginae and levator ani muscles during attempted coitus or during per vaginal examination. Masters and Johnson defined it as "a psychological syndrome affecting woman's freedom of sexual response partially, if not totally, impeding sexual function. Anatomically, it involves all components of the pelvic musculature investing the perineum and outer third of the vagina. Physiologically, these muscles contract spastically as opposed to their rhythmic contractual response in orgasmic experience. This spasm is an involuntary reflex stimulated by imagined, anticipated or real attempts at vaginal penetration.

Kaplan points out that in addition to having the involuntary muscle spasm of the vaginal inlet, patients with vaginismus are usually phobic of any vaginal penetration, and this phobia makes attempt at coitus frustrating and painful. Accompanying the muscle spasm, there is usually adduction of the thighs and frequently the posture assumed is one of opisthotonos. Few authors have compared the vaginismus to the tight blink of the eyelids when a threatening motion towards the eyelids is perceived.

Types

- Primary—when there is no cause.
- Secondary—when some painful lesion is present.

Aetiology

1. Primary impotency of male is many a times associated with vaginismus.
2. Prior sexual trauma.
3. Painful, unhappy first experience with intercourse.
4. Fenichel views vaginismus as a conversion symptom involved in the female "castration complex" and " penis envy". The wife aims to destroy the husband's potency and "castrates" him in retaliation for her own "castration" through aversion to his appeals.
5. However Kaplan interprets vaginismus as a conditioned response that results from the association of pain or fear with attempts at or even fantasies of vaginal penetration. The original noxious stimulus may have been physical pain or psychological distress, including painful vaginal conditions. Once the reflex is established, curing the original condition may not result in extinction of the vaginal response.
6. Poinsard feels that a more inclusive phenomenon than a conditioned reflex is involved. Unwillingness to assume the adult role, fear of pregnancy, fear of venereal disease, fear of being hurt, and other anxiety laden feelings are usually involved.
7. Wolpe points out that fear and anxiety play a major role in the production and maintenance of a symptom.
8. Ellison points to ignorance and misinformation as the major aetiological factors. In his study he found that ignorance and misinformation were present in 90% of the patients. The most widely held apprehension was that the hymen was a completely obstructing barrier that must be broken, accompanied by excruciating pain and bleeding. In many of the patients sexual guilt was often found.

Diagnosis

Usually the presenting complaint is different. It is physical one in most of the cases, which includes difficulty in breathing, abdominal pain, vomiting, diarrhea etc. Only 25% of the patients complain of specific sexual dysfunction.

Diagnosis should be made of primary or secondary vaginismus. Take detail history. Do complete examination. Find out any skin changes at vulva or vagina to rule out any visible cause. If none is found and patient presents typically with vaginismus during attempted vaginal examination, diagnosis of vaginismus should be made.

Treatment

1. Psychological treatment
2. Muscle strengthening exercises
3. Surgery.

PSYCHOLOGICAL TREATMENT

Master's and Johnson's Programme

1. Physically demonstrate the existence of involuntary vaginal spasm to both marital partners.
2. This should be preceded by anatomical illustration of the involved vaginal musculature.
3. Now husband should be taught to insert graduated dilators inside vagina under wife's manual control. Intravaginal retention of dilators for several hours is encouraged.
4. If every thing goes well the couple should be ready to attempt coitus in 3-5 days.
5. After physical symptoms have been relieved psychological aspect should be dealt with.
6. Explain the origin of the symptoms and educate her to overcome the lack of knowledge of sexual responsivity.

Kaplan's Programme

1. Patients' phobic avoidance of vaginal entry must be alleviated.
2. Phobic element can be taken care of by psycho-analysis, hypnosis, and behaviour therapy. The latter two use systematic desensitization.

3. Systematic desensitization involves repeated evocation of imagery of the feared situation while the patient is deeply relaxed. It proceeds gradually while the patient fantasizing the feared sexual situation. As she is able to tolerate this fantasy, she proceeds to more advanced imagery. At last she is able to imagine penetration while remaining relaxed.
4. At this point she should be given graduated vaginal dilators, which should be replaced by husband's finger.
5. After some time sexual intercourse may be attempted.

Muscle Strengthening Exercises

These exercises have been described by Kegel and are to be done daily. The purpose of the exercises is to teach voluntary control over the muscles involved in vaginismus.

1. The patient is asked to sit or lie down.
2. Then she is asked to contract her levator muscles for as long as she can.
3. Once the patient has carried out the programme for two weeks, her husband begins the vaginal dilatation with his fingers. He inserts the finger and does not withdraw until she is able to relax completely, at which point he goes with two fingers with the same technique.
3. This should continue for few weeks and should be replaced by female superior position and then attempt should be made of gradual penile insertion concurrent with the patient doing Kegel exercises to the point of fatigue.

Surgery

Surgery is done if all measures have failed.

Fenton's Operation

If during examinations under anaesthesia a rigid hymen, or tight perineum is found, perineotomy should be done.

- Patient is placed in lithotomy position.
- A longitudinal incision is made in mid line through lower third of the posterior vaginal wall and skin of perineum.
- After cutting the tissues on either side and dividing the superficial muscles of the perineum, the wound is closed transversely.
- After operation vagina should admit three fingers (Fig. 5.16).

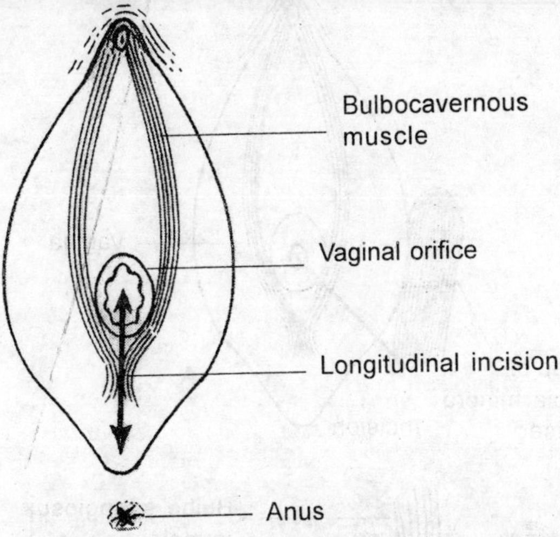

Fig. 5.16A: Fenton's operation: Normal vulva showing longitudinal incision in midline which cuts bulbo cavernous muscles

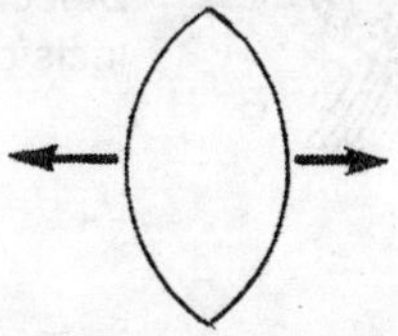

Fig. 5.16B: Fenton's operation: Incision Gaps

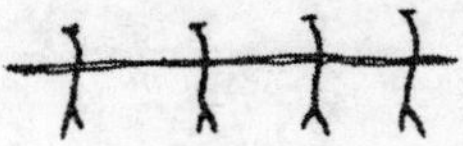

Fig. 5.16C: Fenton's operation: Incision is closed transversely

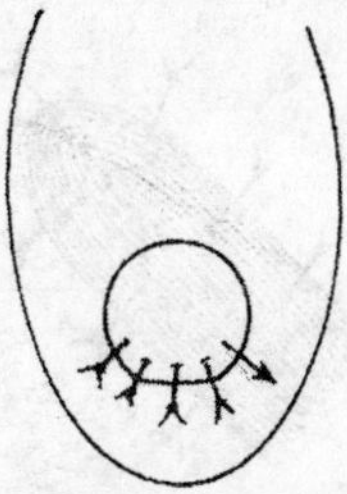

Fig. 5.16D: Fenton's operation: Final closure where vagina admits three fingers

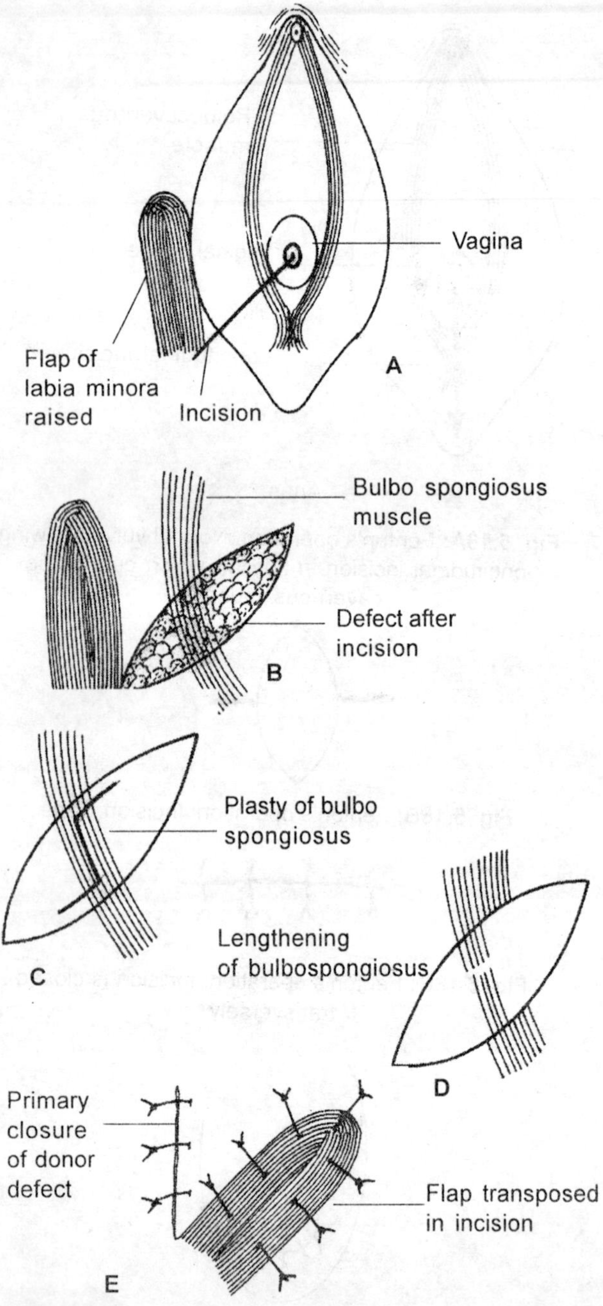

Figs 5.17A to E: Author's operation for vaginismus

Author's approach is to:

- Make incision in lateral position, and
- Resurface with either full thickness skin graft or labial flap.
- It is because author is of opinion that all incisions and scars on posterior mid line should be avoided as they may result in dyspareunia.
- Further direct closure of scar, though transversely, may also result in dyspareunia so. Resurfacing should be done, rather than primary closure (Fig. 5.17).

6

Reconstructive Surgery of Fistulas

VESICOVAGINAL FISTULA

Etiology

- Secondary to prolong obstructed labour.
- Iatrogenic after hysterectomy or anterior colporrhaphy.
- Radiation.
- Carcinoma.
- Infection as in postoperative abscess of the vaginal vault.

Evaluation

1. With the patient in the knee-chest position and using a sim's speculum, a fistula hidden by the vaginal rugae may be visualized. At this time vagina is filled with water, and the bladder insufflated with gas. The resulting bubbles of gas entering the vagina reveal the opening.
2. Endoscopic examination is essential for examination of fistulous tract as well as inside of bladder.
3. Intravenous pyelography.

General Principles of Fistula Repair

- In postmenopausal female, estrogen should be given.
- The catheter is removed one week prior to repair to allow free drainage from the fistula.
- Adequate exposure of the fistula is must. A large episiotomy or Schuchardt's incision may be made if required.
- Wide mobilization is must.

Author is of opinion that well vascularized tissue as dermabraded flap/muscle should be interposed between vagina and bladder.

General Technique of Repair

- Patient kept in lithotomy position.
- Incision is made in vaginal mucosa 1 cm away from fistula margin.
- If fistula is larger than 2 cm in any direction, the fistula should be repaired in two stages.
- Delay of vaginal flap is done in first stage and in second stage vaginal mucosa is raised as flap based on fistulous margins.
- The vaginal mucous flaps are sutured so closing bladder. According to author it is very important stage and if not cared for properly, recurrence takes place.
- The one of the many flaps described in vaginal agenesis is used as interposition tissue. Author does not recommend gracilis because its tendinous portion comes to lie as interposition tissue which is not well vascularized.
- Vagina is closed. If vaginal defect is large, flap's skin may be used to form part of vagina (Fig. 6.1).

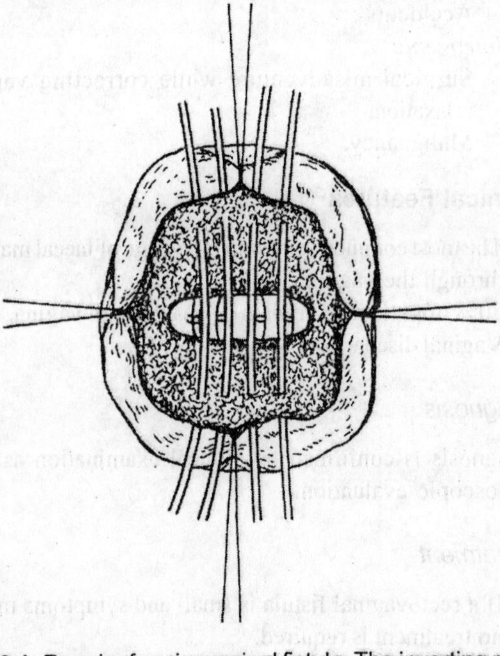

Fig. 6.1: Repair of vesicovaginal fistula: The inverting row of sutures is placed, and the vaginal epithelium is closed with interrupted sutures

Postoperatively

- Suprapubic drainage is must.
- Patient is given stool softeners and advised not to strain.
- Intercourse is delayed for four months.

RECTOVAGINAL FISTULA

A rectovaginal fistula is a communication between the rectum and the vagina, irrespective of the location of the fistulous tract or the cause of the defect.

Etiology

- *Congenital:* This type of fistula may exist in different forms. Usually these are associated with imperforate anus.
- *Inflammatory*
  - Chronic ulcerative colitis
  - Crohn's disease
- *Traumatic*
  - Obstetric
  - Accidents
- *Iatrogenic*
  - Surgical misadventure while correcting vaginal relaxation.
  - Malignancy.

Clinical Features

- The most common symptom is passage of faecal material through the vagina.
- 30% of patients complain of gas through vagina.
- Vaginal discharge.

Diagnosis

Diagnosis is confirmed by clinical examination as well endoscopic evaluation.

Treatment

- If a rectovaginal fistula is small and symptoms minor, no treatment is required.
- If fistula is large, repair is done.
- Repair is done either through vagina or rectum. However vaginal route is preferable. Three types of repairs are

considered—layer by layer anatomic reconstruction, Warren flap type operation and rectovaginal technique of anterior rectal wall advancement.

Preoperative Management

Preoperative management is carried out as:

Two days Preop

- Minimum residue diet
- Two tap water 1000 ml enemas after admission.

One day Preop

- Clear liquid diet.
- Three tap water enemas in morning, afternoon and evening.
- Neomycin, 1g orally at 1.00 pm and erythromycin 1 gm at 11.00 pm.

Day of Operation

- Nil orally after midnight
- No enemas

Operative Technique

- Incision is made around margins of fistula.
- Excision of mucosa from posterior vaginal wall.
- The first line of sutures is placed, inverting the edge into the rectal lumen.
- The second line of sutures is placed into the rectal musculature and fascia.
- Horizontal mattress sutures form the third layer of closure (Figs 6.2 to 6.18).

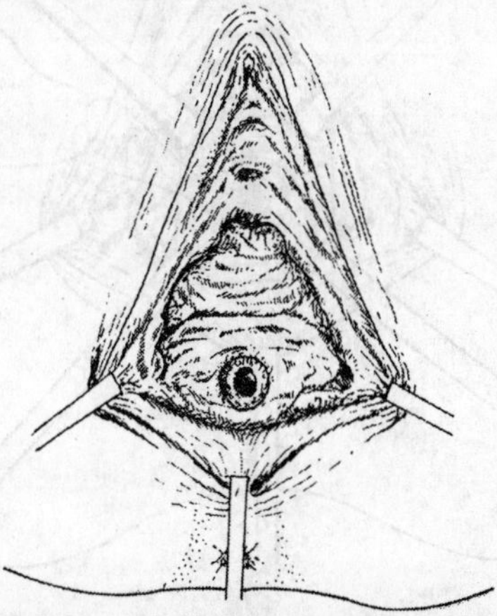

Fig. 6.2: Repair of small rectovaginal fistula: Circular incision

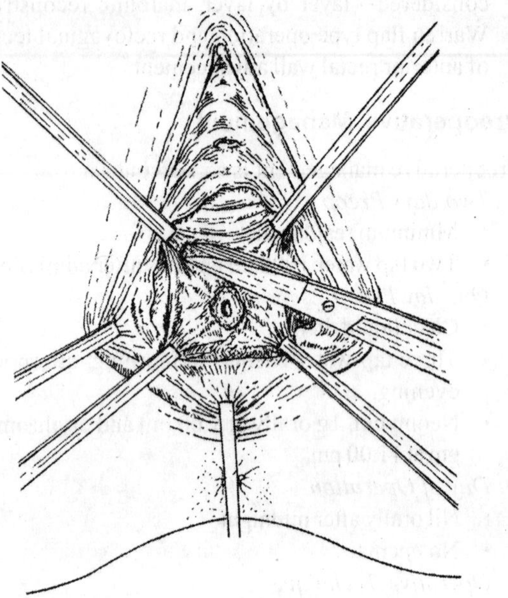

Fig. 6.3: Repair of small rectovaginal fistula: Flaps of vaginal mucosa dissected

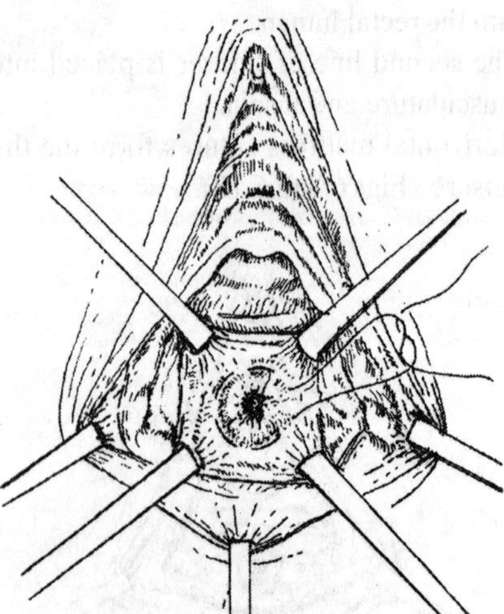

Fig. 6.4: Repair of small rectovaginal fistula: Fistula closed by purse-string suture

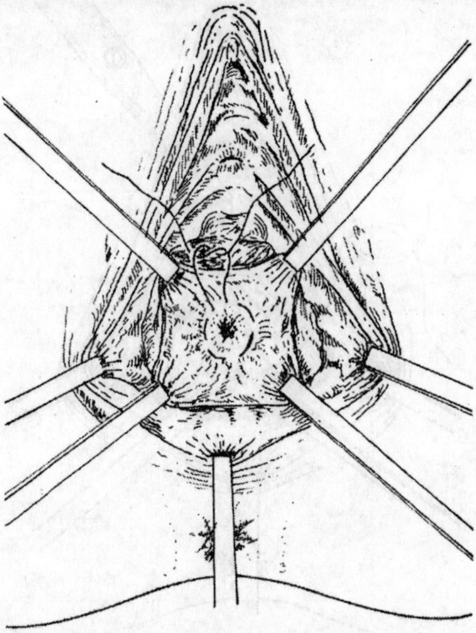

Fig. 6.5: Repair of small rectovaginal fistula: Another purse-string suture

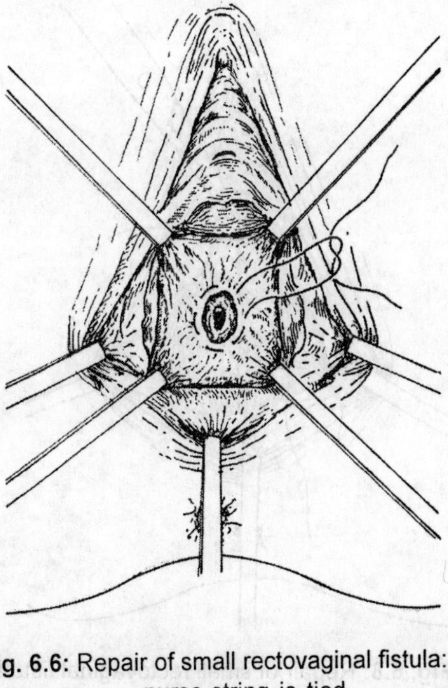

Fig. 6.6: Repair of small rectovaginal fistula: Third purse-string is tied

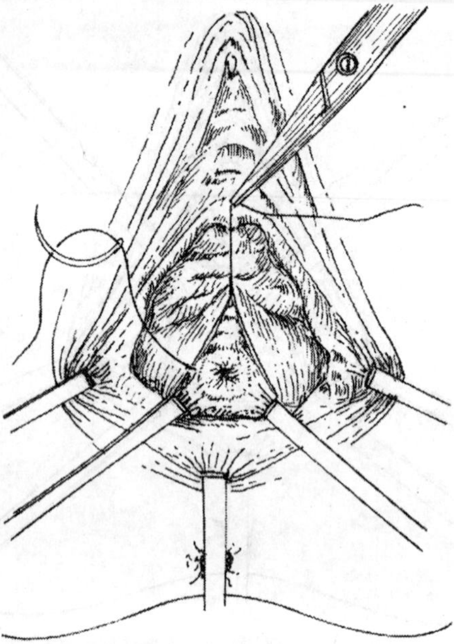

Fig. 6.7: Repair of small rectovaginal fistula: Submucosa sluched

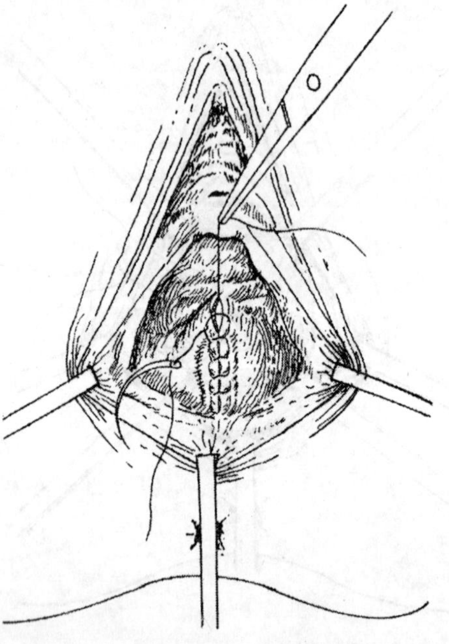

Fig. 6.8: Repair of small rectovaginal fistula: Mucosa is closed

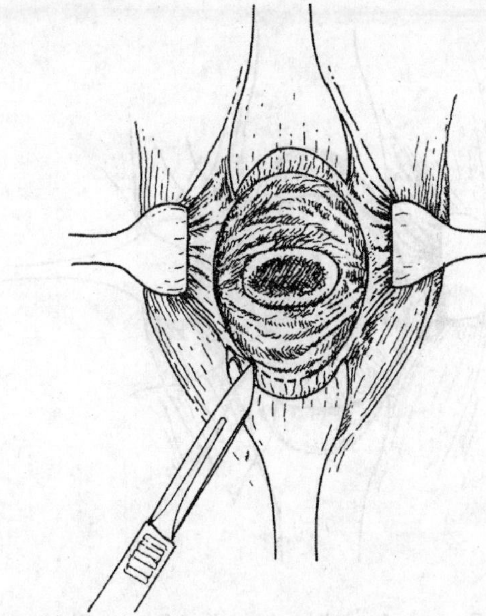

Fig. 6.9: Repair of small rectovaginal fistula: Closure of large fistula (Lalzko technique): Incision around margins of fistula

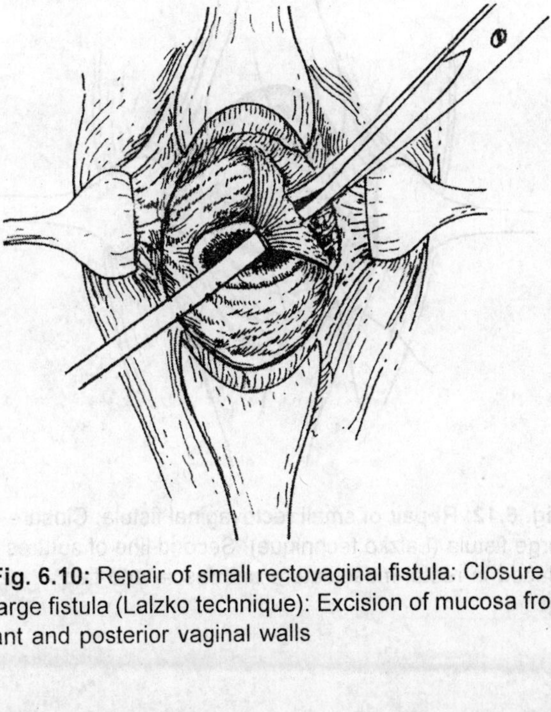

Fig. 6.10: Repair of small rectovaginal fistula: Closure of large fistula (Lalzko technique): Excision of mucosa from ant and posterior vaginal walls

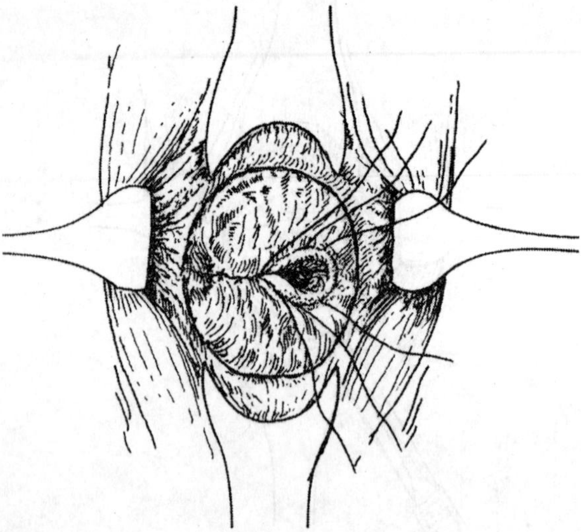

Fig. 6.11: Repair of small rectovaginal fistula: Closure of large fistula (Lalzko technique): First line of sutures inverting edges in rectal lumen

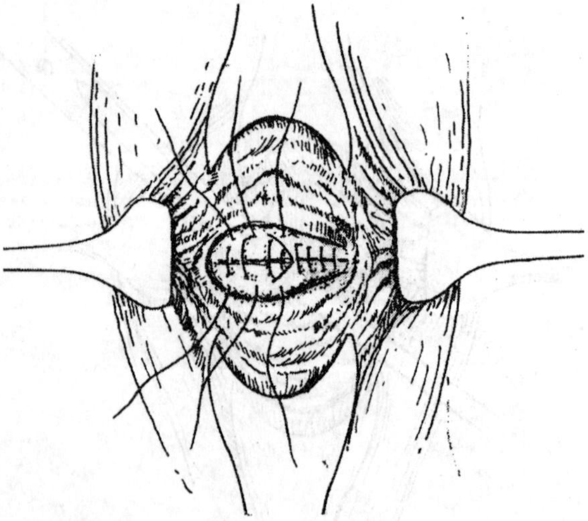

Fig. 6.12: Repair of small rectovaginal fistula: Closure of large fistula (Lalzko technique): Second line of sutures is placed in rectal musculature and fascia and tied

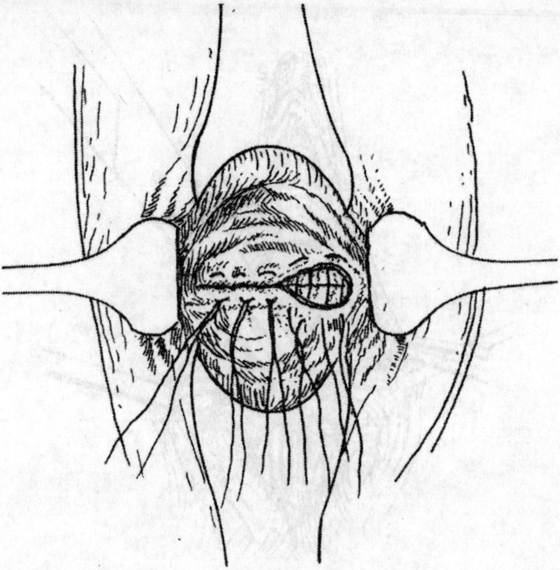

Fig. 6.13: Repair of small rectovaginal fistula: Closure of large fistula (Lalzko technique): Final closure

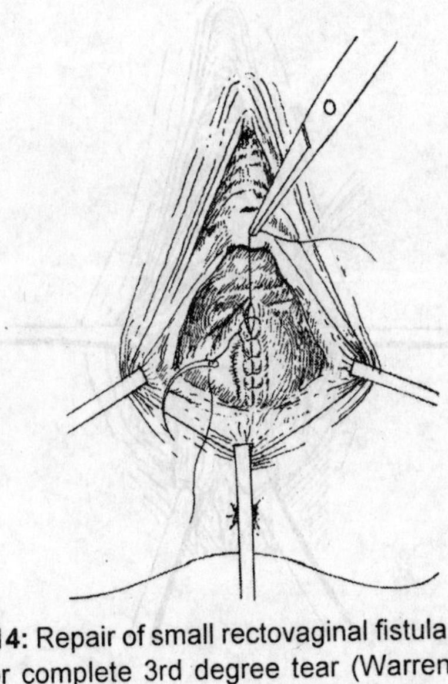

Fig. 6.14: Repair of small rectovaginal fistula: Plastic surgery for complete 3rd degree tear (Warren-flap operation): Line of incision outlining flap of vaginal mucosa

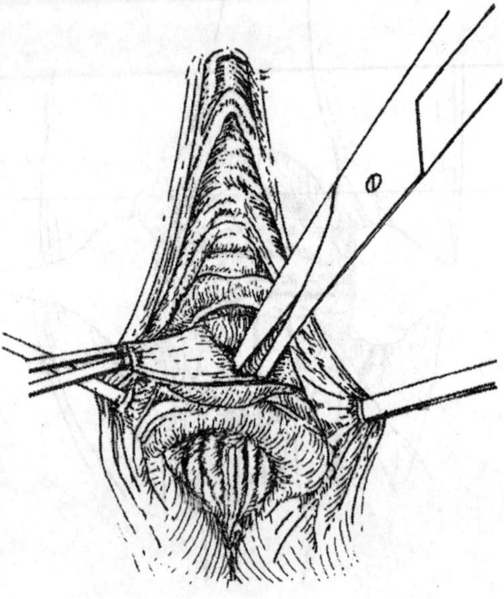

Fig. 6.15: Repair of small rectovaginal fistula: Plastic surgery for complete 3rd degree tear (Warren-flap operation): Flap dissected

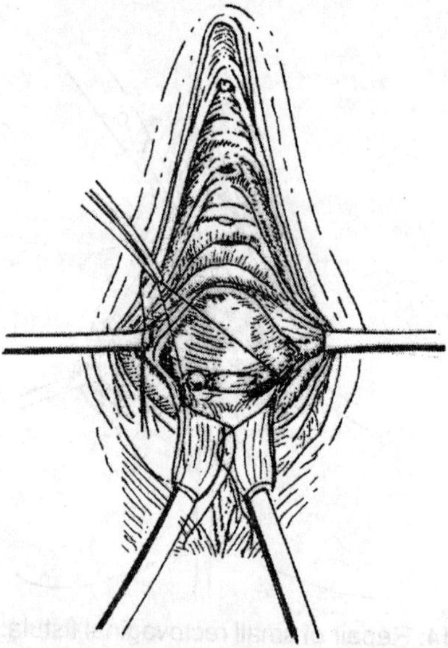

Fig. 6.16: Repair of small rectovaginal fistula: Plastic surgery for complete 3rd degree tear (Warren-flap operation): Ends of sphincter are dissected and sutured

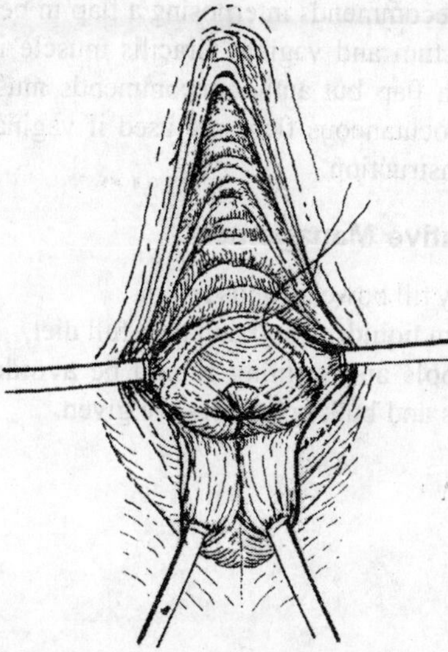

Fig. 6.17: Repair of small rectovaginal fistula: Plastic surgery for complete 3rd degree tear (Warren-flap operation): Puborectalis stitched in midline

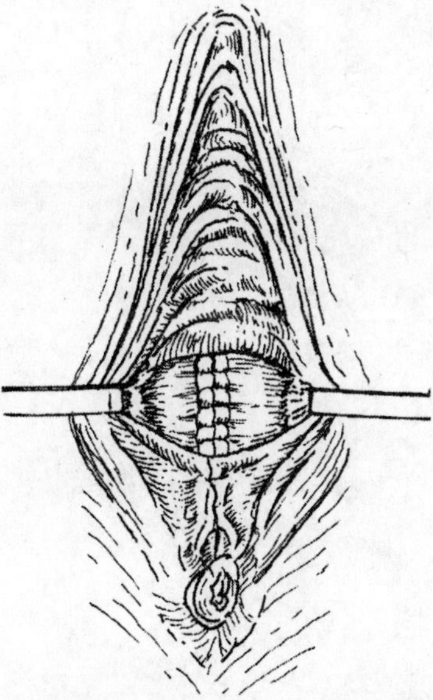

Fig. 6.18: Repair of small rectovaginal fistula: Plastic surgery for complete 3rd degree tear (Warren-flap operation): Vaginal flap is stitched

Author recommends interposing a flap in between the repaired rectum and vagina. Gracilis muscle is used as interposition flap but author recommends muscle flaps. While fasciocutaneous flaps are used if vaginal mucosa needs reconstruction.

Postoperative Management

- Nil orally till bowel sounds return.
- Start from liquids to soft and then full diet.
- Hard stools and staining should be avoided and so softeners and bulk enhancers are given.

7

Reconstructive Surgery of Urinary Incontinence

Storage of urine in the bladder is done under low pressure. The bladder wall muscle is detrusor which has elastic properties, allowing it to expand during filling without increasing the pressure within its lumen upto a certain capacity, at which time the pressure increases as filling continues because the bladder wall is stretched to its limit. Should the pressure within the bladder lumen exceed the pressure within urethral lumen, urine will leak out.

Female urethra is having sphincteric properties consisting of internal smooth muscle component which consists of proximal 2/3rd of urethra, and external striated muscle component.

TYPES OF URINARY INCONTINENCE

- Urge
- Stress
- Overflow
- Functional

Stress Incontinence

In genuine stress incontinence the bladder fills and stores urine normally. When the bladder is subjected to sudden pressure increases as occurs with coughing or straining, the urethra is unable to maintain a closed seal against the pressure within the bladder, and urine leaks.

Causes

1. Sphincteric weakness.

2. Loss of support of urethra.
   Normally the bladder neck and proximal female urethra lie above the female pelvic floor, well suspended behind the pubis. Proximal urethra is in intra abdominal position. In stress incontinence bladder increases its pressure as before but the urethra is no longer subjected to the increased pressures from outside. It may occur in
   - Aging where weakening of all muscular and fascial structures take place.
   - Obesity.
   - Pregnancy and vaginal delivery.
3. Urethral neuromuscular deficiency.
4. Neurologic deficiency.
5. Muscular deficiency.
6. Deficient mucosal seal.
   Effective urethral mucosal seal is very important for preventing incontinence. The female urethral mucosa is richly vascular and appears pliable with redundant longitudinal folds on urethroscopy. The mucosal folds coapt forming a water tight mucosal seal in the normal female. All the conditions which can jeopardize this mucosal seal can lead to incontinence despite normal urethral positioning and neuromuscular sphincteric properties.
   In normal females the urethral mucosa is able to fold into the groove and seal it, preventing incontinence.

Aging is an important cause because post menopausal females, due to lack of estrogens, develop deficiencies in mucosal vascularity and pliability.

Evaluation of a Patient of Urinary Incontinence

Basic evaluation of a patient includes history, physical examination, cough stress test, estimation of post void residual volume, urine analysis, and 24-hour voiding diary.

History should be taken in detail. Physical examination commences with a general examination of mobility, cognition, and manual dexterity. The vulva is assessed for irritation due to urinary leak. Gynecological examination includes a demonstration of pelvic relaxation. Patient is asked to cough and urinary leakage may be observed at this time.

Cough Stress Test

It is done as following:

- Patient is placed in lithotomy position.
- Bladder is filled with 300-350 ml of fluid.
- Patient is asked to cough.
- During coughing the examiner observes for loss of urine from urethra.

Uroflow

Uroflowmetry is a timed measure of voided urine volume. Normally 200 ml of urine is voided in 20 seconds with a residual urine of less than 100 ml. It can be done with the help of stop watch, however electronic equipments are also available. It shows voiding abnormalities, though it can't distinguish between obstruction and detrusor weakness.

Cystometrogram

Cystometry is a test of detrusor function, consisting of an observation and/or recording of the pressure/volume relationship during bladder filling. The main purpose of the CMG is to determine bladder capacity and rule out or confirm motor urge incontinence.

Simplest testing technique is to use the barrel of the syringe and connect it to a catheter that has been used to drain the bladder. The fluid level is maintained 15 cm above the pubic symphysis, and the bladder is filled in increments of 50 ml. The normal bladder capacity should be more than 300 ml. An unstable bladder is suspected when the fluid level rises in the syringe in the absence of increased intra-abdominal pressure. The test has been called urodynamics.

Urethral Closure Pressure Profile

Urethral pressure profile is a record of force exerted along the urethral lumen as a pressure sensor is slowly withdrawn from the bladder through the urethra. Urethral closure pressure profile is a graph of the difference between urethral pressure and simultaneously recorded bladder pressure. As long as the latter measurement remains positive urine can't pass through from the bladder through urethra.

Normal values for urethral closure pressure are greater than 20 cm of water in the sitting posture with subjectively full bladder. Values less than this are associated with surgical failure of SUI and may indicate urethral sphincter weakness.

Profiles are also obtained during coughing. When the bladder pressure exceeds urethral pressure during coughing, urethral closure pressure is zero, and urine generally escapes from urethra. It is urodynamic diagnosis of SUI.

Q-tip Test

Q-tip test is for determining the bladder neck mobility. It is carried out as following:

- A lubricated cotton swab is placed through the urethra into the bladder and gently pulled back against the bladder neck.
- Angle of applicator at rest is measured by comparing the end of the applicator with the horizontal plane.
- The patient strains and coughs vigorously, and the end of applicator moves upward according to the severity of the anatomic defect.
- A measurement of 30 degrees or more indicates UVJ mobility and that defect should be able to be corrected by standard surgery.

Management

A. *Non-surgical therapies*
- Biofeedback therapy.
- Electrical stimulation.

All the above therapies are helpful and have been described in gynecological textbooks.

B. *Surgical therapies*

Standard surgical approach to the correction of stress incontinence is to elevate and support the urethrovesical junction. There are various procedures described for correction of stress incontinence. We would be describing few of those.

Needle Procedures

Needle procedures are based on the principle that retropubic elevation of the urethra vesical junction is an effective means of treating urinary incontinence. So, several procedures were described of passing a permanent suture and elevating the bladder neck.

Surgical Anatomy

Traditionally, the urethra and bladder have been described as resting on a sheet of endopelvic fascia that envelops the vagina and attaches laterally to the arcus tendineus fascia pelvis and the levator ani muscle. Urethral support is provided by the anterior and posterior pubourethral ligaments. Recent studies have revealed these ligaments to be dense band of connective tissue that supports the urethra and is composed of a muscular compartment, which attaches the connective tissue of the vagina to the levator ani muscle, and a fascial component, which connects the endopelvic fascia between the urethra and vagina laterally to the arcus tendineus fascia pelvis.

Surgical anatomy involved in needle bladder neck suspension is described by Fitzpatrick. He did extensive studies on the cadavers and found that point of entry of needle in needle procedures occurs between the levator ani and its superficial fascia, lateral to the arcus tendineus fascia pelvis, the periurethral vascular plexus, and bladder neck. Suspension sutures placed during these types of needle urethropexies incorporate the portion of endopelvic fascia that lies between vagina and urethra.

Indications

Main indication is stress incontinence due to urethral hypermobility. The primary goal of these procedures is to elevate and maintain the bladder neck within the sphere of abdominal pressure during increase in intra-abdominal pressure.

However these procedures do not give long lasting cure therefore, in young patients some other procedure is better.

Techniques

- Modified Pereyra
- Stamey
- Raz
- Muzsnai
- Gittes

Modified Pereyra Procedure (Figs 7.1 to 7.5)

- A midline anterior vaginal wall incision is made through the epithelium beginning 2 cm superior to the external urethral meatus and extending down to just beyond the urethrovasical junction.
- The epithelium is dissected bilaterally to reveal the underlying endoplevic fascia.

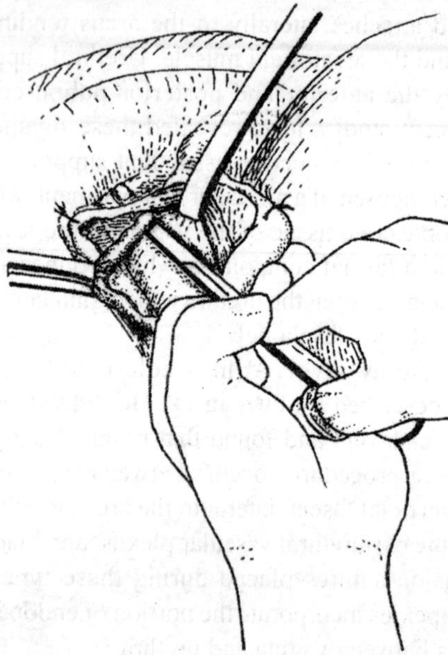

Fig. 7.1: Modified pereyra procedure: Technique of vaginal entrance into the retropubic space using Metzenbaum scissors. Endopelvic fascia is perforated at the inferior margin of pubic bone, as guided by the surgeon's index finger. The blades of scissors are separated, and dissection is completed by inserting one finger into the space created

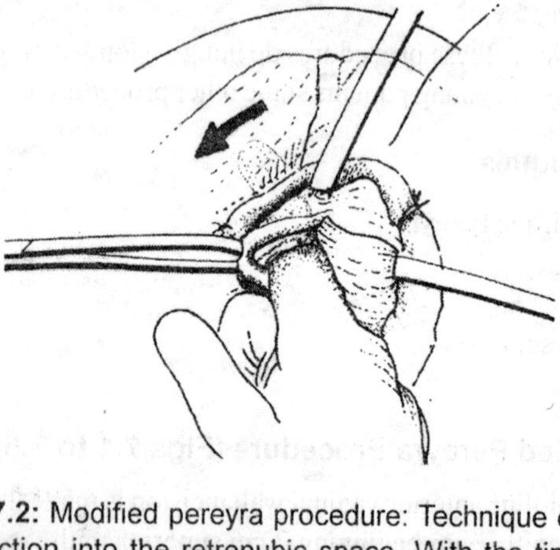

Fig. 7.2: Modified pereyra procedure: Technique of blunt dissection into the retropubic space. With the tip of the index finger flexed anteriorly against posterior symphysis pubis, paraurethral attachment to pubic bone is perforated downward (in direction of arrow) toward ischial spine, completely detaching endopelvic fascia

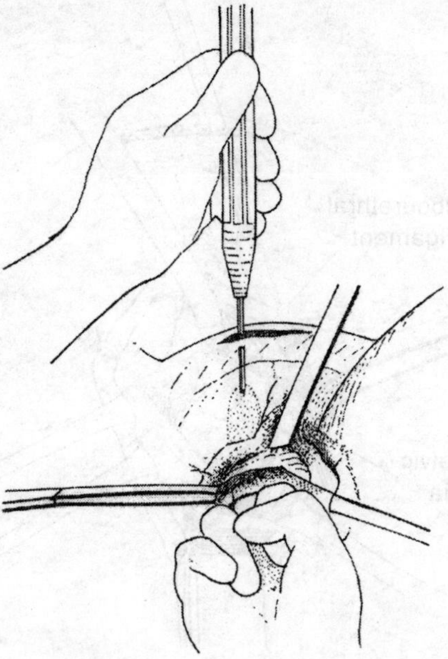

Fig. 7.3: Modified pereyra procedure: Passage of the needle is under direct finger guidance. Finger in vagina is inserted to the posterior aspect of rectus muscle

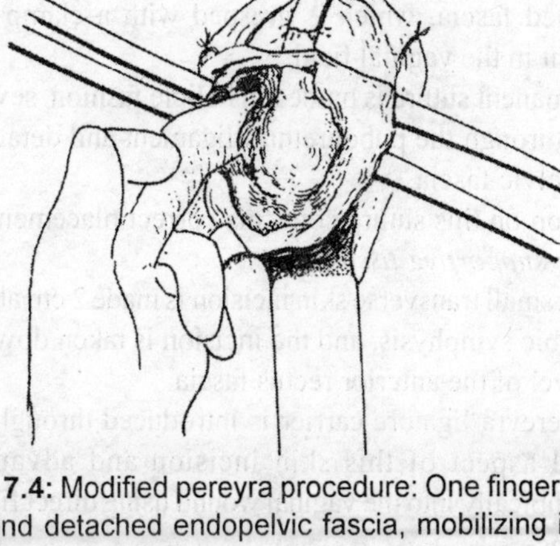

Fig. 7.4: Modified pereyra procedure: One finger is placed behind detached endopelvic fascia, mobilizing it into the vaginal field to facilitate placement of helical suture

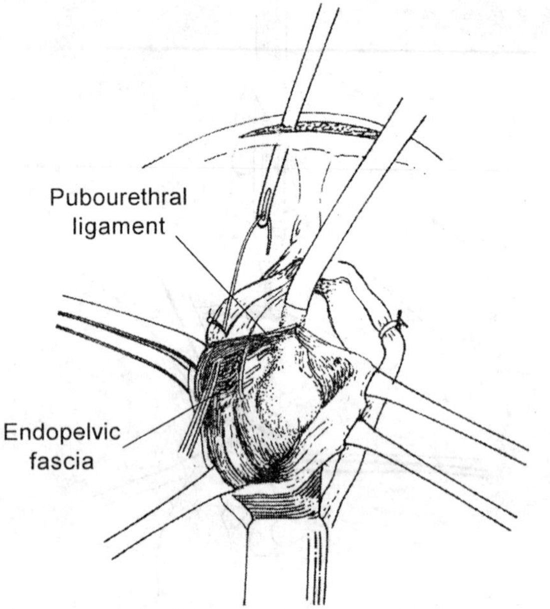

Fig. 7.5: Modified pereyra procedure: Permanent suture is anchored in pubourethral ligament. Numerous passes are taken through detached endopelvic fascia

- At the level of the bladder neck, the dissection is extended laterally to the inferior pubic ramus.
- The anterolateral attachments of the periurethral tissues are released by either sharp or blunt dissection.
- The fingertip is flexed medially to hook the edge of the detached fascia, which is grasped with a clamp and brought in the vaginal field.
- A permanent suture is passed in helicle fashion several times through the pubourethral ligament and detached endopelvic fascia.
- Traction on this suture confirms correct placement in *strong supportive tissue.*
- Now a small transverse skin incision is made 2 cm above the pubic symphysis, and the incision is taken down to the level of the anterior rectus fascia.
- The Pereyra ligature carrier is introduced through the lateral aspect of this skin incision and advanced retropubically into the vaginal wound using direct finger guidance.

- Each suspension suture is passed from the vagina to the suprapubic incision, cystoscopy is done to ensure no bladder injury or stitch penetration.
- Sutures are then tied over the anterior rectus fascia.

Abdominal Retropubic Cystourethropexy

- Lithotomy position.
- Foley catheter is inserted to aid in identification of the vesical neck during surgery.
- Pfannesteil type of transverse incision is made.
- Space of Retzuis is identified.
- No dissection is done near urethra avoiding area between the symphysis and urethra.
- Going beyond 2 cm lateral to each side, fatty tissue is removed from the retropubic area.
- With the surgeon's non-dominant hand in the vagina, the bladder is retracted medially until the white tissue of the muscularis of the vagina is identified.
- Lateral parts of the retropubic area are mobilized down to the muscularis of the vagina.
- Three sutures are placed with the preferred 0 poly-propylene material. The first suture is at urethrovesical junction 2 cm from mid line with the vagina finger placed in the lateral vaginal fornix.
- A mattress suture is placed through the vagina wall's full thickness except vaginal epithelium.
- Suture is brought upto Cooper's ligament.
- Second suture is placed lateral to the first.
- Third suture is placed immediately inferior to the proceeding two sutures.
- Similar procedure is carried out on the opposite side.
- Now bladder is filled to 250 ml and with the urethra at 0°, pressure on the bladder is firmly and sharply produced, while urethral meatus is observed for leakage.
- If there is leakage, the sutures are brought up until it stops.
- The sutures anchored through Cooper's ligament are now tied.
- There are chances of obstruction of urethra in 1% of patients therefore after injecting indigocarmine, bladder must be visualized by cystoscope for urethral function.

Transvaginal Cystourethropexy

Compared to abdominal urethropexy, vaginal procedures have higher failure rates, but these are quicker and may have reduced operative and postoperative morbidity.

- Lithotomy position.
- Marking sutures are placed at least 2 cm lateral to urethra at urethrovesical junction as determined by bulb of foley catheter.
- Inverted U incision is made.
- Apex of inverted U is halfway between urethrovescial junction and the urethral meatus.
- The limbs of U extend at least 4 cm.
- After injecting the tissue with saline an incision is made. Scissor dissection is used to extend the tissue, and on each side of urethra, tissue is penetrated staying close to the symphysis so that finger enters the space of Retzuis.
- Finger should never move medially over urethra.
- An abdominal incision is made 2 finger widths above the symphysis, and passage is made from suprapubic to vaginal position.
- A suture of 0 prolene stitch the vaginal wall and urethral support tissue and brought at abdominal incision.
- Same procedure is repeated on the opposite side.
- Operating table is then kept at 0°.
- Incontinence should be tested before closure.
- Final closure is done with drain in retropubic space.

Sling Procedure

The principle of sling procedure is to suspend the urethra from anterior abdominal wall. For suspension rectus fascia, fascia lata and other synthetic material have been used.

- Abdominal route.
- Vaginal route.

Abdominal Route (Fig. 7.6)

- Pfannestiel incision is made in anterior abdominal wall.
- Space lateral to urethra is dissected.
- Operating vaginally, urethro vesical junction is opened as in vaginal urethropexy procedure, and space of Retzius is entered.

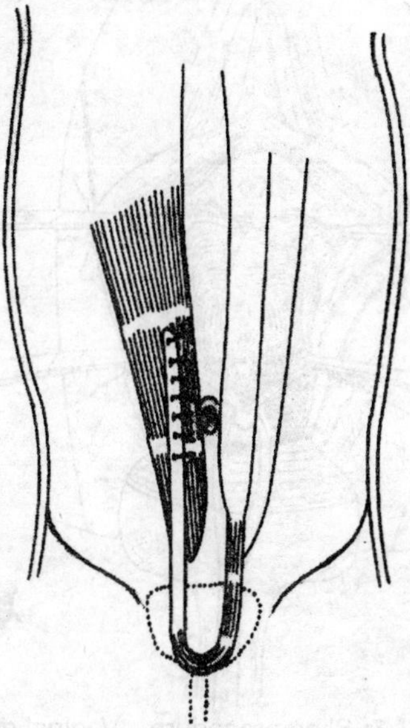

Fig. 7.6: Sling procedure—Abdominal route: Pubourethral sling

- Sling is passed beneath urethrovesical junction and delivered abdominally on both sides going through rectus fascia.
- Incontinence is checked.
- The abdominal ends of the sling are anchored to the rectus fascia with permanent sutures.

Vaginal Route (Fig. 7.7 to 7.9)

- The procedure is same as described in vaginal urethropexy, except that a strip of vagina is left intact.
- The vaginal strip located just beneath the urethra vesical junction extending distally over the proximal urethra for a distance of at least 2 cm.
- Four corners of the vaginal strip are sewn with permanent polypropylene sutures, which are then delivered abdominally, elevating the vaginal bridge of tissue in a sling like manner.
- The vagina is closed over this bridge of vaginal tissue, creating a sling of full thickness vaginal wall.

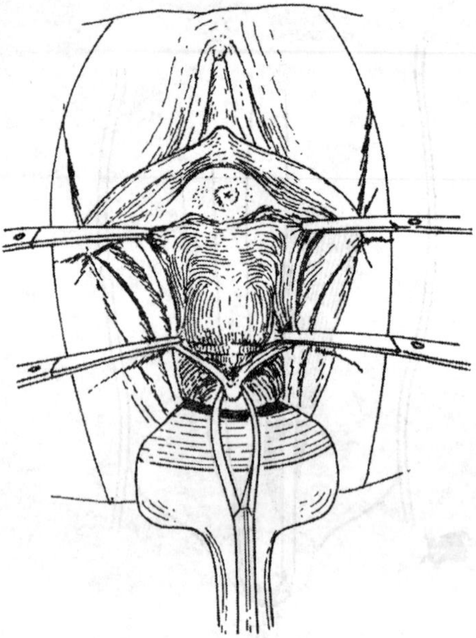

Fig. 7.7: Sling procedure—Vaginal route: Dissection of vaginal flaps

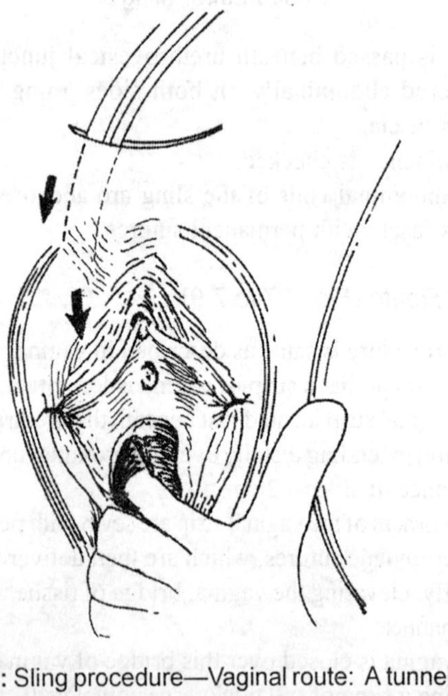

Fig. 7.8: Sling procedure—Vaginal route: A tunnel is made on either side of bladder neck to connect retropubic space with vaginal dissection

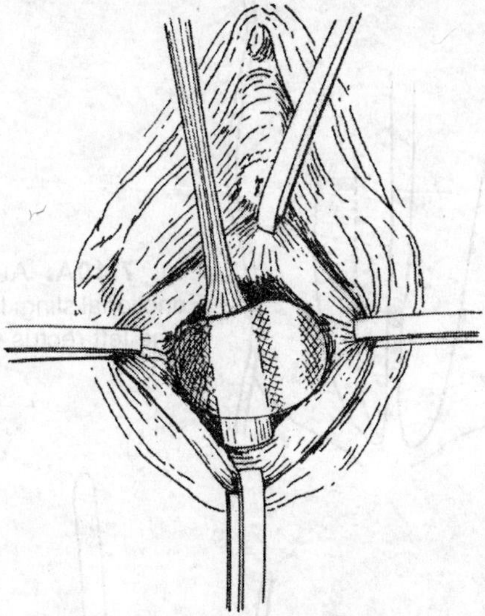

Fig. 7.9: Sling procedure—Vaginal route: Sling is placed before stitching tension is adjusted

Author's Functional Abdominal Sling Procedure

Author has described functional sling for incontinence.

- Abdomen is opened by Pfannenstiel incision.
- Sling of rectus fascia is dissected which is attached to a strip of rectus muscle.
- Sling is passed around urethra vesical junction and stitched to rectus muscle of opposite side (Figs 7.10A to C).

Advantage

Advantage of this procedure is that sling is not static. The female may have voluntary control over sling through rectus muscle.

Peri urethral Injections

Candidates for peri urethral injections to augment bladder outlet pressure are:

- Primary incompetent proximal urethra.
- Incontinence due to surgery on urethra.

Principle of periurethral injection is to enhance the bulk increasing pressure on urethra and reduce urethral lumenal size, so establishing additional urethral resistance to the

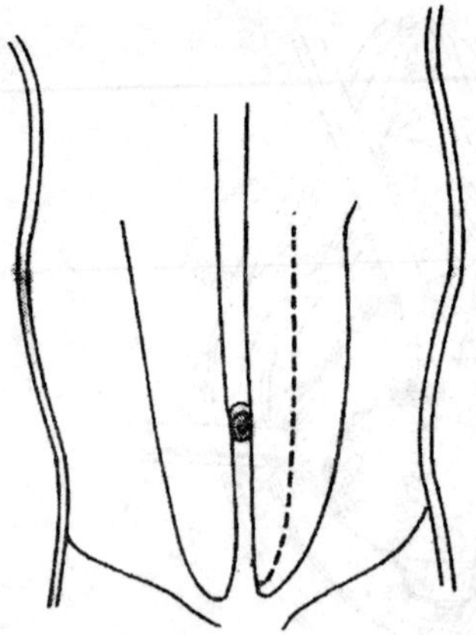

Fig. 7.10A: Author's Functional sling: Incision in the left rectus fascia

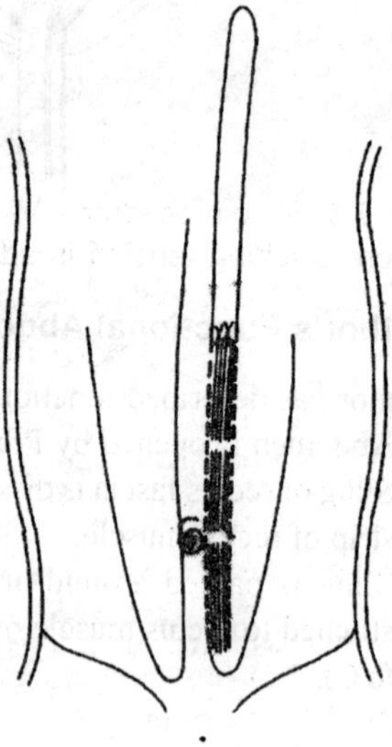

Fig. 7.10B: Author's Functional sling: Left rectus musculo fascial sling raised

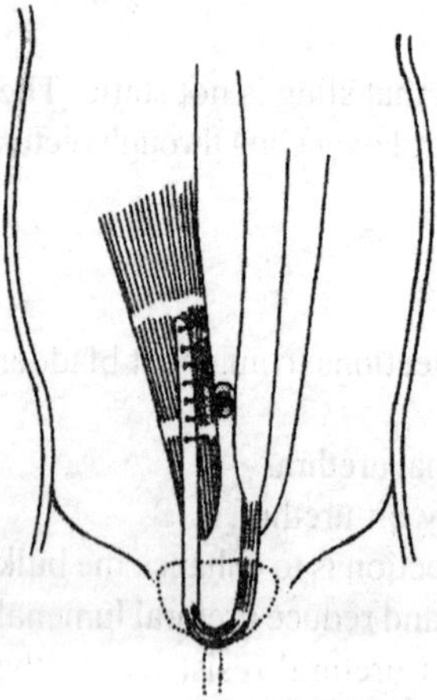

Fig. 7.10C: Author's Functional sling: Rectus musculo fascia sling passed around the bladder neck and sutured to right rectus muscle

flow of urine. The procedure is especially suitable for elderly females.

Various substances have been used like Polytef, contigena etc.

- Cystoscope is passed.
- Needle is placed in correct position.
- Bevel of needle is directed medially.
- Paste is injected.

Author has used autologous fat from pubic area for this. Purpose is that it is autologous tissue and chances of rejection are nil.

Tension Free Vaginal Tape for Surgical Treatment of Stress Urinary Incontinence

The procedure of TVT is based on a series of experimental investigations of the urethral closure mechanisms in the females. The procedure is safe, operating time is less and can be performed with simple training.

Technique

- The patient was operated in local anaesthesia.
- Two minimal incisions were made 5 cm apart in the abdominal skin just above the superior rim of the pubic bone.
  —1.5 cm long sagittal incision was made in the vaginal wall, starting 1 cm from the external urethral meatus.
- After minimal bilateral paraurethral dissections of the vaginal wall a specific prolene tape covered by plastic sheath is introduced, using two component needle instrument.
- The tip of the first perforated the urogenital diaphragm, and within space of Retzius the needle tip was brought upto the abdominal incision.
  –the procedure was repeated on the contralateral side.
- Tape is almost placed in U shape around urethra.
- After cystoscopy to ensure an intact bladder, the tape is adjusted without tension around urethra.
- During adjustment patient is asked to cough to check that she had become continent by the procedure.
- Now the plastic covering is removed.
- Though no fixation is recommended, author opines to fix the tape to subcutaneous tissue.
- The abdominal and vaginal incisions are closed.

8

Reconstructive Surgery of Fecal Incontinence

Fecal incontinence is under reported, under-recognized, and poorly understood. It is defined as involuntary excretion or leakage of feces in inappropriate places or at inappropriate times twice or more in past one month.

About 40-60% of women with anal incontinence report a difficult childbirth. It is found that innervation to the external anal sphincter is damaged during vaginal delivery. It may result due to:

- Prolonged second stage of labour.
- Forceps application.
- Large fetus.

Usually there is recovery in 2 months' time

Not all patients with nerve injuries present immediately after child birth, but may present several years later when additional denervation takes place as a result of aging.

Surgical Repair (Figs 8.1 to 13)

Position of the patient is lithotomy, if the injury is in anterior midline of anal circumference. However it is prone jackknife for all other injuries.

- Overlying scar is excised.
- Skin incision extended in a curvilinear direction along the anal margin.
- Subcutaneous scar tissue is excised, and the ends of divided muscle external sphincter are identified.
- Be careful to damage the nerve supply which enters in posterolateral quadrant.
- Sphincter is repaired.
- Anal mucosal repair is done.

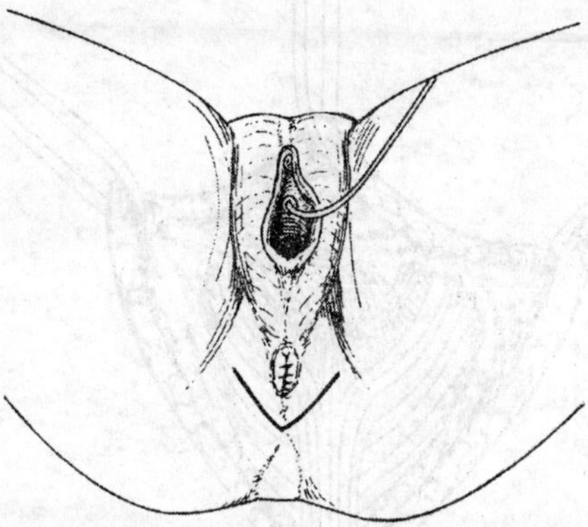

Fig. 8.1: Fecal incontinence—Surgical repair: Patient who was previously catheterized is placed in the lithotomy position and a V-shaped incision created posterior to the anus with the apex directed toward the coccyx

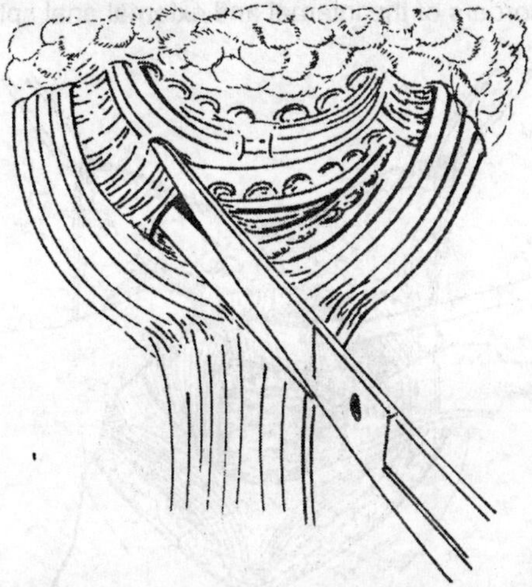

Fig. 8.2: Fecal incontinence—Surgical repair: The commencement of the dissection of the intersphincteric space using scissors

- Skin flaps are advanced medially and skin bridge is made between anus and vagina.

Silastic Anal Sling (Figs 8.14 to 8.18)

Indications

1. Failed repair.
2. Not amenable to repair.

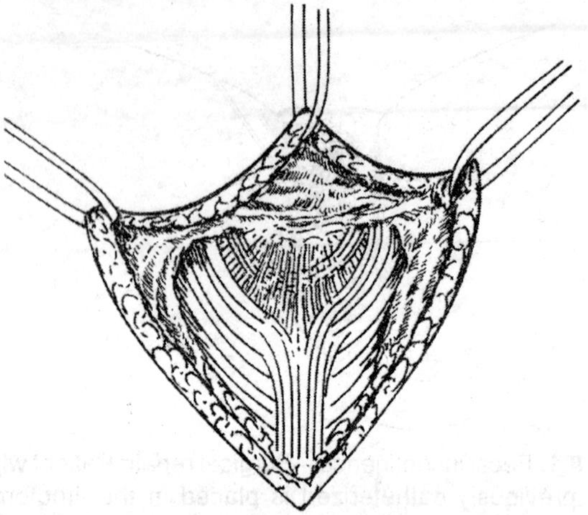

Fig. 8.3: Fecal incontinence—Surgical repair: An anterior flap was created and is reflected forward to expose the lower borders of the internal and external anal sphincters

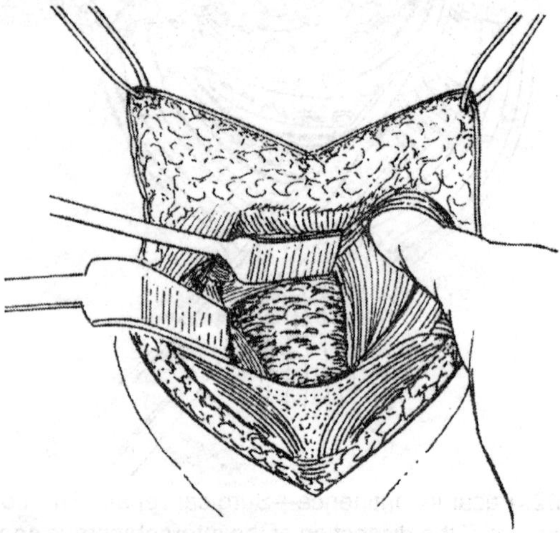

Fig. 8.4: Fecal incontinence—Surgical repair: The dissection continues using blunt dissection. The internal anal sphincter (anterior) is dissected free from the external anal sphincter (posterior)

The procedure is performed as following:

- Done under local anesthesia.
- Patient is placed in prone jackknife position.
- Curvilinear incision are made overlying the ischiorectal fossa.

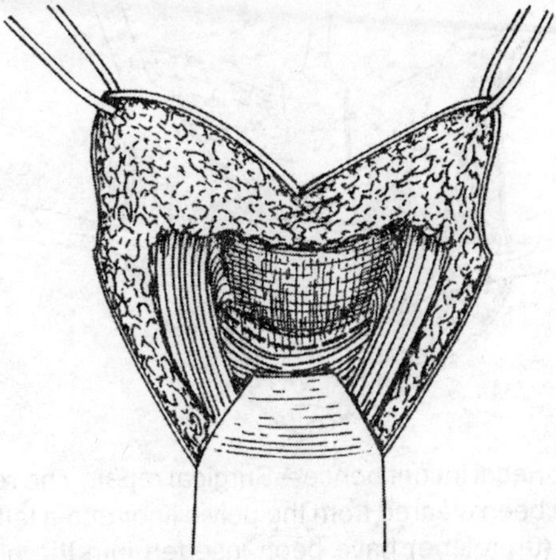

Fig. 8.5: Fecal incontinence—Surgical repair: At the level of the anorectal junction a dense layer of fascia is encountered within the intersphincteric space (Waldeyers fascia). This must be divided by sharp dissection in order to gain access to the pelvis

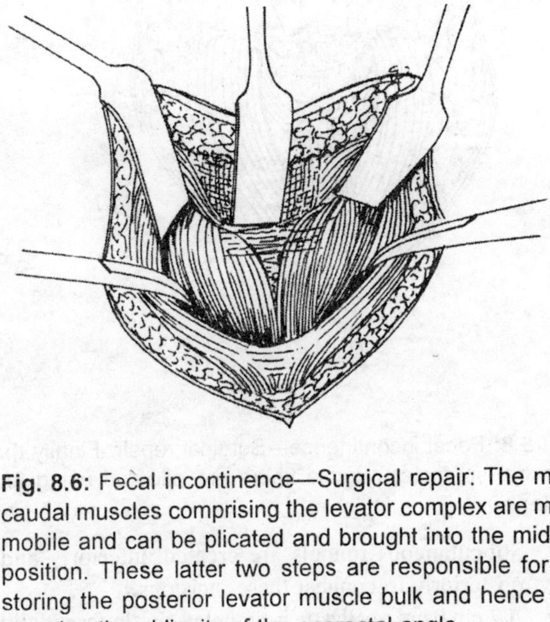

Fig. 8.6: Fecal incontinence—Surgical repair: The more caudal muscles comprising the levator complex are more mobile and can be plicated and brought into the midline position. These latter two steps are responsible for restoring the posterior levator muscle bulk and hence decreasing the obliquity of the anorectal angle

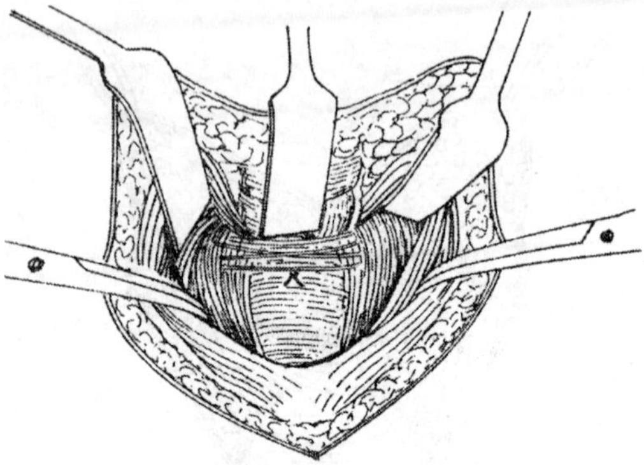

Fig. 8.7: Fecal incontinence—Surgical repair: The rectum has now been cleared from the pelvic floor and a lattice of sutures (0 prolene) have been inserted into the highest component of the levator muscle complex (ileococygeus)

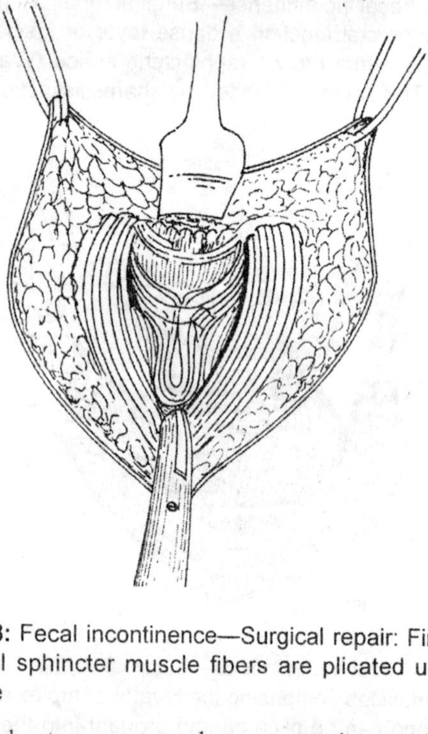

Fig. 8.8: Fecal incontinence—Surgical repair: Finally the external sphincter muscle fibers are plicated using 2/0 prolene

- Subcutaneous tunnels are created anteriorly and posteriorly to connect these incisions.
- A 2 cm band of silastic is tunneled circumferentially to encompass the remaining sphincter muscle and perianal soft tissue.

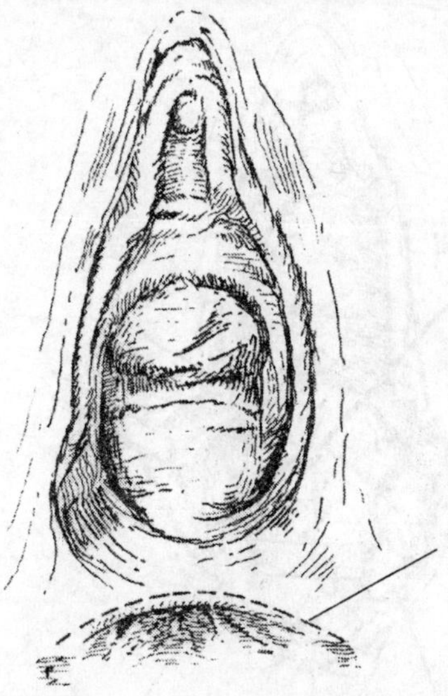

Fig. 8.9: Fecal incontinence—Surgical repair

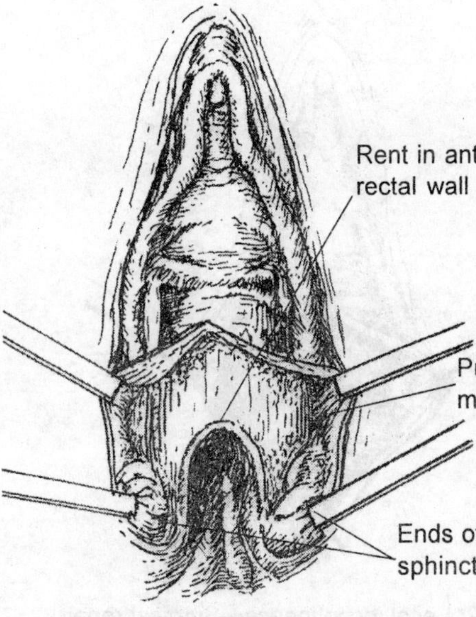

Fig. 8.10: Fecal incontinence—Surgical repair

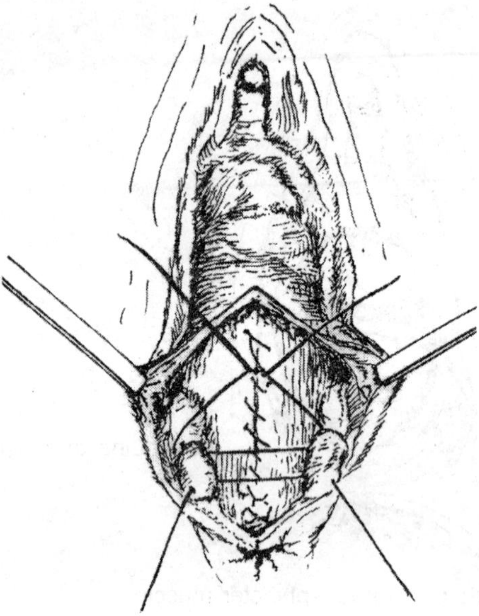

Fig. 8.11: Fecal incontinence—Surgical repair

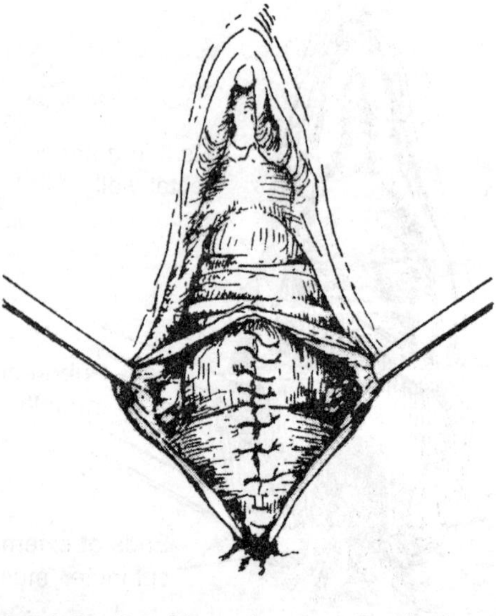

Fig. 8.12: Fecal incontinence—Surgical repair

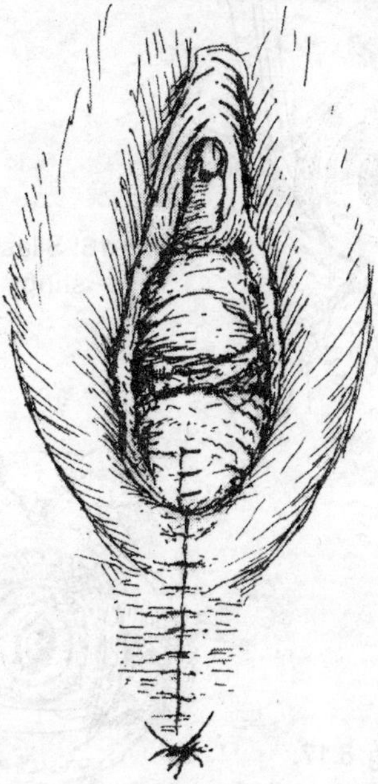

Fig. 8.13: Fecal incontinence—Surgical repair

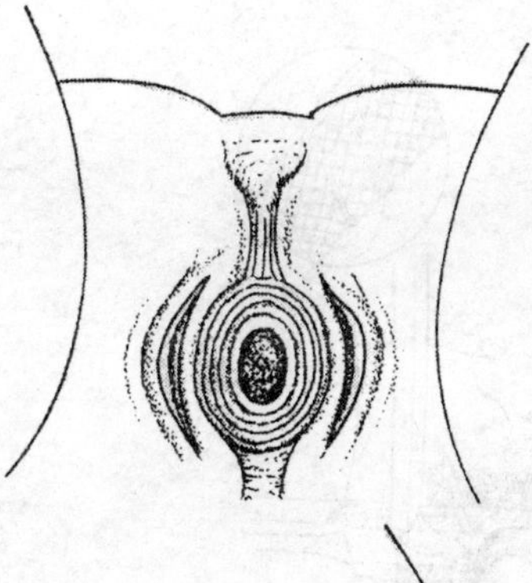

Fig. 8.14: Silastic anal sling

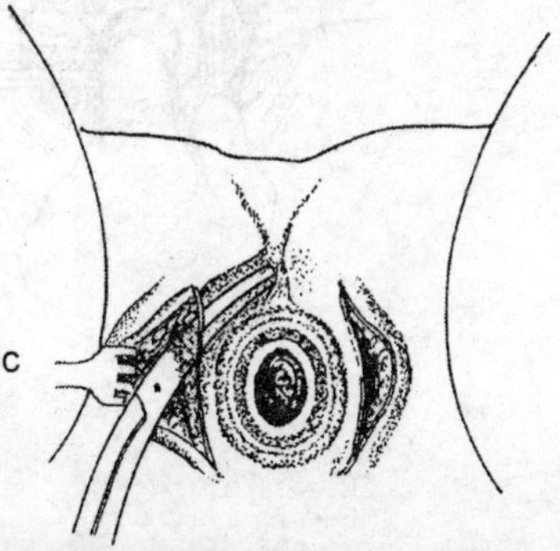

Fig. 8.15: Silastic anal sling

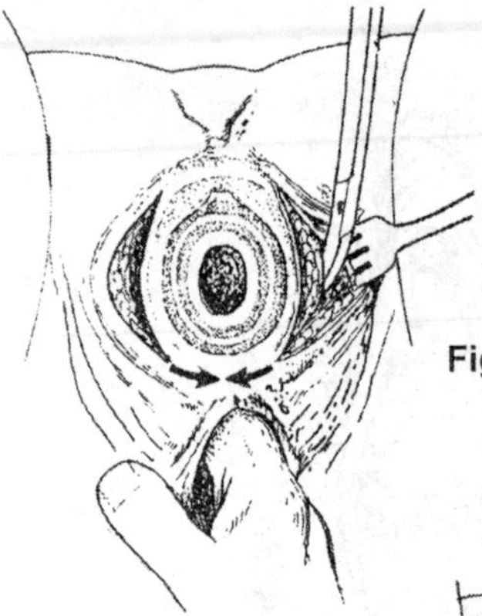

Fig. 8.16: Silastic anal sling

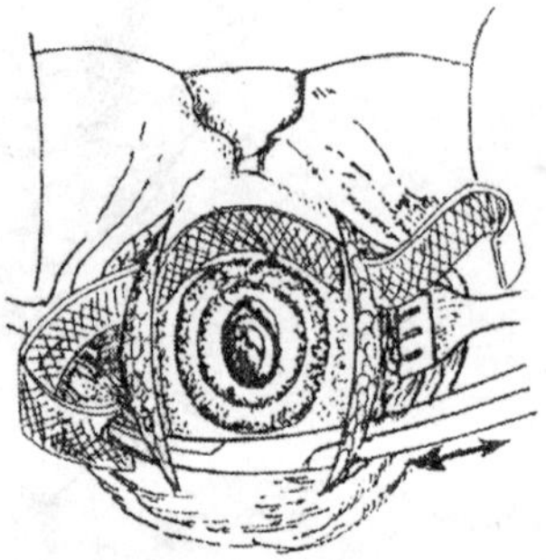

Fig. 8.17: Silastic anal sling

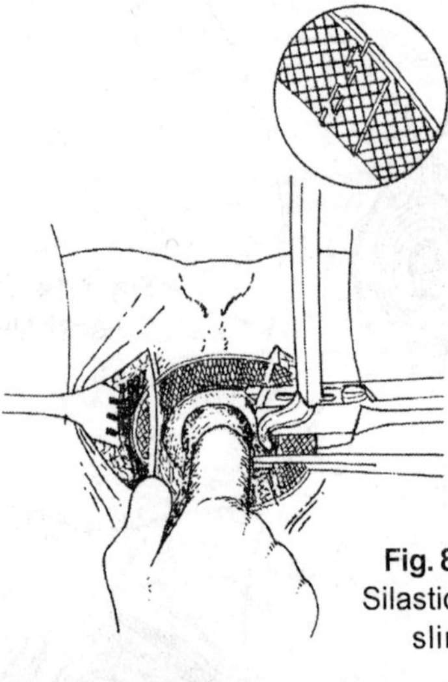

Fig. 8.18: Silastic anal sling

- The ends of the bands are overlapped and secured with non-absorbable monofilament sutures.
- The silastic band should be sufficiently lax to permit insertion of the distal interphalangeal joint of index finger in the anus the incision are closed.

Postanal Repair

The indication of this procedure are same as of insertion of silastic ring.

Procedure is performed as following:

- The patient is placed in lithotomy position.
- Subcutaneous tissue posterior to anus are infiltrated with weak adrenaline solution.
- A V-shaped incision is made approximately 1 cm posterior to the anus with the apex at the tip of coccyx.
- Flap of skin is lifted forward to expose the inferior border of the internal and external sphincters.
- The intersphincteric space is identified between the two muscles.
- Upper surface of the levator ani muscles is exposed by diving the Waldeyers fascia.
- Once the levator muscle is exposed, suturing can be done.
- At the highest level, a lattice is constructed across the ileococcygeus muscle with 0 prolene.

Below this level the puborectalis muscle is approximated, ensuring that the sutures are not subject to undue tension.

Postoperative Care

Excessive straining is avoided so stool softening is advisable.

9

Microsurgery of Tubal Blockage

Tubal blockage is common cause of infertility in about 20% of patients.

ETIOLOGY OF TUBAL BLOCKAGE

- Infectious tubal damage.
- Endometriosis.
- Tubal surgeries.
- Tubal diverticulosis, salpingitis isthmic nodosa, tubal polyps.
- Congenital abnormalities.
- Myometrial tumours.

Preoperative Evaluation

Tubal occlusion is best diagnosed by hysterosalpingography. Rubin's transcervical tubal insufflation with oxygen is also important diagnostic tool.

Tubal blockage can also be diagnosed by instilling methylene blue in uterus and visualizing escape of dye on laparoscopy.

One must not end evaluation of infertility once tubal abnormality is discovered. Following diagnostic procedures are required before tubal surgery.

- Proof of male fertility.
- Proof of ovulation.
- Proof of luteal phase adequacy.
- Absence of genital infections.

Microsurgical Technique and Principles

Microsurgery is a principle, rather than a technique. It permits precise cutting, accurate hemostasis, anatomically correct apposition of tissues, and use of fine sutures. After being trained in microsurgery one can give superior pregnancy results.

For microsurgery magnification can be obtained with loupes or an operating microscope placed over the operating field.

Along with loupe/microscope special microsurgical instruments are required. The delicate, miniaturized microsurgical instruments are designed for accurate maneuvering and precise handling of tissues under magnification. The essential microsurgical instruments are micro needle holder, microscissors, and a couple of jeweller's forceps.

The tip diameter of the microforceps is between 0.1 and 1.5 mm; the 0.5 mm tip is most commonly used. The length of the instruments ranges from 9-22 cm. All needle holders and scissors must be spring loaded to allow smooth digital opening and closing.

Microelectrodes: The monopolar microelectrode is used for cutting the tube and adhesions and for coagulation of small bleeders. An insulated microelectrode with a 0.1 to 0.2 mm pointed tip inserted into the ubiquitous electrosurgical handle is suitable for work under the microscope.

Bipolar coagulation is the essence of hemostasis in microsurgery.

Irrigators and Aspirators: Continuous irrigation to avoid desiccation and to identify bleeders is essential in microsurgery.

Retracting rods: Retracting rods are used for traumatic tissue holding. Most of them are L-shaped and 17-23 cm long, have a cylindrical tip, and are made of glass, quartz, teflon or titanium.

Probes: Probes are used to sound the tubal lumen, facilitate reanastomosis, or introduce a splint. Lacrimal duct probes are extremely useful for this purpose. These are available in sizes 00 to No. 10 have blunt tips, and are made of malleable materials. Hollow flexible probes facilitate the introduction of tubal splints.

Size 1 or 2 Nylon or Prolene suture materials are flexible enough to be introduced through the convoluted intramural tubal segment.

Fine blades and reamers: Fine and sharp blades are required. Sometimes special blades are necessary to pare and gouge out intramural oviduct.

Tubal clamps: Clamps that encircle the tube and compress the subtotal vasculature are useful for both steadying the cut ends of the tubes during anastomosis, and helping hemostasis.

Suture materials: Sutures traumatize the tissues and leave temporary or permanent foreign materials in the wound. Therefore, the finest and least reactive sutures appropriate for each particular tissue should be employed. In gynecological microsurgery ethilon, nylon /prolene between 7- and 10-0 are used. Black monofilament nylon is the recommended suture if a non-absorbable suture is chosen.

Mesothelial Re-epithelialization and Prevention of Post Surgical Adhesions

The smooth peritoneal membrane covering both the coelomic cavity and the intra-abdominal organs permits unrestricted movement and allows the organs to slide against each others.

Areas where the mesothelial lining is irreversibly damaged become covered by the peritoneum of the nearest organ and heal by retaining the donated peritoneum and the organ. The fusion of the two surfaces leads to the most severe form of adhesions with restricted function of the organ.

Different types of infection through peritoneal tubal opening; as well as mechanical, chemical and infectious damage inflicted during laparotomies, invariably leads to mesothelial damage, periadnexal adhesions, and restricted tubal motility and function.

Adhesion formation is the major factor in post infectious tubal infertility and the principal reason for failure after tubal reconstructive surgery.

So, avoidance of adhesion formation is most important component of tubal surgery. Further, prevention of unwanted adhesion formation should not only be limited to tuboplasty, but must include all conservative pelvic surgery (e.g. ovarian cystectomy, myomectomy, metroplasty, and resection of endometriosis).

Pathogenesis of Adhesions

The development of adhesions is the consequence of excessive fibrin deposition, which overwhelms the fibrinolytic activity. The persistent coagulated inflammatory exudate is invaded by the subperitoneal fibroblasts, which deposit the connective tissue matrix, allowing new vessels to sprout from the existing capillary endothelium. New mesothelial cells arising from mesenchymal cells, will ultimately cover the organized fibrin matrix to create an established fibrous adhesion.

PREVENTION OF PERITONEAL ADHESIONS

Surgical techniques with minimal tissue trauma, the prevention of infection and employment of pharmacological agents are the aspects under the surgeon's control.

Surgical Technique

- Reapproximation of serosal edges under tension should be avoided.
- Application of free peritoneal or omental grafts should be avoided.
- Placement of transperitoneal sutures for hemostasis or uterine suspension should be avoided.
- Use of thick non-absorbable sutures should be avoided.

Contrary to usual concept, peritoneal defects should be left unrepaired if reperitonealization produces ischemia because they usually heal without adhesions regardless of their size.

Pharmacologic Adjuvants

Steroids act by minimizing the inflammatory response to injury. Combination of dexamethasone and promethazine has been advocated by Horne et al.

Single dose

- Dexamethasone 20 mg
- Promethazine 25 mg.

Treatment Schedule

1. 2-3 hours before surgery.
2. Intraoperatively before peritoneal closure.
3. Postoperatively every 4 hours for total of 12 doses.

Separation of serosal surfaces would prevent fusion of fibrin-covered surfaces while healing occurs. Ideally, such a substance should be inert, distribute, over all potential adhesion sites, remain until the complete healing takes place, and not facilitate bacterial growth. Dextran is commonly used substance for this purpose. Dextran 70 is instilled intraperitoneally which results in temporary ascites for 5-10 days. Dextran 40 is less effective as it is resorbed rapidly. The dose of Dextran 70 is 1-5 ml/kg. The 32% Dextran 70 in 10% dextrose in the volume of 100-250 ml is relatively safe.

PROXIMAL TUBAL OCCLUSION

The intra mural portion of the tube begins at the tip of an endometrial funnel and ends at the outer border of uterus, where it becomes the isthmus. The length of this segment is 8-20 mm, whereas the diameter of the lumen varies from 0.2 mm to 2 mm. Its course, as it traverses the myometrium is usually curved or convoluted, straight in only one fourth of cases. A branch of the ascending uterine artery and vein supply the interstitial portion of the tube.

This uterotubal barrier is functional only when eggs are present in the tube, and is non-functional for the rest of the cycle.

Etiology of Proximal Tubal Occlusion

Destruction of the tubal epithelium by infections is the most common etiological factor in proximal tubal occlusion. Extensive deciliation. Alteration of non-ciliated cells, and focal destruction of epithelial cells result in both post inflammatory fibrosis and follicular salpingitis.

The bacterial etiology is Neisseria gonorrhoea, Chlamydia trachomatis, Escherichia coli, Hemolytic streptococci etc. in postpartum and post abortal endometritis.

Intrauterine contraceptive devices are associated with a three- to five-fold increased risk of pelvic inflammatory disease.

A list of etiological factors is given in below:

1. Infections—Chronic salpingitis and follicular salpingitis.
2. Salpingitis—Isthmica nodosa- and tubal diverticulosis.
3. Heterotopic endometrium, intraluminal endometriosis, and tubal polyps.
4. Iatrogenic tubal occlusion
   - Sterilization.
   - Occlusion during uterine suspension and other procedures.

5. Non-infectious obliterative fibrosis.
6. Cornual leiomyomas and adenomyomas.
7. Functional or false tubal occlusion.

Diagnosis

Accurate diagnosis of proximal tubal occlusion is little difficult due to several reasons.

- Patency of the proximal oviduct sometimes depend on the hormonal status of the endometrium and endosalpinx.
- A functional sphincter is present at the uterotubal junction.
- Luminal size is 0.2 mm.
- The intramural tubal segment is not visible by laparoscopy.

Hysterosalpingography is the best method. Normal hysterosalpingography shows a constriction at the junction of the endometrial funnel and the beginning of the tube, followed by a club-shaped dilatation of intramural tube called pretubal bulge.

Obstruction at the level of physiological constriction are seen with intrauterine synechiae.

Demonstration of proximal 2 cm of tube only or unilateral cornual occlusion might indicate tubal spasm.

In salpingitis, isthemica nodosa, the proximal tube has money comb appearance.

Intravasation in a localized area represents a large adenomyoma.

Laparoscopy and tubaloscopy are some investigations required before surgery.

Surgery

Surgical procedures available are:

- Cornual anastomosis (Figs 9.1 to 9.4).
- Tubal reimplantation (Figs 9.5 to 9.19).

Cornual anastomosis is always preferred over tubal reimplantation. In most of the patients, at least part of the intramural portion of the tube is patent, and a cornual anastomosis following resection of the obstructed segment is feasible. Lack of expertise with the operating microscope should not be an excuse for choosing reimplantation over anastomosis. Both procedure are described in details in figures.

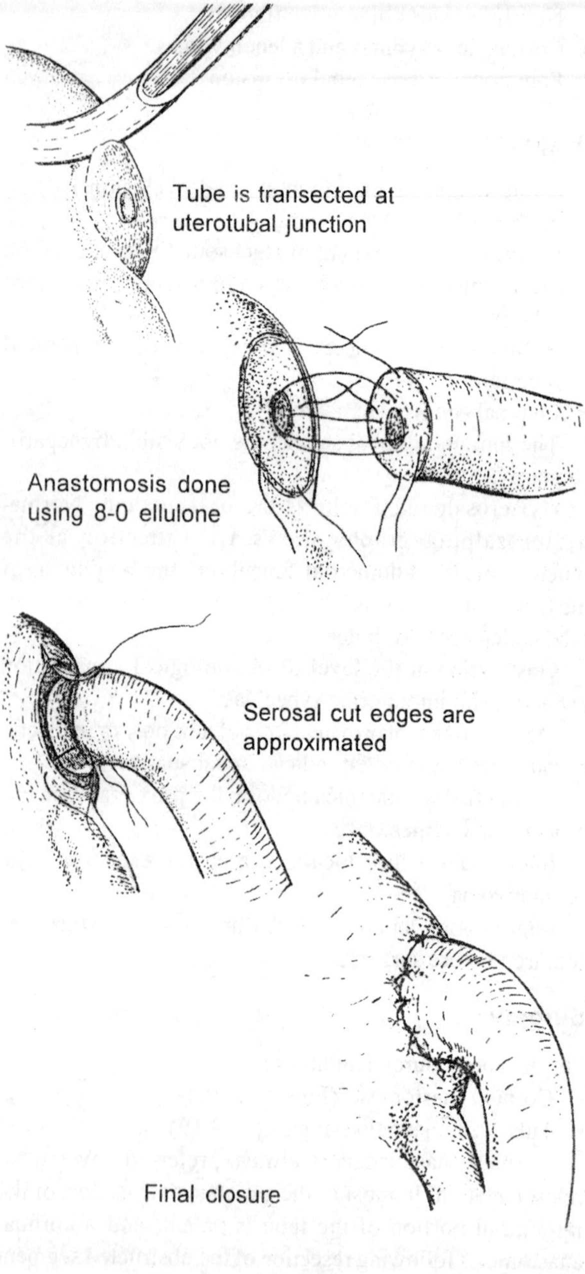

Figs 9.1 to 9.4: Cornual anastomosis: Preoperatively No. 8 Foley Calhela is introduced into uterine cavity inflated with 3–5 ml saline and connected to dilute dye solution

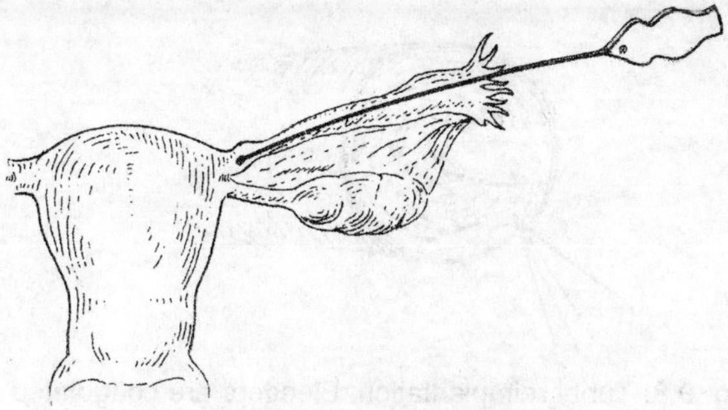

Fig. 9.5: Tubal reimplantation: A lacrimal sound is passed in tube from distal end

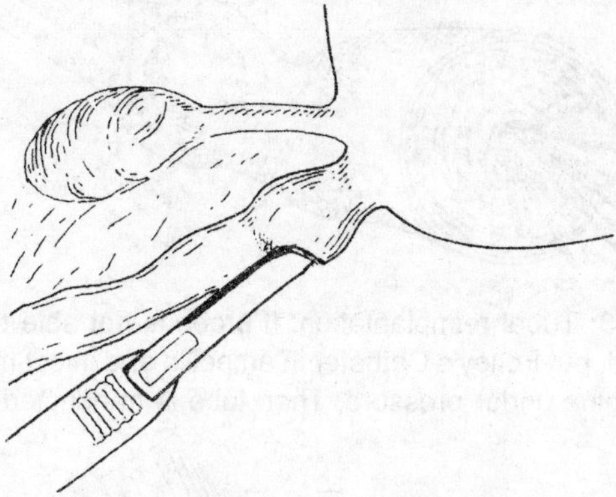

Fig. 9.6: Tubal reimplantation: Isthmic portion of tube is and transected

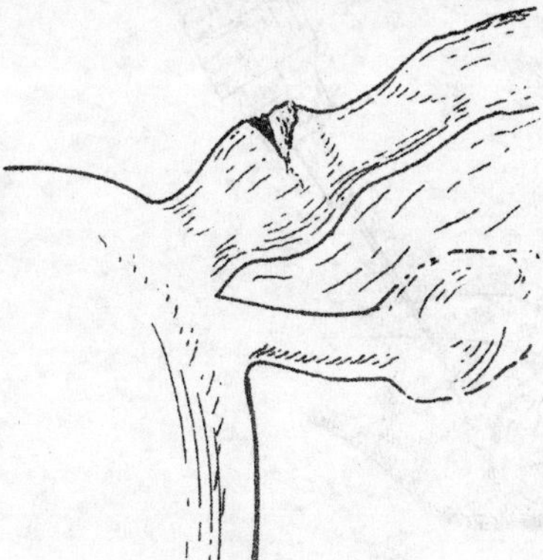

Fig. 9.7: Tubal reimplantation: Isthmic portion of tube is and transected

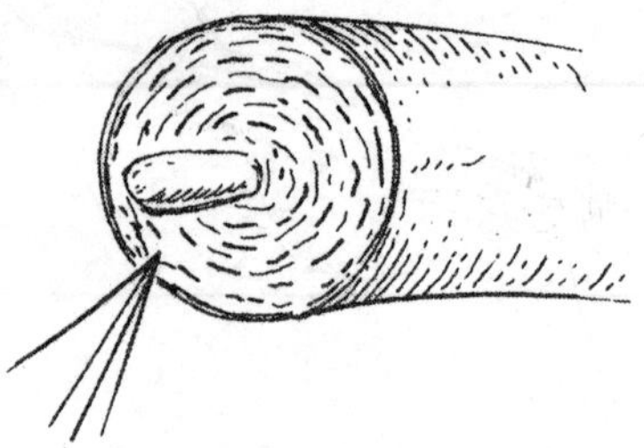

Fig. 9.8: Tubal reimplantation: Bleeders are coagulated

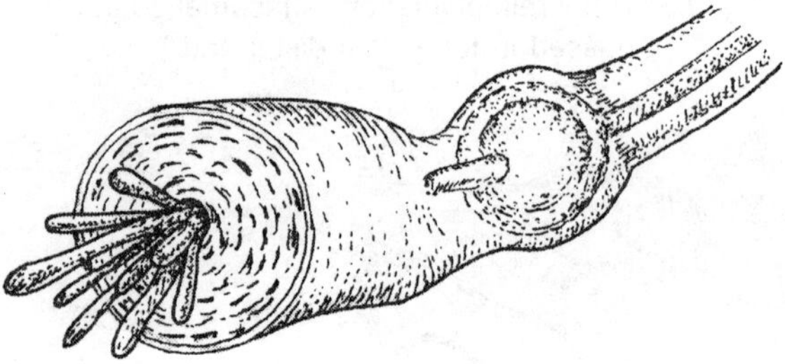

Fig. 9.9: Tubal reimplantation: If probe is not able to be passed, put Folley's Catheter in ampeilla and inject methylene blue under pressure. Then tube is transected

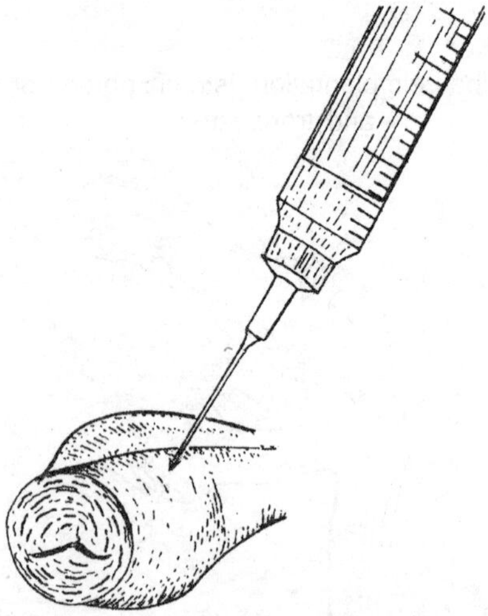

Fig. 9.10: Tubal reimplantation: Subserosa is infiltrated with 1:2 lac adrenatine solution

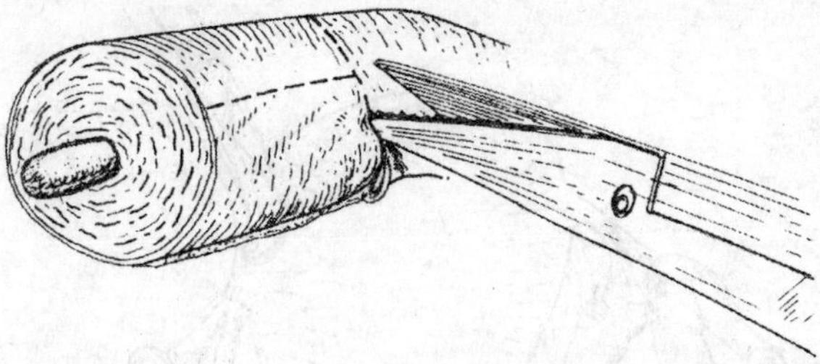

Fig. 9.11: Tubal reimplantation: At about 1 cm a circular cut through tubal peritoneum is made

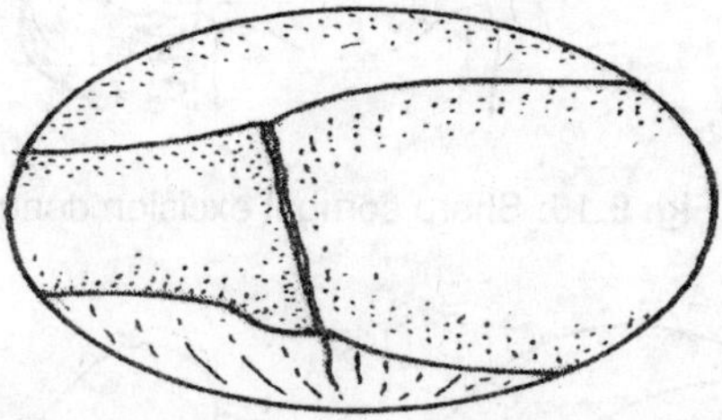

Fig. 9.12: Tubal reimplantation: Peritoneum removed from distal 1 cm of tube

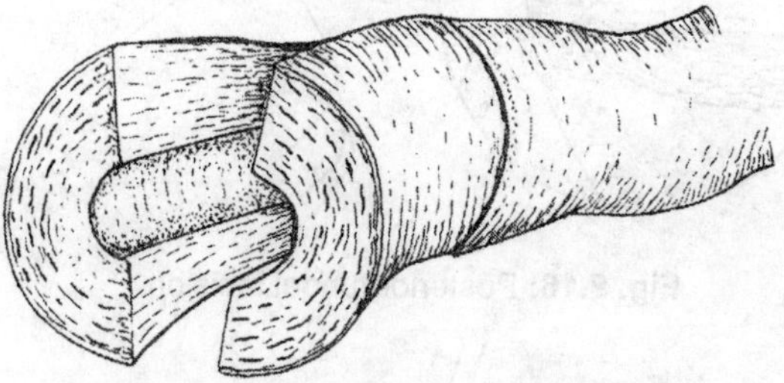

Fig. 9.13: Tubal reimplantation: Tube is slit

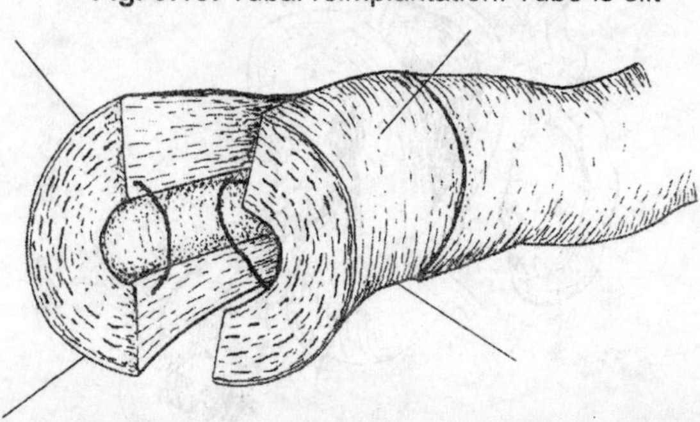

Fig. 9.14: Tubal reimplantation: Sutures passed

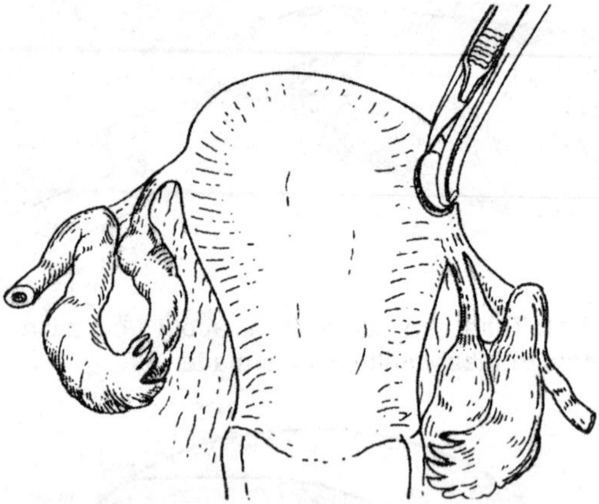

Fig. 9.15: Sharp cornual excision done

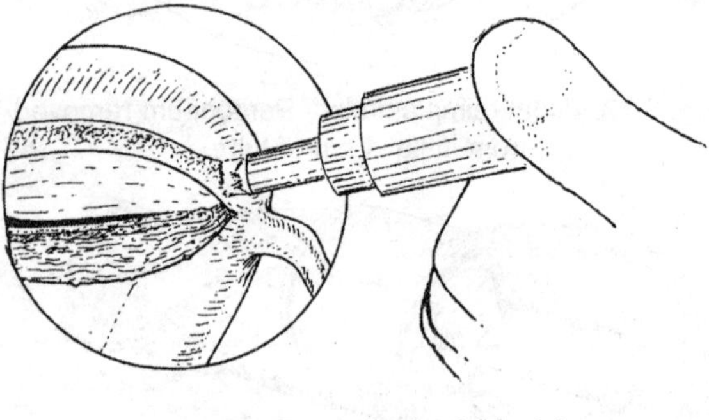

Fig. 9.16: Posterior fundal incision

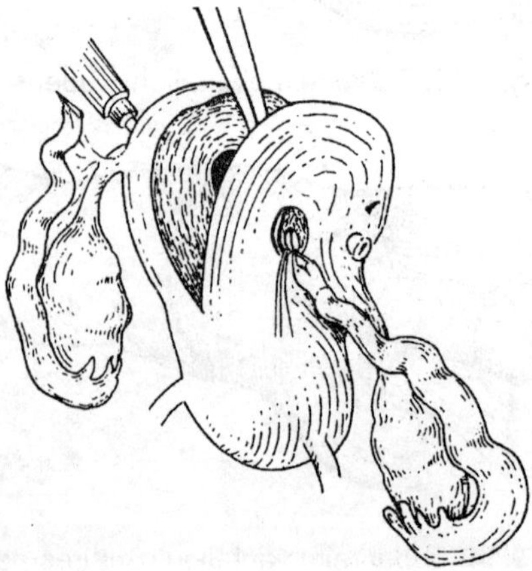

Fig. 9.17: Transverse fundal incision

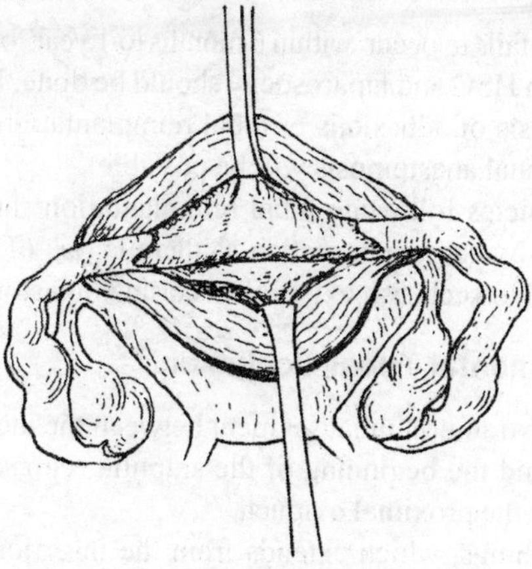

Fig. 9.18: Reimplantation done

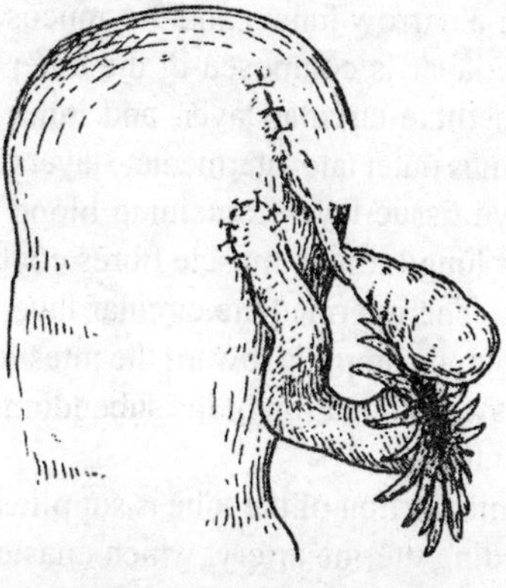

Fig. 9.19: Final closure

Once the patient is under anaesthesia an intrauterine irrigation device (Foley catheter) should be inserted. Transfundal tubal lavage is impractical. After this vagina should be packed tightly with bandage soaked in paraffin-betadine lotion. It results in elevation of uterus along with tubes out of pelvis, facilitating microsurgical work over tubes.

Upon opening the abdomen, bowels are packed into the upper abdomen and placing the retractor pelvis is examined. Any adhesion is lysed.

Success and Failure Following Surgical Treatment of Proximal Tubal Occlusion

Patency rate of anastomosis following procedures is 70-100%, however pregnancy rate may not be so high. If pregnancy fails to occur within 6 months to 1 year following surgery, an HSG and laparosocpy should be done. In some patients lysis of adhesions or tubal reimplantation after a failed cornual anastomosis will be possible.

Pregnancies following tubal reimplantation should be delivered by caesarean section as there is risk of rupture of uterus. No such risk exists after cornual anastomosis.

Mid Segmental Tubal Occlusion

The thin extramural tubal segment between the uterotubal junction and the beginning of the ampulla represents the isthmus or the proximal oviduct.

The isthmus, which extends from the insertion of the tube into the uterus distally, is characterized by heavy musculature, a narrow lumen and 3-5 mucosal folds. The thick muscle layer is composed of the outer longitudinal layer, intermediate circular layer, and inner longitudinal layer. In isthmus outer and intermediate layers are separated by connective tissue layer containing blood vessels.

The outer longitudinal muscle fibres continue into the mesosalpinx. The intermediate circular layer increases in thickness from the ampulla toward the intestinal tube. The inner layer is a continuation of the subendometrial muscle layer of the uterus.

The isthmic portion of the tube is supplied by a branch of the ascending uterine artery, which anastomose with a branch of the ovarian artery forming a subtubal vascular arcade.

Following successful fertilization in the ampulla, the arrival of the embryo in the uterus is synchronous with the maturation of endometrium. In humans, the time from ovulation to arrival in the endometrial cavity is 80 hours. Propulsion of ovum through the isthmus is a combination of increased luminal diameter and increased peristalsis.

Etiology of Mid Segmental Tubal Occlusion

Previous sterilization performed by salpingectomy, tubal diathermy, or tubal clipping is by far the most common indication for mid tubular anastomosis. Etiology factors for mid segment tubal occlusion are given below.

Etiology of Mid Segment Occlusion

A—Sterilization by tubal ligation
B—Segmental salpingectomy for ectopic pregnancy
C—Congenital segmental absence of the tube
D—Tubal endometriosis
E—Tubal polyps and diverticula
F—Segmental intraluminal adhesions.

Tubotubal Anastomosis

Classification of operative procedures are:

- Intramural isthmic anastomosis
- Intramural ampullary anastomosis
- Isthmic—isthmic anastomosis
- Isthmic—ampullary anastomosis
- Ampullary—ampullary anastomosis
- Ampullary—infundibular anastomosis

All the operative procedures are described in (Figs 9.20 to 9.27).

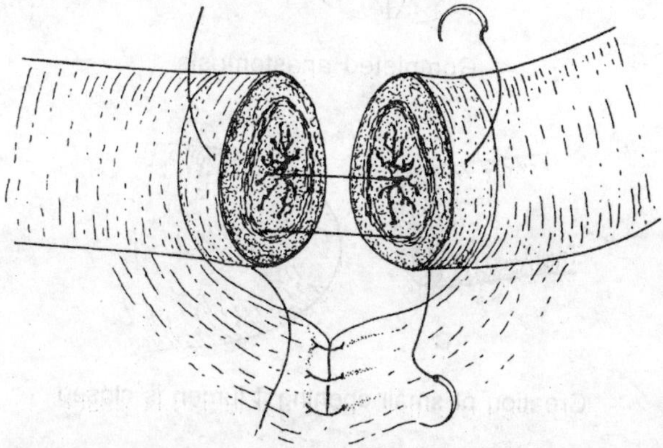

Fig. 9.20: Ampullary-Ampullary Anastomoses. At this site a teflon or any other probe should always be passed to avoid pecking up mucosal folds of opposite wall. First suture at 6 O'clock position including muscularis and mucosa

Successes and Failures

From recent series of over 1800 microsurgical tubal reversals, an overall cumulative intrauterine pregnancy rate of 64% and an ectopic pregnancy rate of 4% has been found.

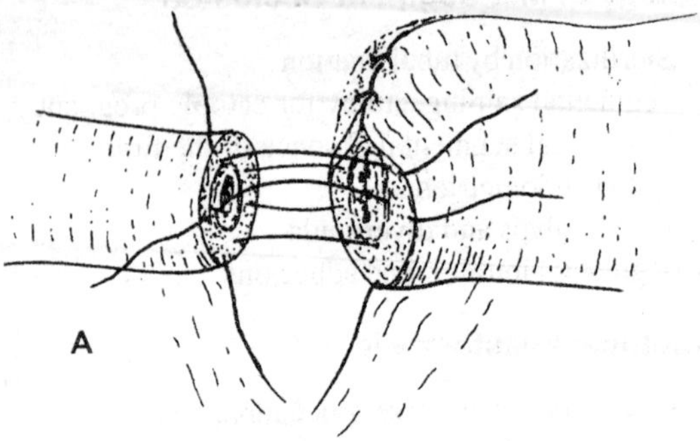

Reduction of distal lumen

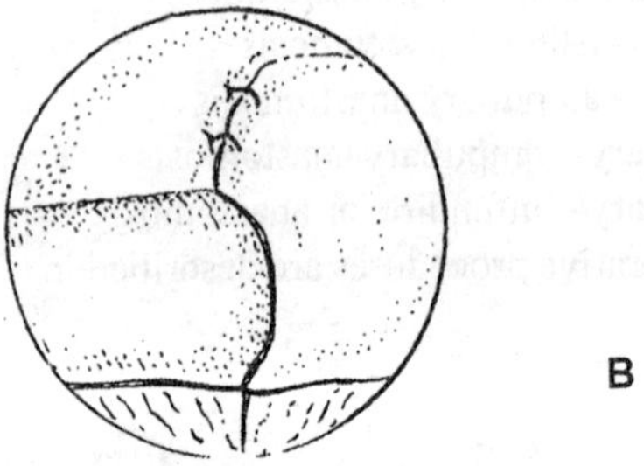

Completed anastomosis

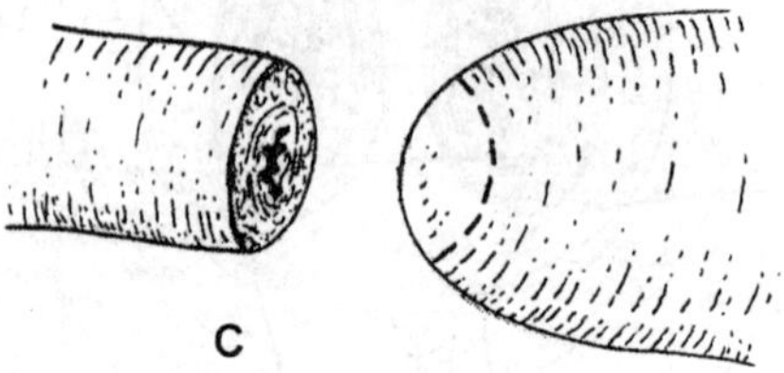

Creation of small opening if lumen is closed

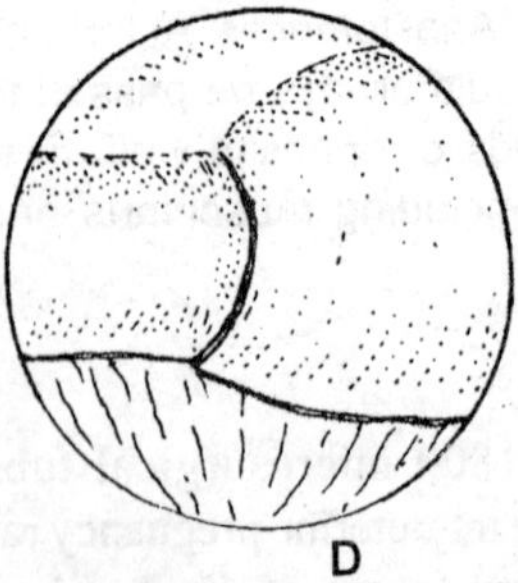

Completed anastomosis

Fig. 9.21: Isthmic-Ampullary Anastomosis (unequal lumen)

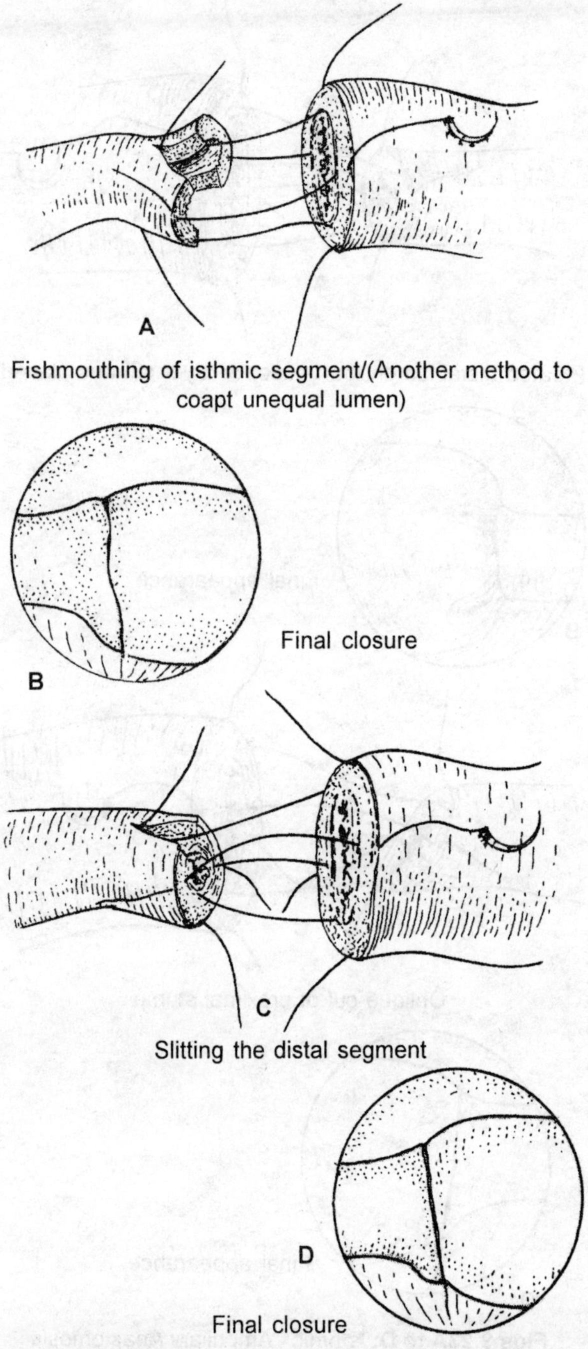

Figs 9.22A to D: Isthmic-Ampullary Anastomosis

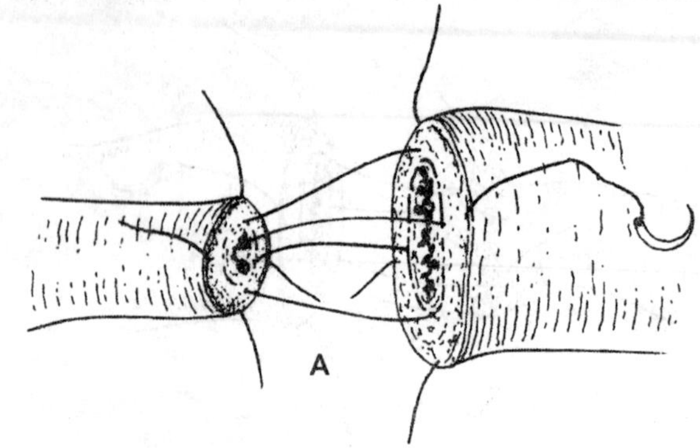

Pleated distal lumen four muscular layer sutures placed

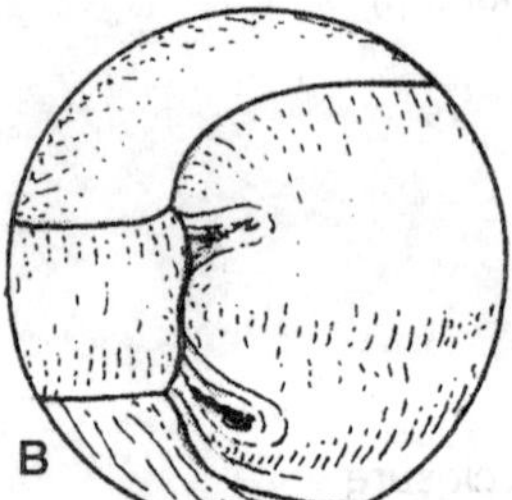

Final appearance

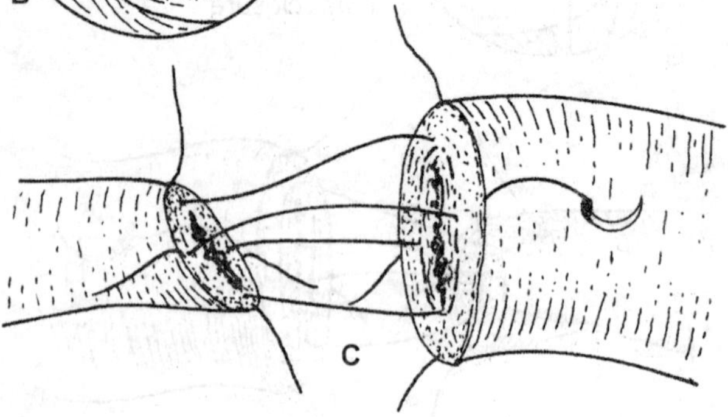

Oblique cut of proximal stump

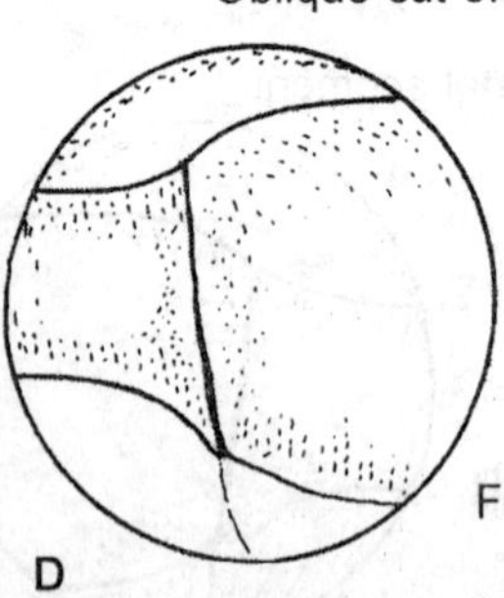

Final appearance

Figs 9.23A to D: Isthmic - Ampullary Anastomosis (Coaptation of unequal lumen)

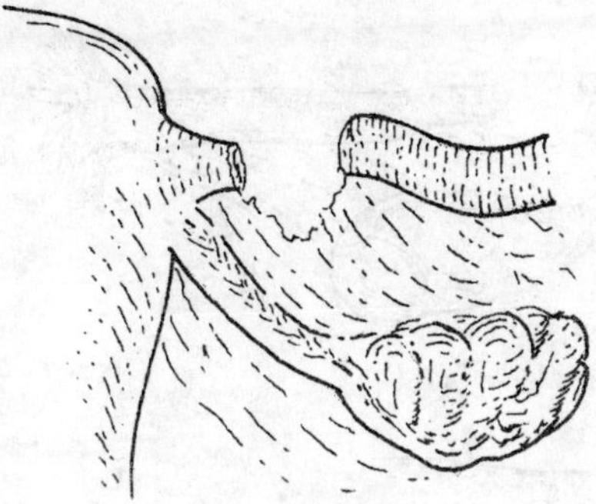

A. Tubal stumps

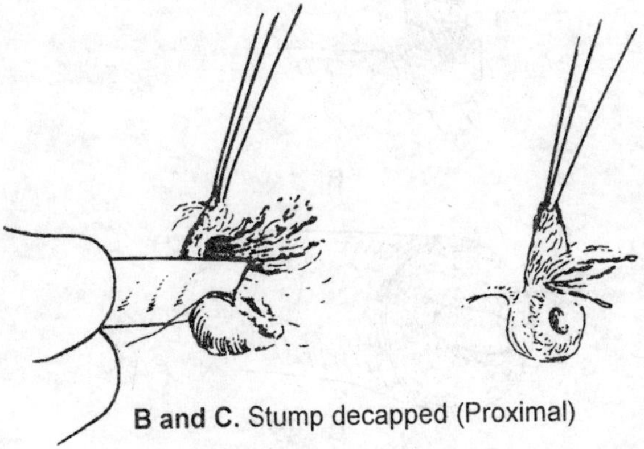

B and C. Stump decapped (Proximal)

D. Hemostasis of cut surface

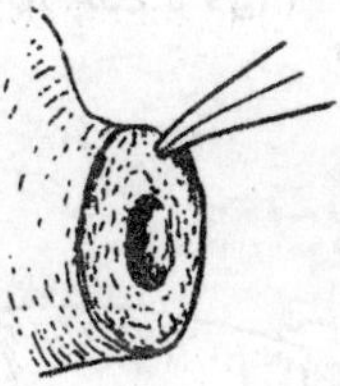

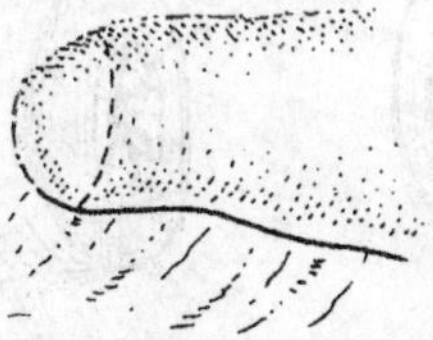

E. Stumps decapped (distal)

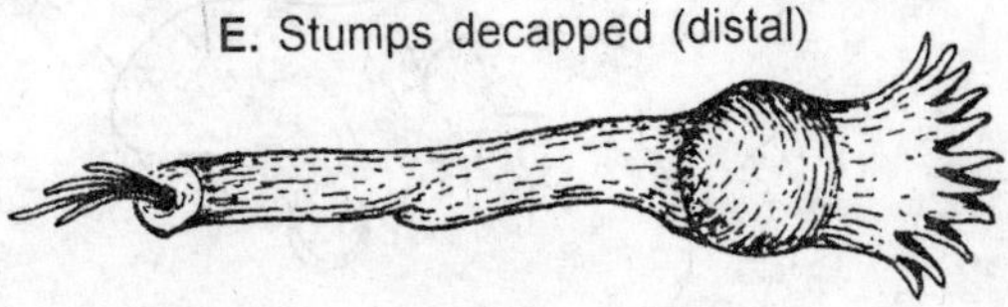

F. Stumps decapped (distal)

Figs 9.24A to F: Isthmic - Isthmic Reanastomosis

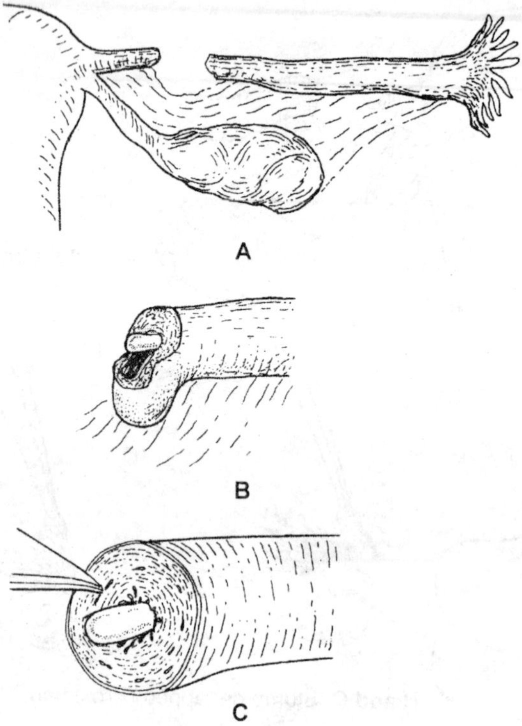

Figs 9.25A to C: Isthmic - Ampullary reanastomosis: Stumps prepared

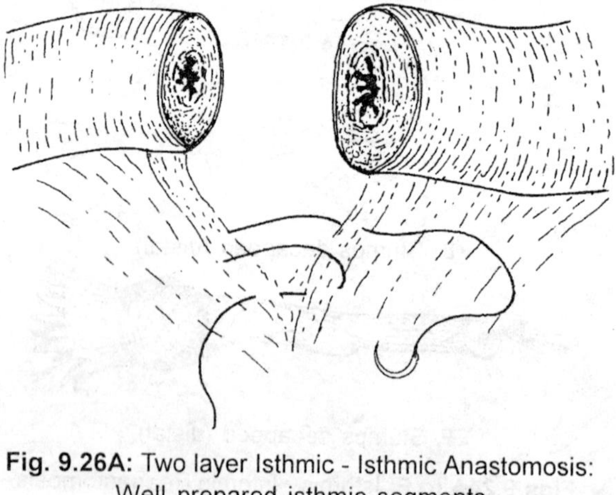

Fig. 9.26A: Two layer Isthmic - Isthmic Anastomosis: Well prepared isthmic segments

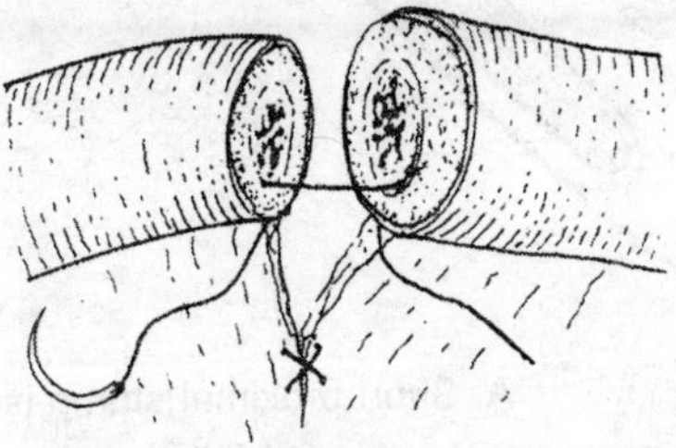

Fig. 9.26B: Two layer Isthmic - Isthmic Anastomosis: Placement of 6 O'clock muscular layer

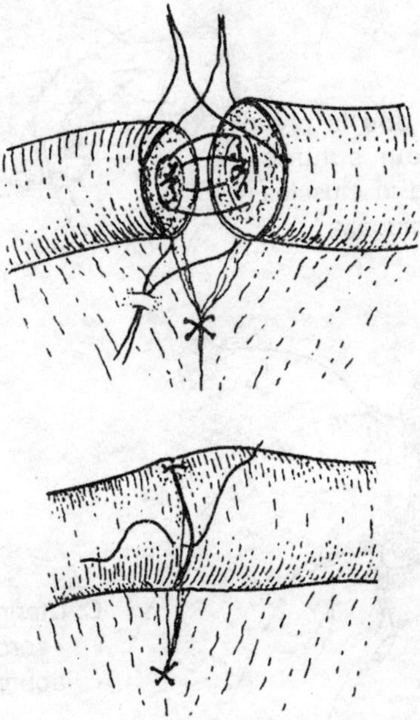

C

D

Figs 9.26C and D: Two layer Isthmic - Isthmic Anastomosis (C) Placement of three muscular sutures. Each suture is left untied and sutured at end (D) Approximation of tubal serosa

Among other factors, the feasibility and ultimate success of tubal reanastomosis depends on the type of previous tubal ligation, length of remaining tube, and the location of the anastomosis.

Irrespective of the method of sterilization, tubal length is critical for success, although it is not known what represents the minimal length beyond which the pregnancy

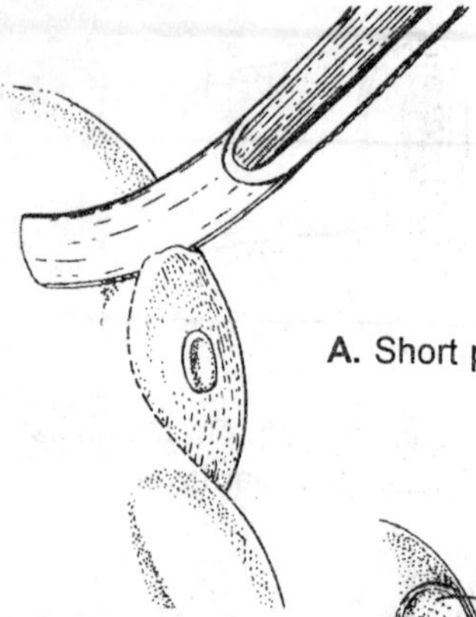

A. Short proximal stump is pared away

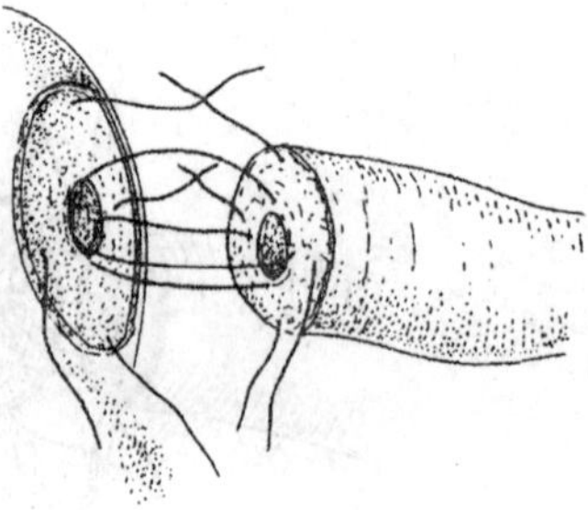

B. Distal end is prepared. Four sutures are placed in muscles avoiding mucosa

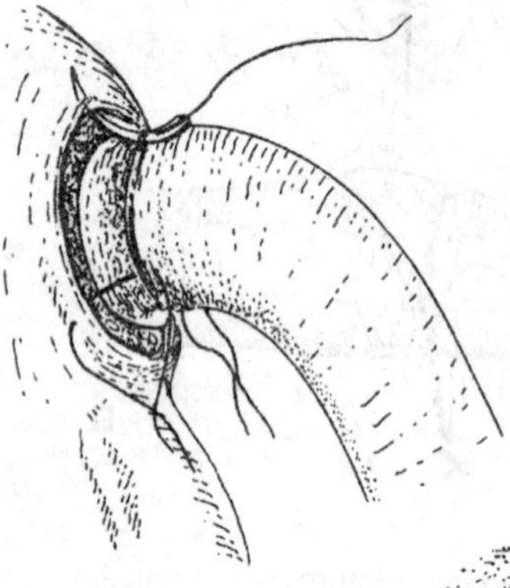

C. Uterine and tubal serosa are approximated

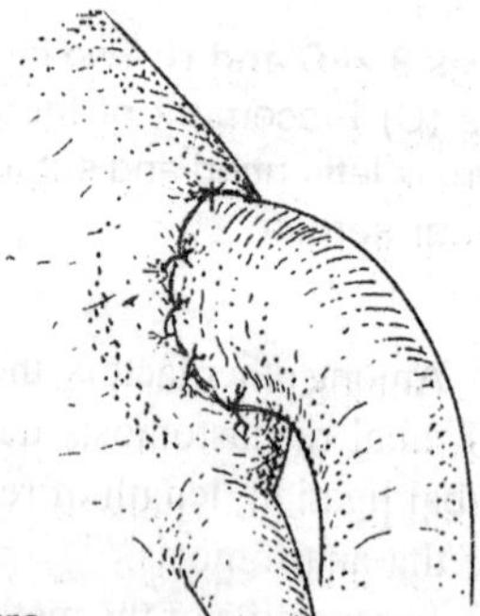

D. Final closure

Figs 9.27A to D: Intramural isthmic anastomosis

rate is unacceptably low. Several studies has proved that pregnancy rate is significantly lower with an extramural tube less than 4 cm long. A critical drop in pregnancy rate occurs with a tubal length 3 cm or less.

Causes of Failure of Tubal Reanastomosis

- Unrecognized proximal stump pathology
- Distorted or nonpatent anastomotic site
- Postoperative adhesions
- Foreshortened fallopian tubes
- Ovarian dysfunction.

DISTAL TUBAL OCCLUSION

The tubal segment lateral to the ampullary-isthmic junction is considered the distal oviduct. It consists of 5-8 cm long ampulla ending in a funnel shaped infundibulum with an abdominal opening and numerous slender processes called fimbriae. The relaxed abdominal tubal ostimum is about 3 mm in diameter, although the stretched luminal diameter of ampulla is about 1 cm. The mesosalpinx ends short of the infundibulum, allowing the terminal end of the tube to move freely while the fimbriae embrace the ovary.

The arterial supply of the distal oviduct is derived from a vascular anastomosis between the ovarian and uterine arteries.

The functional role of the abdominal tubal ostium and fimbrae is to facilitate ovum transit from the ovary to the ampulla. Several speculations on ovum pick up have been brought forward, however the oldest and most prominent theories are fimbrio-ovarian approximation, embracement of the ovary by the infundibulum and fimbriae, fimbrial ciliary activity, and tubal peristalsis with tubal suction.

Etiology of Distal Tubal Occlusion

Sequelae of pelvic infections is by far the most common etiological factor in distal tubal occlusion. The etiological factors for distal with tubal occlusion are following:

A: Pelvic inflammatory diseases

B: Endometriosis

C: Pelvic and abdominal surgery

D: Tubal surgery
E: Parovarian and ovarian cysts
F: Pelvic hemoperitoneum.

Morphological sequelae of the infectious tubal damage are:

- Intraluminal and fimbrial adhesions (follicular salpingitis and fimbrial conglutination).
- Infundibular constriction ring or tubal phimosis.
- Fimbrial encapsulation by the ampullary or other visceral peritoneum.
- Complete occlusion of the terminal tubal opening with accumulation of tubal fluid and formation of hydrosalpinx.
- Fibrosis of the tubal wall or thick wall hydrosalpinx (interstitial salpingitis).
- Pelvic and tubo-ovarian adhesions.
- Complete fusion of the pelvic organs or the formation of a tubo-ovarian complex.

Morphological Classification of Distal Tubal Occlusion

Morphological classification of distal tubal occlusion is following:

Distal Tubal Occlusion

Status of Fimbria

A: Preserved fimbria
- Fimbrial conglutination
- Fimbrial concealment
- Tubal phimosis (mild)

B: Absent fimbria
- Tubal phimosis (severe)
- Thin-wall hydrosalpinx
- Thick-all hydrosalpinx

Adhesions

A: Nature of adhesions
Velamentous, filmy, fibrous, vascular, dense, fixed.

B: Extent of adhesions
Limited: Covering less than 50% of ovarian surface.
Extensive: Covering more than 50% of ovarian surface.

Status of Endosalpinx and Myosalpinx

A. Deciliation, pressure atrophy
B. Defective ciliary function
C. Complete loss of the epithelium
D. Intraluminal adhesions
E. Atrophy of myosalpinx
F. Sclerosis of myosalpinx.

Diagnosis of Distal Tubal Occlusion

An HSG followed by laparoscopy is indispensable.

Dilated ampulla without any peritoneal spillage is seen in thin walled hydrosalpinx.

Luminal contours are straight or rigid in thick walled hydrosalpinx.

Distension of ampulla, followed by spillage is found in phimosis.

Pooling of dye about the ends of tubes, a peritubal halo, indicates periadnexal adhesions.

Microsurgical Correction

Classification of Operative Procedures

A. Fimbrioplasty for cases with preserved fimbria.
   1. Fimbrial conglutination.
   2. Fimbrial encapsulation.
   3. Mild tubal phimosis.
B. Terminal salpingostomy for cases without visible fimbria.
   1. Severe tubal phimosis.
   2. Thin-walled hydrosalpinx.
   3. Thick-walled hydrosalinx.
C. Adhesiolysis for periadnexal adhesions (Figs 9.28 to 9.37).

Success and Failure

Intra uterine pregnancy rate following surgical treatment of distal tubal occlusion is 25-50%, though tubal patency rate is twice as high.

Reasons of failures following surgery of distal tube are:

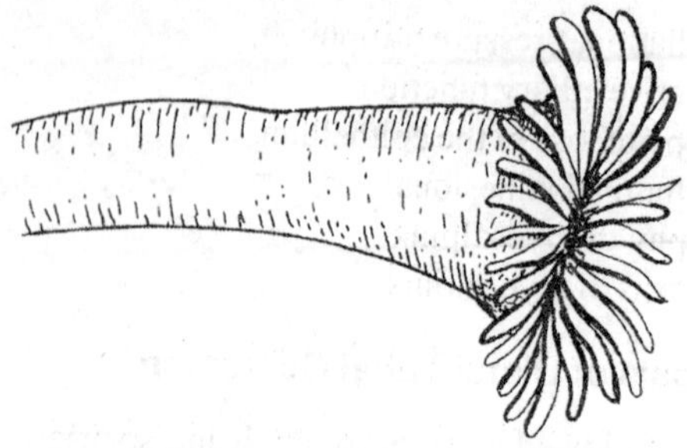

Fig. 9.28: Normal tubal fembria

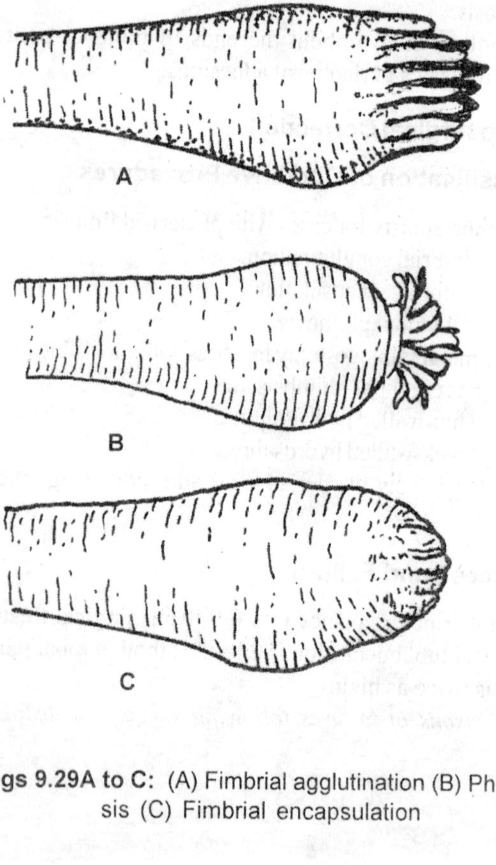

Figs 9.29A to C: (A) Fimbrial agglutination (B) Phimosis (C) Fimbrial encapsulation

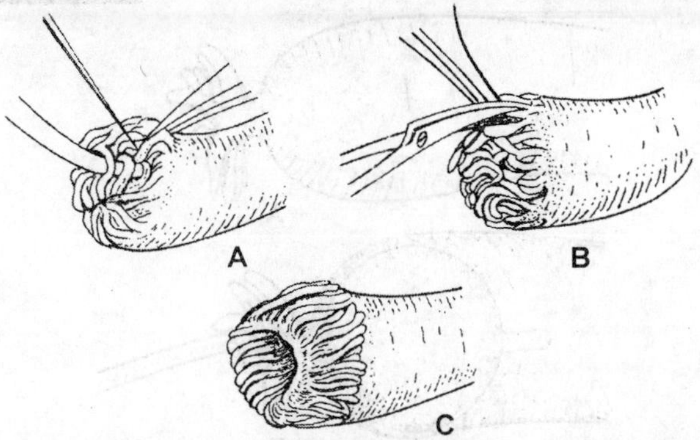

Figs 9.30A to C: Fimbrial conglutination **(A & B)** Adhesions are identified and separated **(C)** Separated fimbria are folded back and sutured to serosa

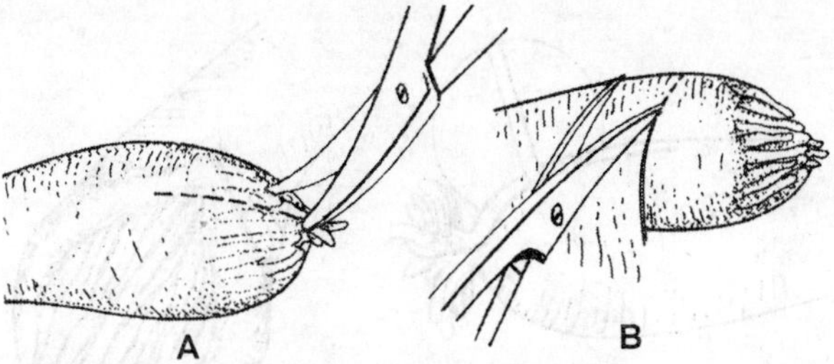

Figs 9.31A and B: Fimbrial encapsulation: (A) Longitudinal Incision of peritoneum over fimbria (B) Peritoneum is circumcised at a distance of 1–2 cm from tubal end

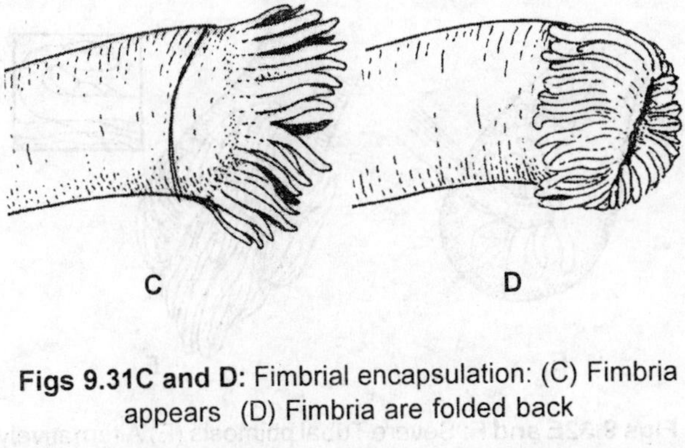

Figs 9.31C and D: Fimbrial encapsulation: (C) Fimbria appears (D) Fimbria are folded back

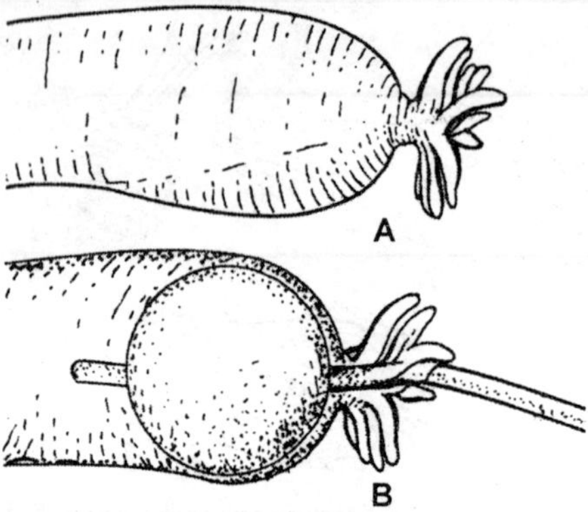

Figs 9.32A and B: Severe Tubal phimosis (A) Peritoneal constriction ring (B) Pediatric foley catheter is passed and balloon inflated

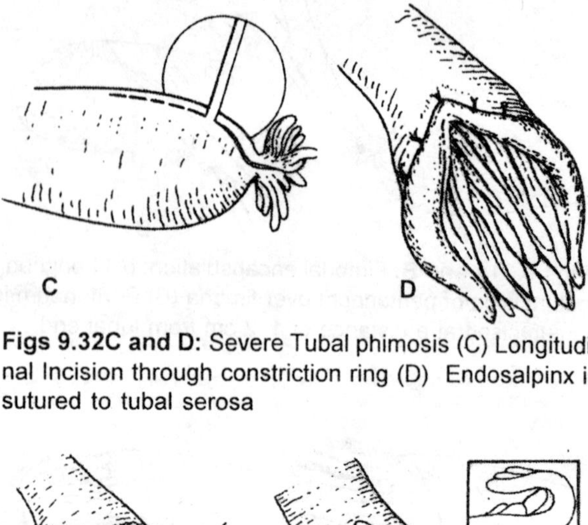

Figs 9.32C and D: Severe Tubal phimosis (C) Longitudinal Incision through constriction ring (D) Endosalpinx is sutured to tubal serosa

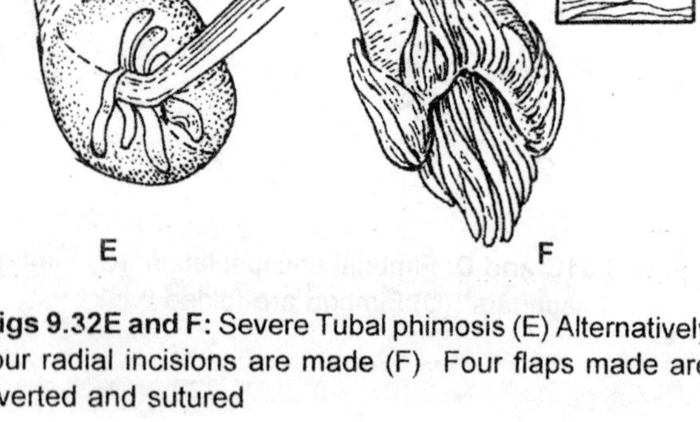

Figs 9.32E and F: Severe Tubal phimosis (E) Alternatively four radial incisions are made (F) Four flaps made are everted and sutured

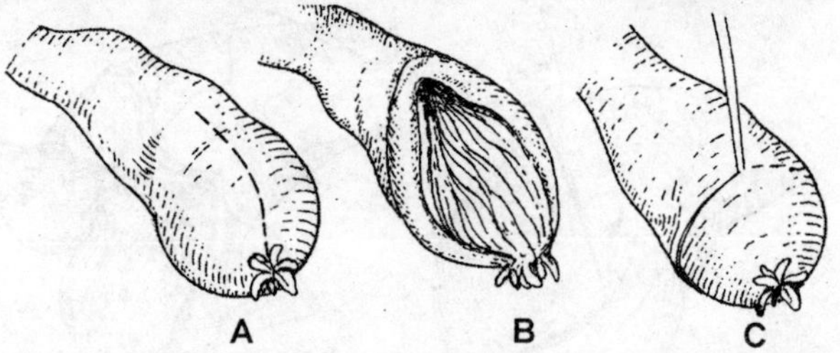

Figs 9.33A to C: Severe Tubal phimosis (A) Longitudinal Incision (B) Tube opened (C) Ampulation of tubal end

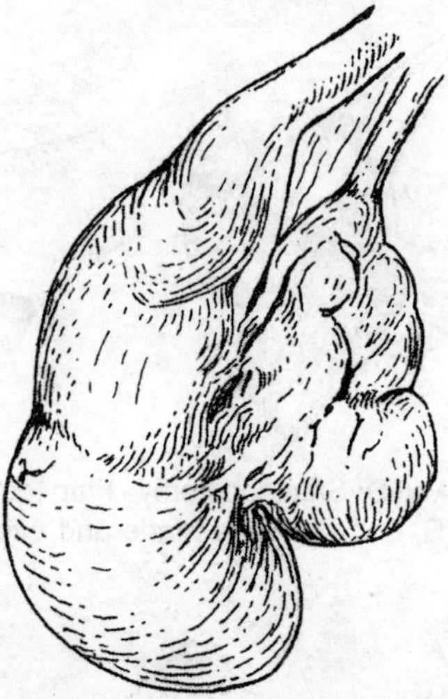

Fig. 9.34: Hydrosalpinx

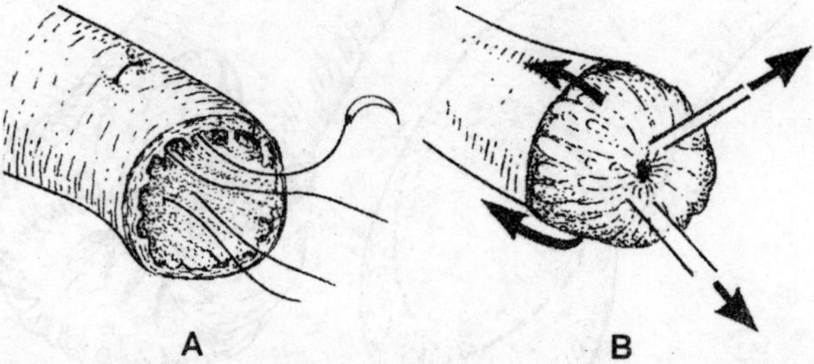

Figs 9.35A and B: Salpingo neostomy (A) Removal of terminal cap (B) Two-three sutures placed and cut edges everted

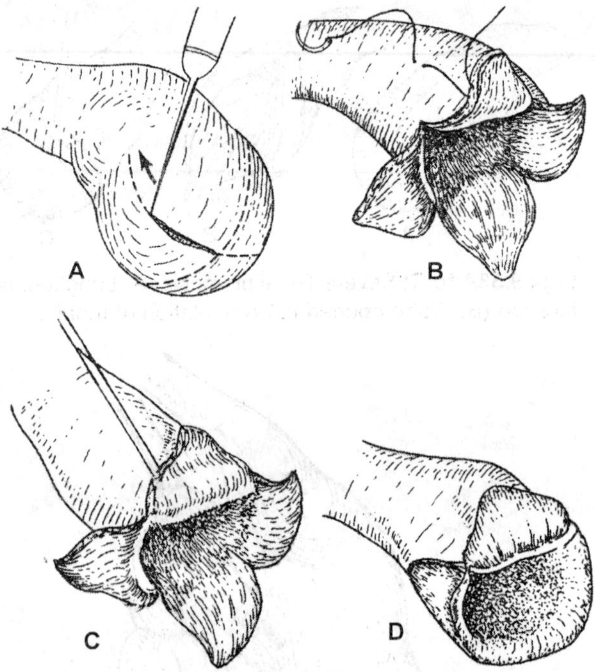

Figs 9.36A to D: Salpingostomy - Flap technique (A) Four incisions (B, C & D) Flaps made and everted

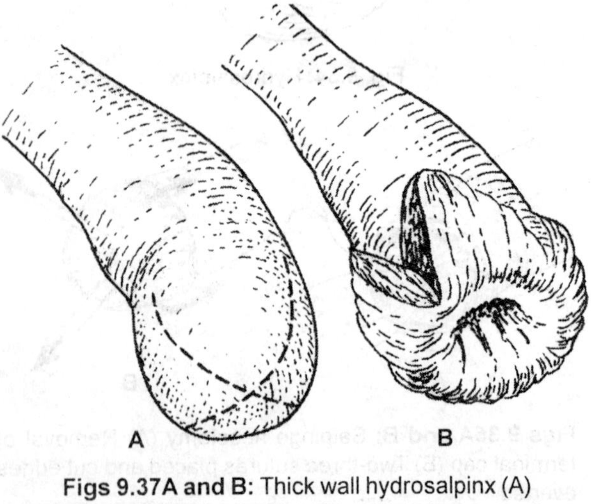

Figs 9.37A and B: Thick wall hydrosalpinx (A) Four radial incisions (B) Flaps may be everted

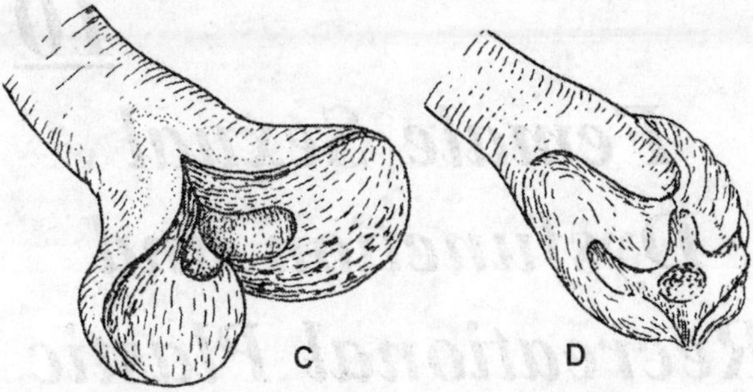

Figs 9.37C and D: Thick wall hydrosalpinx (C) In very thick wall only one incision is made (D) Flaps everted

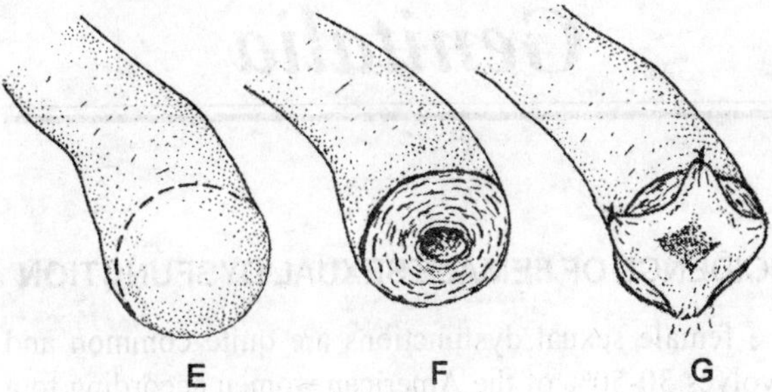

Figs 9.37E to G: Thick wall hydrosalpinx (E & F) In severely thick wall termine end of tube is amputated (G) Mucosal and serosal cut edges are approximated

- Faulty surgical technique
- Postoperative adhesions formation
- Unrecognized pre-existing tubal damage
- Subsequent inflammation or PID
- Other unrecognized infertility factors.

10

Female Sexual Dysfunction and Recreational Plastic Surgery of Female Genitalia

INCIDENCE OF FEMALE SEXUAL DYSFUNCTION

The female sexual dysfunctions are quite common and involves 30-50% of the American women according to a study. Ongoing epidemiological studies in the women suggest that the same disease processes and the risk factors that are associated with male erectile dysfunction, including aging, hypertension, cigarette smoking, hypercholesterolemia, and pelvic surgeries, are responsible for female sexual dysfunction.

THE FEMALE SEXUAL RESPONSE CYCLE

Masters and Jonson first described the female sexual response in 1966 as consisting of four successive phases:

- Excitement
- Plateau
- Orgasmic
- Resolution.

During sexual arousal, the clitoris and labia minora become engorged with blood, and vaginal and clitoral length and diameter increases. Labia minora are increased 2-3 times and are everted exposing the inner surface.

However **Kaplan** proposed three-phase model consisting of desire, arousal and orgasm. This three-phase model is the basis for classification system proposed by American Foundation of Urologic Disease in 1998. The Foundation has classified the female sexual disorders as:

- Hypoactive Sexual Desire Disorder
- Sexual Aversion Disorder
- Sexual Arousal Disorder
- Orgasmic Disorder
- Sexual Pain Disorder.

ETIOLOGIES OF FEMALE SEXUAL DYSFUNCTION

The etiological factors of female sexual dysfunctions are:

- Vasculogenic
- Neurogenic
- Hormonal
- Musculogenic
- Psychogenic.

Plastic surgeons are usually interested in musculogenic causes of female sexual dysfunctions.

MUSCULOGENIC FACTORS FOR FEMALE SEXUAL DYSFUNCTION

The pelvic floor muscles, in particular, the levator ani and perineal muscles, participate in female sexual function and responsiveness. The perineal muscles, consisting of the bulbocavernosus and ischiocavernosus muscles, when voluntarily contracted contribute to and intensifies sexual arousal and orgasm. In addition these muscles are responsible for the involuntary rhythmic contractions during orgasm. The levator ani muscles also modulate motor responses during orgasm and vaginal receptivity

When these muscles are hypertonic, vaginismus can develop, leading or causing dyspareunia and other sexual pain disorders. When hypotonic, vaginal hypoanesthesia, coital anorgasmia, or urinary incontinence during sexual intercourse or orgasm can develop.

CIRCUMVAGINAL MUSCULATURE AND FEMALE SEXUAL FUNCTION

One of the nature's remaining secret is the nature of orgasm. This is associated with series of convulsive contractions, suddenly erupt during the orgasmic process in a series of convulsive contractions, involuntary localized to a specific area, with a rhythmic unreproducible by voluntary efforts. The circumvaginal musculature consists of ischiocavernosus and bulbocavernous muscles, the external urethral sphincter and the anal sphincter. Superficial transverse perinei and the deep transverse perinei together with connective tissue comprise the urogenital diaphragm. Lying beneath these perineal muscles are the muscles of the pelvic diaphragm

It is proved that an external stimulus, usually representing more of as pressure response such as squeeze, can increase the electrical activity of these muscles and induce contraction in various perineal muscles.

A number of investigators have and continue to look at the actions of these muscles during sexual response. Cambell, using a pressure transducer, demonstrated an increase tone in the lower vagina which he felt was from the smooth muscles of the vagina and the surrounding levators which was followed by rhythmic contractions of the superficial muscles and not include the levators. Clinically Kline-Graber and Graber reported on objective measures of strength using the perineometer as well as subjective evaluation of atrophy both of which showed significant differences between women, with the muscle condition being best in coitally and nonçoitally orgasmic women.

Following procedures are done for enhancing the sexual pleasure in females:

- Aesthetic vaginoplasty
- Creation of super female
- Fat implant behind clitoris
- Labioplasty
- Bells implantation inside vagina.

Aesthetic Vaginoplasty

Aesthetic vaginoplasty is needed with the aim to tighten the relaxed vagina so as to restore the gripping effect over the penis.

The vagina starts relaxing after the first act of sexual intercourse. During pregnancy and delivery it relaxes further. It is due to relaxation of ligaments and the fascia. As the female grows older the vagina relaxes further.

Main pathological factors responsible for relaxation of vagina are:

1. During sex passage of penis acts as expander and expands the vagina making it looser. It is due to stretching of bulbospongiosus and surrounding fascia and ligaments.
2. During pregnancy and delivery the same effect is increased manifold. Bulbospongiosus may be torn if vaginal delivery has been carried out and the repair of muscle has not been done properly during stitching of episiotomy.
3. During aging there is loss of generalized tone of muscles and fascia. As a result the bulbospongiosus relaxes which is the external sphincter and hold the perineal body closer to symphysis. As the muscle starts losing the tone the perineal body starts descending down and sphincteric action starts diminishing. Along with this the levators also starts losing the tone and second sphincter of the vagina also starts losing its grip and the vagina becomes a hollow tube without sphincter. At this stage passage of penis is without any grip over the penis and both partners feel loss of sexual pleasure as sexual pleasure is more by gripping effect and not by mere passage of penis inside the vagina.

Diagnosis

Aesthetic vaginoplasty is the patient's requirement. However one should assess the losses:

1. Assess the tone of bulbospongiosus by passing a finger at vaginal orifice and pressing the perineal body downwards. Normal female should exhibit spring action with two fingers whenever the perineal body is pushed down.
2. Ask the female to contract the bulbospongiosus, and find the sphincteric action.
3. Now insert the finger further about 2 cm and again ask the patient to contract the muscles and assess the gripping effect of muscles over the finger.
4. Assess for any cystocele and rectocele.

Plastic Surgery

Plastic surgery depends upon the different deficiencies.

- Patient is put in lithotomy position.

- Incision are marked in the vagina. In the vagina it is in the form of inverted V and over the perineum it is in the form of V.
- Bulbospongiosus is exposed.
- Muscle is reefed. This reefing will elevate the perineal body which has descended down due to decrease in tone.
- Further levator ani muscles are identified.
- These muscles are also reefed in the midline.
- Extra skin is excised.
- Closure is done.

Creation of Superfemale

Aim of this operation is enhancement of sexual pleasure. In the operation a third sphincter is created at vaginal orifice which can compress the glans in the way that he cries in ecstacy.

Operation

The operation can be done by two methods:

1. A piece of fascia lata is taken from the thighs and placed in a way that vaginal orifice is encircled. It makes the vaginal orifice very narrow but resilient. Whenever the glans penis is inserted inside the vagina, the vagina grips the penis so tightly that he screams with joy.
2. In another method gracilis muscle is taken from the thigh and encircled around the vaginal orifice. The muscle can contract and compress the glans penis. So whenever the penis is inserted inside the vagina, the lady contracts the vaginal orifice and male screams with joy.

Second operation is better than the first, because in second operation the lady can contract the vaginal orifice and so compress the penis in any way she likes. While in first operation there is narrowing of vaginal orifice, which is static in nature.

Fat Implant Behind the Clitoris

The aim of this operation is to make the clitoris protuberant so that it rests in the position of protuberance and is stimulated a lot resulting in immensely pleasurable sexual act.

Operation

1. Small incision is made in the mons pubis.
2. By syringe suction the fat is aspirated.
3. It is injected beneath the clitoris.

Labioplasty

Labioplasty is done in those females in whom the labia are very much enlarged. On account of enlargement there are two problems:

1. Vaginal orifice is not visible.
2. There is frequent trauma to labia during the sexual act. So the operation is done.
    1. Avoiding the trauma to the labia during the sexual act.
    2. In professional models and the call girls in whom the show of the vaginal orifice is supposed to be beauty. In such females if labia are large, the vaginal orifice is not visible and so the beauty of genitals is lost.

Operation

- Patient is kept in lithotomy position.
- Excess length of labia is marked, in a way that after removal of labia, remaining labia should lie flush with vaginal orifice.
- The excess labia are removed and remaining labia are sutured.

Bells Implantation Inside Vagina

Aim: The operation is done in those females who are severely anorgasmic.

Operation

Special bells are fabricated of gold.

Now-a-days special chips can also be inserted. These are inserted in the vagina on the posterior vaginal ball.

Whenever she walks these bells twinkle and arouse the female. She has arousal whole day and then enjoys the sex at last. Once she is cured the bells are removed.

If she does not want the bells to be inserted inside the walls of vagina, then the bells may be kept in vaginal cavity whenever she want stimulation.

11

Microsurgery in Ectopic Pregnancy

ECTOPIC PREGNANCY AND ROLE OF MICROSURGERY

Recent advances in diagnostic technology have radically changed the treatment of tubal pregnancy. Now the trend is for planned microsurgical tubal repair which preserves and even enhances future fertility. With the development of new diagnostic tools (serum β sub unit of human chorionic gonadotrophin, ultrasound, laparoscopy) the diagnosis of ectopic pregnancy can be made in 60-80% of patients before life-threatening circumstances develop.

The new conservative surgical approach in cases of ectopic tubal pregnancy, should preserve fertility as well as recognize and correct factors that lead to the pregnancy's development. The occurrence of ectopic pregnancy is an indication that there is some underlying defect in tube, which must be corrected to avoid the relapse of the condition.

Etiology of Ectopic Pregnancy

The etiological factors for ectopic pregnancy are described as following:

- Abnormal tubal morphology
  - Inflammatory changes
  - Previous tubal surgery
  - Salpingitis isthmica nodosa, polyps, diverticula etc.
- Tubal dysfunction
  - Inappropriate estrogen/progesterone levels
  - Exogenous estrogens/progesterone.
- Uterine abnormalities or foreign body, congenital abnormalities, polyps, fibroids, IUD.

- Ovum transmigration; delayed ovulation.
- Intrinsic abnormalities of the fertilized ovum.

Abnormal Tubal Morphology

Infection results in destruction of the tubal epithelium resulting in adhesions between plical folds and leads to the morphologic picture of chronic follicular salpingitis. The resulting endosalpingeal labyrinth prolongs the travesty of the fertilized ovum and implantation occurs before the journey to the uterus is completed.

Same type of morphologically disordered tube due to any reason predisposes a patient for ectopic pregnancy.

Tubal Dysfunction

Tubal dysfunction due to changes in hormonal atmosphere predisposes for ectopic gestation. It is seen during ovulation induction with human menopausal gonadotrophins and clomiphene.

Rationale for Conservative Surgical Treatment

According to a study data was complied of 1630 patients who had salpingectomy for treatment of tubal pregnancy and 434 patients who had conservative surgery with the preservation of the involved tube. The subsequent intrauterine pregnancy rate was 40.9% for the radical surgery group and 66% for the conservative surgery group. Repeat ectopic pregnancy rates were 14.2 and 10% respectively. Repeat ectopic pregnancies following conservative surgery, happened as often in conservatively operated tube as in the contralateral tube. So one should attempt to preserve and possibly repair the tube with ectopic pregnancy, because the other tube is also diseased.

Conservative Microsurgical Techniques

Procedures are:

- Segmental salpingectomy.
- Linear salpingotomy/salpingostomy.
- Fimbrial expression (Figs 11.1 to 11.5).

Results of Conservative Tubal Surgery

Conservative tubal surgery does not appear to increase the chances of subsequent ectopic pregnancy in the

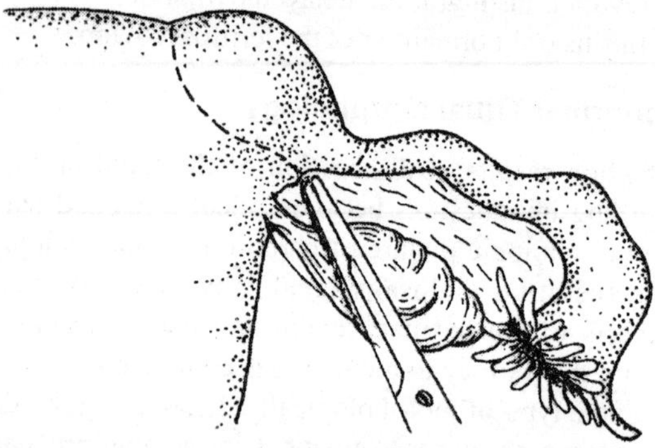

Fig. 11.1: Segmental salpingectomy - Intramural pregnancy: Distended uterine cornua is identified

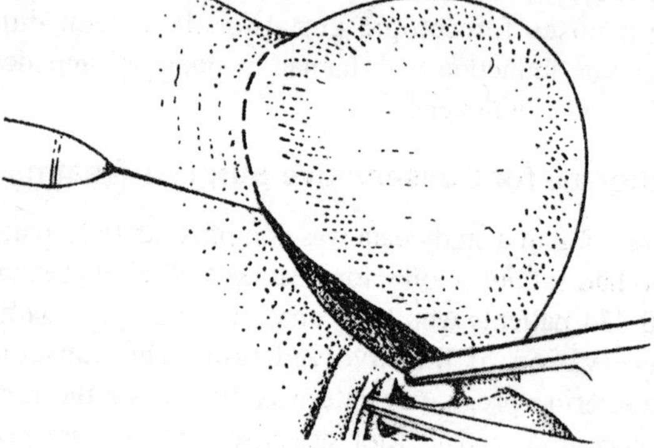

Fig. 11.2: Segmental salpingectomy - Intramural pregnancy: Involved part of tube is removed

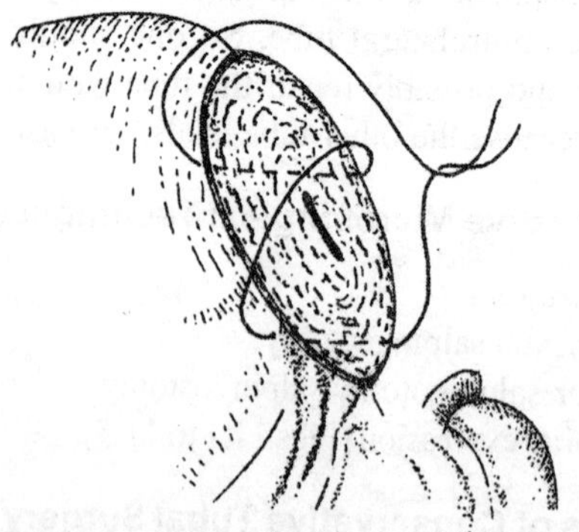

Fig. 11.3: Segmental salpingectomy - Intramural pregnancy: Microsurgical tubocornual anastomasis is done at later date

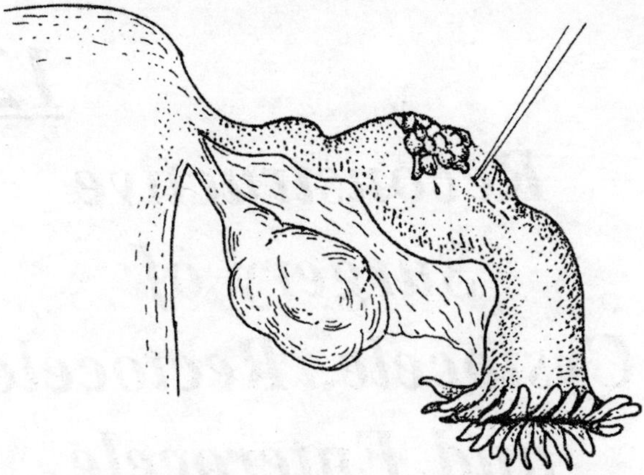

Fig. 11.4: Segmental salpingectomy - Intramural pregnancy: Linear salpingectomy

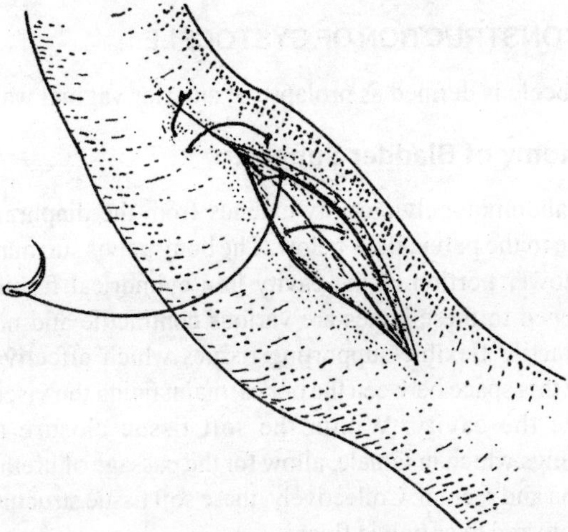

Fig. 11.5: Segmental salpingectomy - Intramural pregnancy: Microsurgical closure

operated tube. Furthermore, the intrauterine pregnancy rate following conservative surgery is superior to the rate following salpingectomy. However, one should not opt for another conservative surgery following second ectopic pregnancy in the same tube.

12

Reconstructive Surgery of Cystocele, Rectocele and Enterocele

RECONSTRUCTION OF CYSTOCELE

Cystocele is defined as prolapse of anterior vaginal wall.

Anatomy of Bladder Support

The abdominopelvic cavity extends from the diaphragm above to the pelvic floor below. The bony pelvis surrounds this lower portion of the cavity in a cylindrical fashion. Attached to these bones are various contractile and non-contractile flexible supporting tissues which effectively close this space between the bones, maintaining the viscera inside the cavity. Within the soft tissue closure are openings which in female, allow for the passage of urethra, vagina and rectum. Collectively, these soft tissue structures are referred to as pelvic floor.

The pelvic floor consists of three layers:

- Endopelvic fascia
- Levator muscles and
- Perineum.

Endopelvic Fascia

The network of fibro muscles tissue immediately beneath the peritoneum is usually referred as endopelvic fascia. This network surrounds the viscera and fills the space between peritoneum above and the levators below.

It extends from symphysis to sacrum and ischial spine to ischial spine, providing a continuity of support from front to back and side to side.

In places it is referred to as ligaments (uterosacral cardinal etc.). In other areas it is called fascia or covering.

Levator Muscles

Levator muscles are made up of pubococcygeus (including puborectalis), iliococcygeus, and coccygeus muscles. The endopelvic fascia above fuses with and/or merges into the fascial covering of the levator group.

Perineum

The outer most layer of pelvic floor is urogenital diaphragm (urogenital membrane, deep transverse perinei muscle) and its attached underlying intrinsic striated perineal muscles, with their fascial covering.

The bladder, vagina and rectum are essential extra-territorial structures that rest on and are contained within this pelvic floor. Whenever there is defect in the integrity of soft tissue closure, one of the viscera is pushed outward. The defect is then named according to the displaced viscera, such as urethrocele, cystocele, uterine prolapse, enterocele and rectocele.

Bladder Support

Bladder rests on pubocervical fascia which is a part of endopelvic fascia. It extends from pericervical tissue in midpelvic ventrally to pass under the symphysis and merge with urogenital diaphragm. Laterally on each side it fuses into fascia covering of muscles of pelvic side wall. The urethra traverses the layer tangentially.

All operations for cystocele repair revise the pubocervical fascia. It is either plicated from below (classic anterior vaginal wall repair and kelly urethroplasty) or pulled upward and reattached to some structure from above (in Marshall-Marchetti Krantz procedure).

The continuity of endopelvic fascia can be interrupted compromising support to the bladder at four places:

- Lateral or paravaginal
- Distal
- Central
- Transverse.

Diagnosis of each defect is of paramount importance because each anatomic defect requires a different operative procedure.

Paravaginal Defect

- Lateral attachment of the pubocervical fascia separates from its attachment to the fascial covering of the obturator interns and levator muscles.
- It may be unilateral or bilateral.
- It results in urethrocystocele.

It is thought usually that cystocele result from a generalized stretching or attenuation of the pubocervical fascia. But in paravaginal defect if the superior sulcus is supported during examination the bladder and urethra don't descend. Which means that supporting tissue has been broken off its attachment to the lateral pelvic wall. AC Richardson has done extensive studies and found that break is not always at the pelvic side wall. Four areas have been identified in which the continuity can be interrupted- lateral or paravaginal, distal, central and transverse.

- **Diagnosis** is made by supporting superior vaginal sulcus, which should result in diappearance of cysto urethrocele.
- If defect is unilateral then support of the sulcus on that side alone corrects the cystourethrocele.
  1. In paravaginal defect lateral attachment of the pubocervical fascia separates from its attachment to the fascial covering of the obturator internus muscles and levator muscles. Because the vagina is attached to the pubocervical fascia, when the break is in this area lateral superior vaginal sulcus descends, the bladder neck becomes hypermobile, and often there is stress incontinence. For correction of this defect paravaginal repair is most appropriate.
  2. In Transverse Defect the pubocervical fascia separates transversely from its attachment to the pericervical ring of fibromuscular tissue, into which not only the pubocervical fascia but also the cardinal uterosacral ligaments merge. It yields large cystocele, however the bladder neck is well supported. Bladder descends downwards, obliterating the anterior fornix. Vaginal approach works well for these patients. The

defect should be repaired anteroposteriorly and not side to side.

3. In central defects there is break in the central part of fascia. Isolated central defects are not very common. The treatment in these patients is careful reapproximatiom of the edges of fascia.
4. In distal defect the distal urethra is avulsed or separated from its attachment by way of urogenital diaphragm. From its attachment to symphysis pubis. These patients have severe stress incontinence and the sling procedure is the procedure of choice.

Surgical Technique of Paravaginal Repair

- Pfannenstiel incision is made.
- Peritoneum is freed from the undersurface of the rectus muscles and recti are retracted.
- Retropubic space is entered by incising the transversalis fascia which is then wiped off of superior pubic ramus laterally until the obturator notch is palpated or seen.
- The bladder is drawn medially away from the side wall of the pelvis.
- Left hand is inserted in vagina and laterally superior sulcus as identified by prominent veins are exposed.
- Lateral sulcus of vagina with its overlying pubocervical fascia to pelvic side wall is attached.
- The procedure is repeated on the opposite side.
- Drains are put in retropubic space.
- Closure is done (Figs 12.1A to D).

Vaginal Approach to Cystocele Repair (Figs 12.9A to 12.9H)

A cystocele developing from stretching of the anterior vaginal wall past the point of accommodation is termed pulsion cystocele. However cystocele resulting from loss of the lateral vaginal wall support is termed as traction cystocele.

Cystocele has also been divided into different grades.

Grade 1: If during Valsalva maneuver in the upright position the cystocele does not reach the introitus.

Grade 2: If cystocele reaches the introitus.

Grade 3: If during the same maneuver the cystocele protrudes beyond introitus.

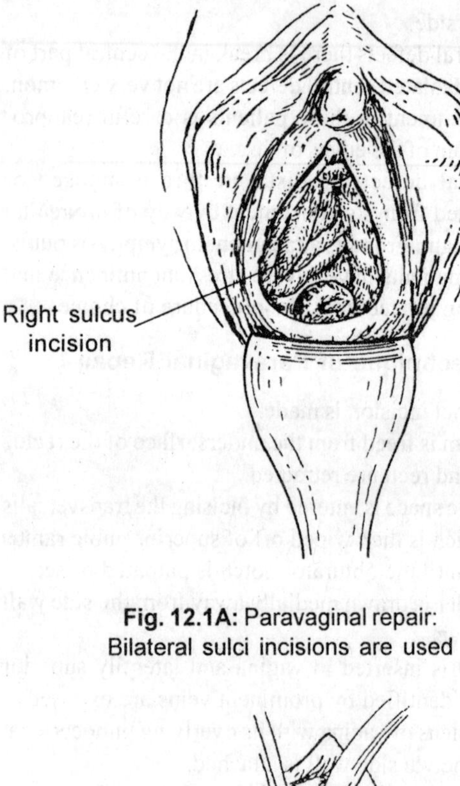

Fig. 12.1A: Paravaginal repair: Bilateral sulci incisions are used

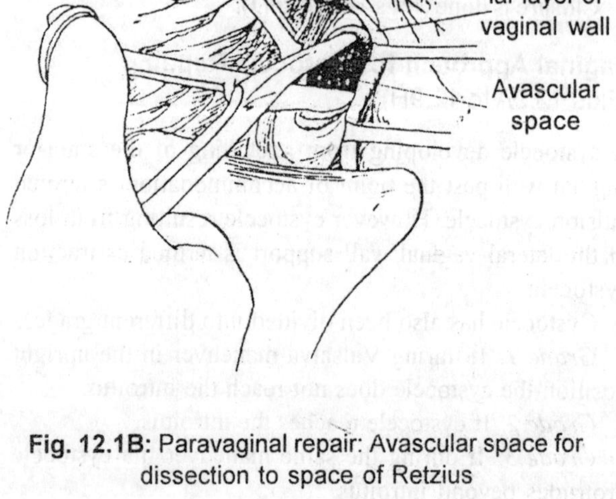

Fig. 12.1B: Paravaginal repair: Avascular space for dissection to space of Retzius

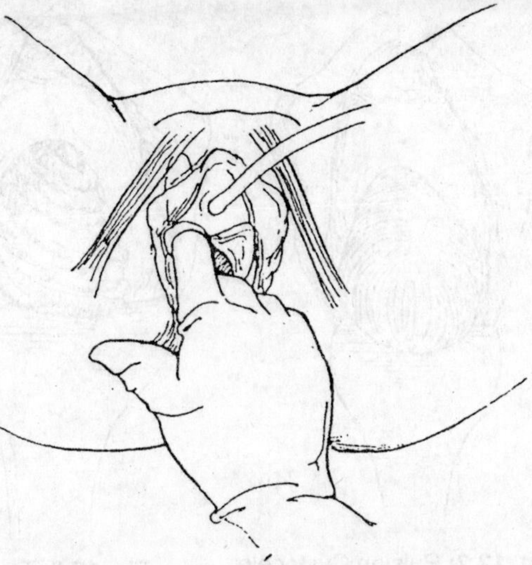

Fig. 12.1C: Paravaginal repair: Operator's finger passed to space of Retzius

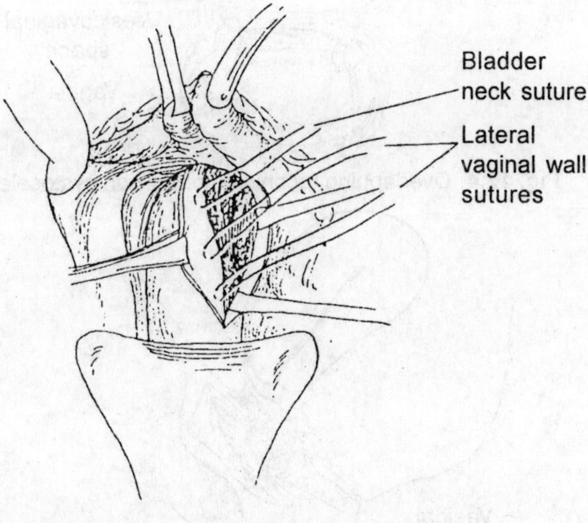

Fig. 12.1D: Paravaginal repair: Vaginal wall anchoring to obturator internus fascia

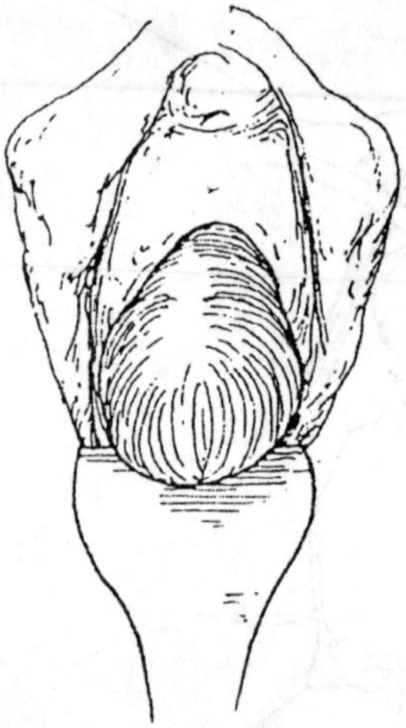

Fig. 12.2: Pulsion Cystocele

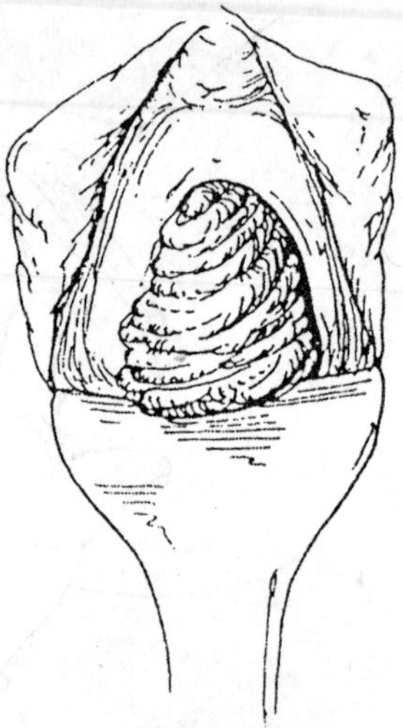

Fig. 12.3: Traction cystocele

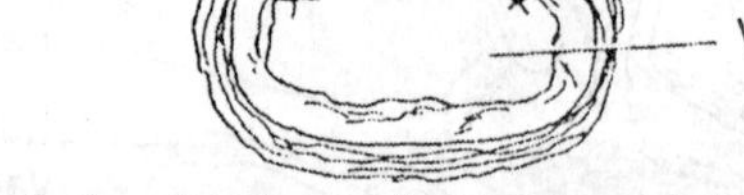

Fig. 12.4: Overlapping technique for pulsion cystocele

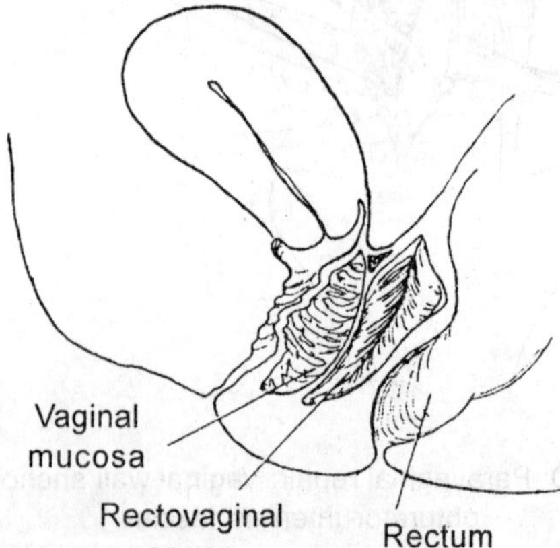

Fig. 12.5: Rectovaginal space

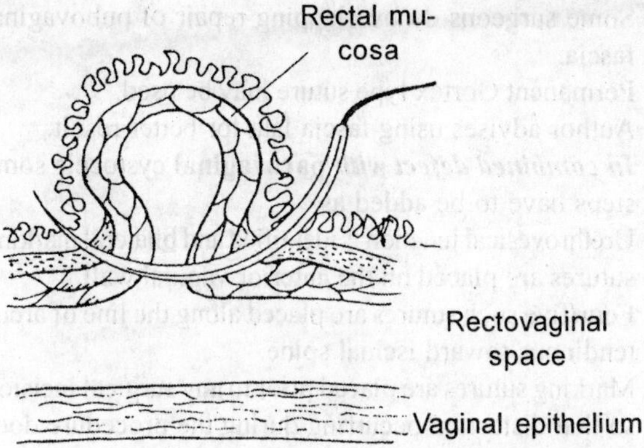

Fig. 12.6: Imbricating suture on rectal wall during posterior colporrhaphy

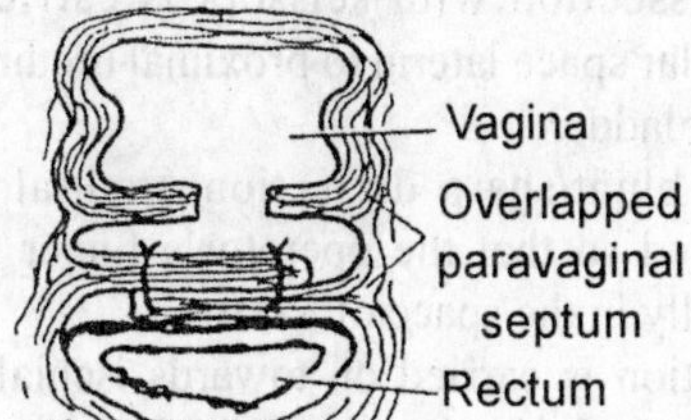

Fig. 12.7: Overlapping closure of rectovaginal septum during posterior colporrhaphy

Grade 4: If the cystocele protrudes beyond introitus during rest.

Surgical Technique

- Area of Pulsion defect is identified and Allis clamps are placed in the sagittal line at the superior and inferior aspect of the defect.
- Entire thickness of the vagina wall is incised so that vesicovaginal space in entered. For ease of dissection saline may be infiltrated.
- Fibromuscular bladder capsule is then plicated using 3-0 catgut.
- Full thickness of vaginal wall is either resected or closed with full thickness sutures.

- Some surgeons do overlapping repair of pubovaginal fascia.
- Permanent Gortex type suture may be used.
- Author advises using fascia lata for better result.
- ***In combined defect with* paravaginal** cystocele some steps have to be added as:
- Urethrovesical junction is identified and bilateral marking sutures are placed on the anterior vaginal wall.
- Four/five such sutures are placed along the line of arcus tendinous toward ischial spine.
- Marking sutures are placed prior to any surgical incision so that distortion occurring during the procedure does not lead to improper suture placement.
- After injecting the muscularis of the vaginal wall with saline an inverted U incision is used.
- The fibromuscular layer of the vaginal wall is opened and dissection with scissors is carried out in the avascular space lateral to proximal urethra and inferior to the bladder.
- Using blunt/sharp dissection urethral supports are traversed so that the operator's finger is now retro-pubically in the space of Retzius.
- Dissection is carried on towards ischial spine, being careful to avoid the obturator nerve and vessels by remaining posterior and inferior to them.
- Bladder is then reflected medially and with direct visualization, a Deschamps ligature carrier is used to place cortex sutures in the obturator interus fascia. These sutures are anterior to internal pudendal vessels and nerves and lateral to inferior hypogastric nerve plexus overlying the iliococcygeal muscle.
- At least 4 sutures are used beginning near the ischial spine and extending along the arcus tendinous to the symphysis.
- They are then serum into the vaginal on the lateral aspect of U-shaped incision line, a line indicated by the previously placed markers.
- Next Pereyra procedure is performed in patients of urinary incontinence (it has been described in chapter of urinary incontinence).
- If there is loss of supported at the superior aspect near ischial spine (i.e. a vaginal vault inversion prolapse) a Mc Call culdoplasty and/or a bilateral sacrospinous

ligament suspension is performed. (It is described elsewhere).

- The anterior vaginal wall is then closed with running continuous 2-0 polyglactin sutures.
- Now bladder is filled to 300 ml of sterile saline and tested for continence by direct application of force over the suprapubic region. The pereyra sutures are then elevated until continence is established.

ANTERIOR COLPORRHAPHY REINFORCED WITH MARLEX MESH FOR THE TREATMENT OF CYSTOCELES (Fig. 12.8A to E)

Anterior wall is the Achilles heel of pelvic prolapse surgery. Long term follow-up reports are scarce, but the rate of recurrence of anterior wall defects may be as high as 37%. The use of artificial mesh may improve the success of the anterior vaginal wall repair as described by Flood and Waja in 1998.

Technique

1. The patient is placed in lithotomy position.
2. The anterior vaginal wall is incised vertically in the midline from the vaginal vault to the external urethral meatus.
3. The bladder is mobilized off the lateral walls of the vagina.
4. Periurethral tunnels are created through the urogenital diaphragm into the space of Retzius. These are created with sharp and blunt dissection between the plane of the vaginal mucosa and the periurethral fascia
5. The cystocele is reduced with interrupted plicating 00 Dexon sutures.
6. A piece of marlex mesh approximately 4 cm long and 1 cm wide is placed under the vesicourethral junction extending up into the periurethral tunnels.
7. The mesh is secured at the level of the bladder neck with four interrupted sutures of 0 chromic, in order to prevent migration of the mesh in the immediate postoperative period.
8. Excess vagina is trimmed.

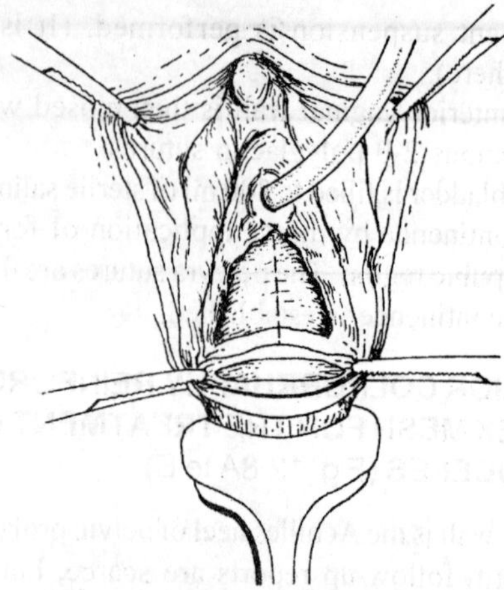

Fig. 12.8A: Marlex mesh to treat cystocelle

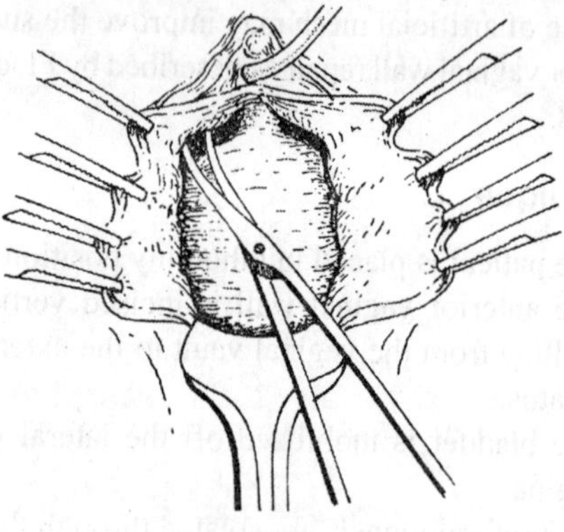

Fig. 12.8B: Marlex mesh to treat cystocelle

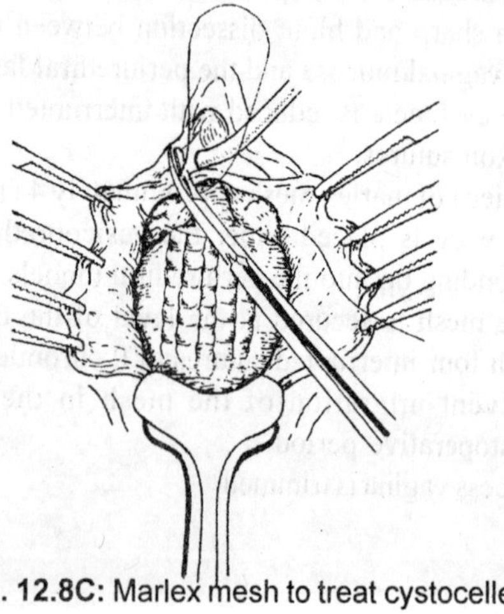

Fig. 12.8C: Marlex mesh to treat cystocelle

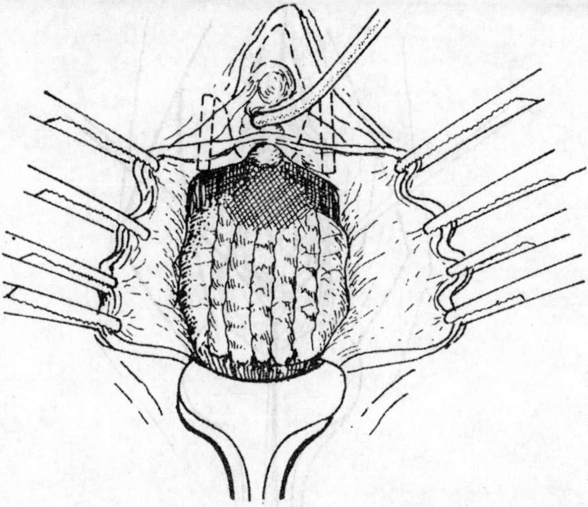

Fig. 12.8D: Marlex mesh to treat cystocelle

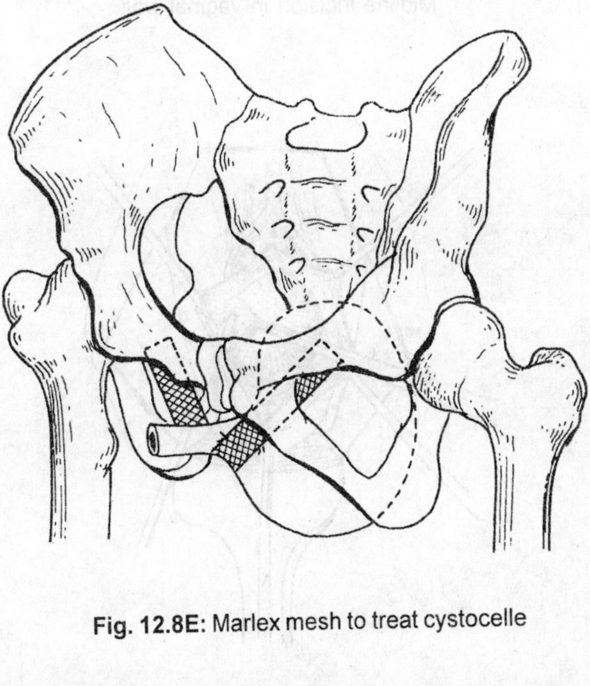

Fig. 12.8E: Marlex mesh to treat cystocelle

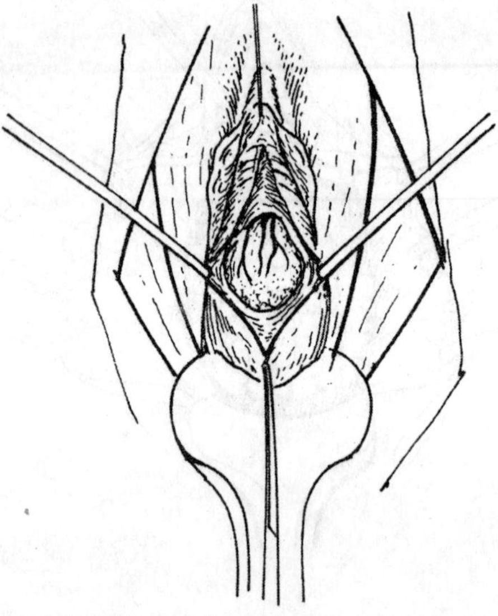

Fig. 12.9A: Vaginal approach to cystocele repair: Midline incision in vaginal wall

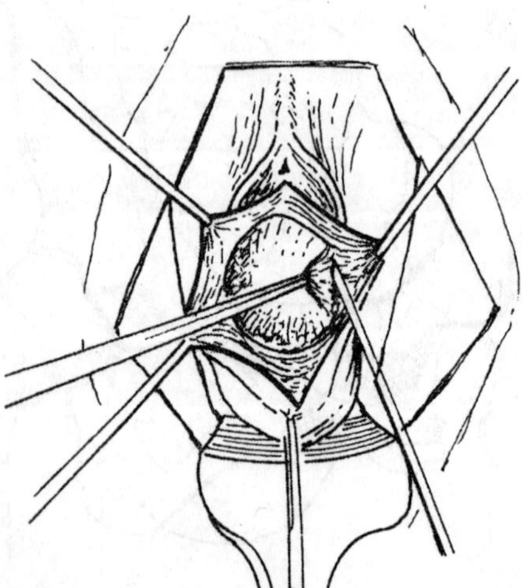

Fig. 12.9B: Vaginal approach to cystocele repair: Vesicovaginal space opened

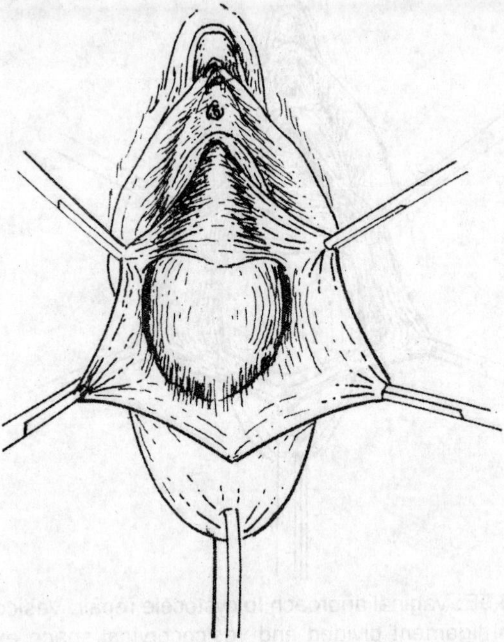

Fig. 12.9C: Vaginal approach to cystocele repair: Vaginal flaps dissected

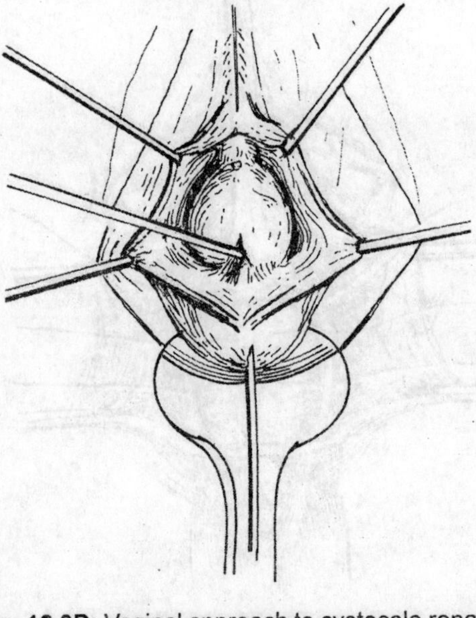

Fig. 12.9D: Vaginal approach to cystocele repair: Vesicocervical ligament is held up with forceps

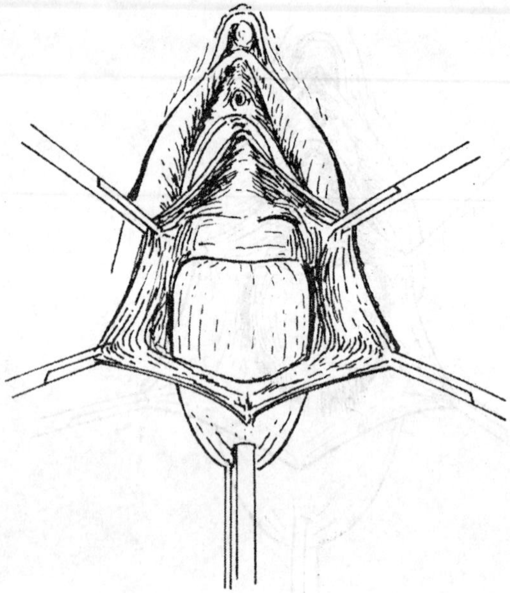

Fig. 12.9E: Vaginal approach to cystocele repair: Vesicocervical ligament divided and vesicocervical space exposed

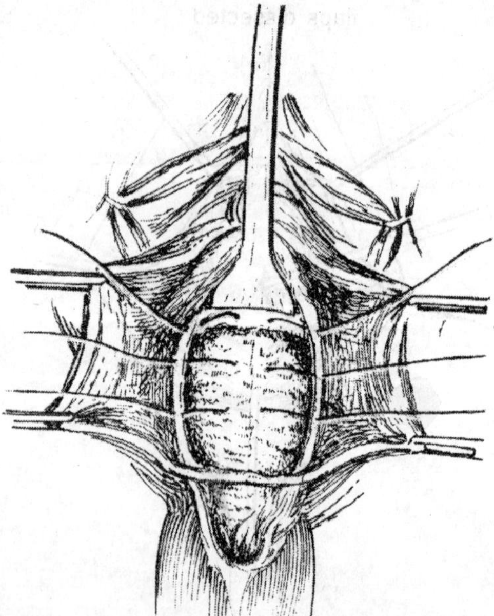

Fig. 12.9F: Vaginal approach to cystocele repair: Lateral pillars of pubocervical fascia suture together

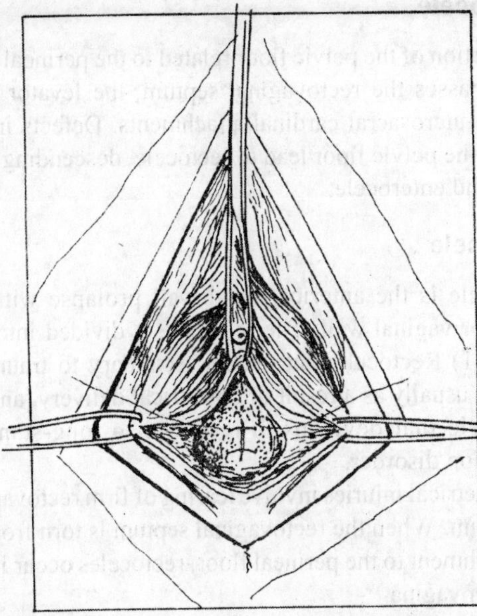

Fig. 12.9G: Vaginal approach to cystocele repair: Levator ani muscles sutured in midline after removal of triangular piece of vagina

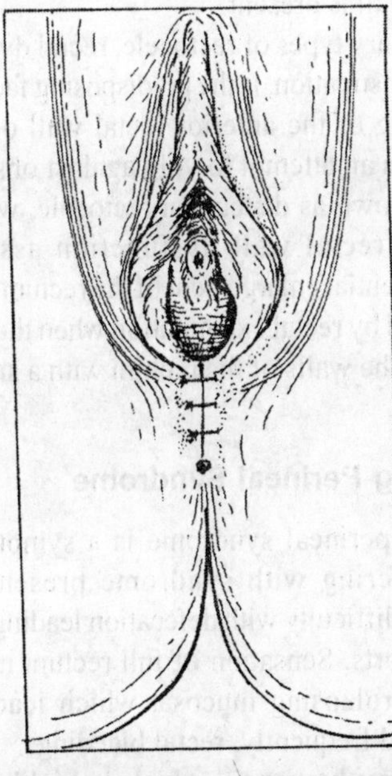

Fig. 12.9H: Vaginal approach to cystocele repair: Completion of celpoperineorrhaphy

Enterocele

The portion of the pelvic floor related to the perineal body encompasses the rectovaginal septum, the levator plate and the uterosacral cardinal attachments. Defects in this area of the pelvic floor lead to rectocele, descending perineum and enterocele.

Rectocele

Rectocele is the anterior rectal wall prolapse with the posterior vaginal wall. The rectocele is divided into two types: (1) Rectocele that occurs secondary to traumatic change, usually as a result of obstetrical delivery, and (2) Rectocele that develops in response to long-standing defecation disorder.

- Obstetrical injuries involve tearing of firm rectovaginal septum. When the rectovaginal septum is torn from its attachment to the perineal floor, rectoceles occur in the lower vagina.
- Mid or high rectocele when posterior vaginal wall and recovaginal septum are attenuated.
- Pulsion type rectocele. If the attenuation of the posterior vaginal wall is present.
- In secondary types of rectocele, rectal dysfunction, primarily constipation, is the predisposing factor. Continual weakening of the anterior rectal wall occurs in these patients in an attempt to void against obstruction. This is also known as distension rectocele, which is due to intrinsic rectal wall dysfunction associated with circumferential enlargement of the rectum. It is clinically diagnosed by rectal examination when there is failure to touch all the walls of the rectum with a single sweep of the finger.

Descending Perineal Syndrome

Descending perineal syndrome is a symptom complex. Patient suffering with syndrome presents as having pronounced difficulty with defecation leading to prolonged straining efforts. Sensation of full rectum may be in part caused by prolapsing mucosa, which leads to mucous discharge and frequently, rectal bleeding.

Patient may have pain which is highly problematic component of the syndrome. It is a poorly localized deep discomfort precipitated by prolonged standing and relieved by lying down or sleep.

Surgical Correction

Posterior Colporrhaphy with Perineorrhaphy

- Allis clamps are placed wide apart at posterior introitus at a width which, when approximated, still allows coital functioning.
- A third Allis clamps is placed above the anal verge and a triangular segment of skin overlying the perineum is removed.
- With the finger in rectum a sagittal incision is made in the posterior vaginal wall.
- Once the rectovaginal place is entered, complete vaginal wall should be incised.
- Any adhesion in the rectovaginal space are lysed.
- Usually by blunt dissection the rectum can be freed from its attachments.
- Ballooning defect in anterior rectal wall is corrected by absorbable suture running the entire length of rectal wall.
- Denonvillier's fascia and the entire vaginal wall thickness is now trimmed.
- Fascia should be repaired.
- If fascia is torn and flimsy, repair should be enforced with fascia lata, marlex mesh or dermal layer.
- Posterior vaginal wall is closed.
- Perineorrhaphy is then completed.
- The suture closing Denonvillier's fascia is approximated to the perineal musculature.
- If there is large, attenuated pulsion defect in the posterior vaginal wall, the wall is dissected from the rectovaginal septum, which is then overlapped and closed in a multilayer fashion.

Posterior Colporrhaphy without Perineorrhaphy

In this initial incision is different and perineal musculature is not addressed.

- The initial incision enters the rectovaginal space and may be either transverse or longitudinal.
- Rest steps are same as described above.

Fascial Technique for Surgical Repair of Isolated Posterior Vaginal Wall Prolapse

As we have already described that rectocele may result from tears in the rectovaginal septum, detachment from the perineal body, or attenuation and thinning of the septum. Various surgical techniques have been used in the past for the repair of rectocele. Maerek in 16 proposed a transverse repair of rectovaginal septum for midvaginal rectoceles found more commonly in younger females. Cortes and reid said in a report in obstetrics and gynecology that levator ani plication hides rather that cures the prolapse.

- Whereas the technique of fascial repair of the recto-vaginal septum appears anatomically more rational and improves the accompanying symptomatology. They evaluated consecutive women presenting with a symptomatic rectocele, having the symptoms of vaginal protrusion, defecatory symptoms and sexual dys-function.

  After evaluation they performed the operation as described below.
- A transverse incision was made in the vagina at the level of hymen.
- Rectovaginal space was sharply dissected with a finger in the rectum.
- The vaginal flap was raised until the area of maximal bulge was reached.
- The tears in the septum were either obviously visible or bimanually palpated by rectovaginal examination.
- The edges of the septum were grasped with Allis forceps and approximated in the direction of the tear.
- If the septum was detached from the perineal body, it was reattached.
- If there were no clear defects but only attenuation of the septum, then thick septal tissue was grasped from its lateral edges and buttressed in the center
- External plication of the rectal wall was done if there was obviously dilated rectum.
- Perineorrhaphy was done to reconstruct the perineal body if that appeared to be thin and flattened.

Enterocele

Hernia of intestine through vagina, located posterior to the uterus and anterior to the rectum in the pouch of

Douglas. In the absence of uterus, herniation may occur at the vaginal apex.

Enterocele is usually associated with cystocele, rectocele, vaginal vault prolapse, and levator hiatal defects.

Treatment

Principles of treatment are:

- Excision of hernial sac
- High ligation of hernial sac
- Adequate structural support.

Approaches

Abdominal approach/vaginal approach. Author is of opinion that both approaches used simultaneously gives best result.

COMPLETE EXTROVERSION OF VAGINA

This problem is difficult to correct. Mostly extroversions develop after total abdominal hysterectomy, but may also develop after vaginal hysterectomy for prolapse, when the technique for closing the aperture between the bladder and rectum has been defective.

The treatment depends upon whether the vagina is to be left functional or non-functional.

The extroversion can be corrected by vaginal route as well as by abdominal route.

Vaginal Operation

- Incision is made in midline along the whole length of the anterior wall of the vagina.
- Lateral flaps so formed are stripped away so that the vaginal wall is separated from the bladder and urethra.
- Peritoneal cavity is now opened.
- Posterior vaginal wall is then incised longitudinally and the lateral flaps are dissected away to expose the anal canal, and anterior wall of the rectum.
- Prolapsed bladder is reduced and series of reefing sutures are applied.
- If the round ligaments can be identified they should be sutured together to make a shelf below the bladder.

- Posteriorly the redundant peritoneum is excised, rectum is pushed up and prerectal fascia is sutured to the shelf of tissue formed below the bladder.
- Then a layer of tissue derived from both the levator fascia and prerectal fascia should be stitched in front of the rectum and suture this layer anteriorly to the shelf of tissues formed below the bladder.
- Afterwards the levator ani must be stitched together
- Redundant vaginal wall is excised.
- Closure is done.

Abdominal Route

After total abdominal hysterectomy prolapse of the vaginal vault is relatively uncommon, but if it occurs may lead to complete extroversion of the vagina as the vaginal vault cannot be usually stretched to the sacral promontory and so a graft or prosthesis is used for this purpose. The operation is done as follows:

- Pfannenstiel incision is made.
  - External oblique aponeurosis is cleared.
  - Two fascial strips are made and are cut and freed at the midline from the linea alba, but left attached where the aponeurosis fuses with the muscle fibres of the external oblique.
  - Now abdomen is opened in the midline.
  - The vault of the vagina is now identified and pulled up.
  - The fascial strips are taken inside after piercing the muscles along the course of the round ligament and between the leaves of the broad ligament.
  - The fascial strip is attached to the peritoneum at the lateral angle of the vagina and taken back to the site of origin.
  - Similar procedure is carried out on the opposite side.
  - Uterosacrals are now shortened by reefing sutures and attached to the posterior fornix.
  - Closure is done.

Michighan Four-Wall Sacrospinous Suspension

Sacrospinous suspension is an established technique successful in treating vaginal vault eversion. However proper selection of the points on the vagina to be suspended is critical. A point on the vaginal wall too near the introitus may not allow the selected length of vagina to reach the ligament. Selecting a point on the vagina too far from the introitus results in too long a length of suspended vagina that may continue to prolapse after suspension.

The place on the sacrospinous ligament to which the vagina will be suspended averages 9 cm from the vaginal introitus. In women with large vaginal prolapse the vagina is often longer than this distance. In this situation, simply attaching the posterior vaginal wall to the sacrospinous ligament does not always leads to satisfactory suspension of the anterior or lateral vaginal walls.

To avoid sagging, points should be chosen on anterior and the posterior walls which should be same distance from the ligament as the distance between introitus and the ligament. Although traditional sacrospinous suspension attaches only the posterior wall to the ligament, it is possible to attach the anterior and lateral walls also as described by Michighan.

Technique

1. At the preoperative visit the standardized pelvic organ prolapse quantification score are used to measure the prolapse.
2. In this system measurements are made of the location of predefined points along the anterior and posterior vaginal walls relative to the hymenal ring. Negative values lie cephalad to the hymen and positive values caudal. Point Aa is 3 cm from the hymen on the anterior wall, and point Ba is the most dependent point on the anterior wall above this point. Point Ap and SBp are analogous points on the posterior wall. Point C is the cervix.
3. Identify the points on each wall of the vagina that comfortably reach the ligament yet eliminates sagging.
4. The intervening vagina is then removed.
5. A point on the anterior vaginal wall that is estimated to be same distance from the introitus as the distance to the ligament is grasped with an Allis forceps.
6. Test the exact point by elevating the tip of the clamp and it included vagina to the sacrospinous ligament to confirm that this point on the vaginal wall reaches the ligament comfortably.

7. A similar point is chosen on the posterior wall and both lateral walls.
8. The intervening tissue between these points is then excised.
9. A right unilateral sacrospinous suspension is then performed by using previously placed sutures in the sacrospinous ligament to sew the anterior and posterior margins of this open cuff to the ligament.

13

Constipation

Patients moving their bowels twice a week are diagnosed as having constipation.

AETIOLOGY

1. Primary (Idiopathic)—hereditary
2. Secondary
   - Inadequate dietary fibre
   - Drug therapy
   - Metabolic/endocrine
     - hypothyroidism
     - diabetes
     - hypercalcemia
     - hyperparathyroidism
     - hypokalemia
   - Infiltrative
     - scleroderma
     - amyloidosis
   - Neurologic

     CNS

     Peripheral–pudendal neuropathy
   - Intestinal

     Chaga's disease.
     - Psychological

       Irritable bowel syndrome

Pelvic Floor and Anorectal Abnormalities

Pelvic floor and anorectal anomalies are one of the important group of causes causing constipation.

Anismus is a condition in which anal sphincter musculature contracts on attempted defecation rather than relaxes. Anismus is associated with pelvic floor dyssynergia.

In addition, damage to the pudendal nerves is found in constipated women with chronic defecation straining.

Perineal descent may result from chronic defecation straining and contribute to pudendal neuropathy.

Treatment

- Medical
- Surgical

Surgical

- Subtotal colectomy
- Section of part of puborectalis muscle
- Section of posterior and lateral division of the puborectalis muscle.

14

Urethral Diverticula

Etiology

Diverticula develops secondary to obstruction of the duct between the urethra and the paraurethral gland, which may lead to abscess formation, and rupture back into the urethra.

Location

Majority of female urethral diverticula are located in the middle or distal third of the urethra.

Clinical Features

- Postmicturition dribbling.
- Chronic urinary tract symptom like dysuria, difficult in voiding following intercourse.
- Palpable sub urethral mass and expression of pus from a tendon urethra is diagnostic.

Investigations

- Voiding cystourethrogram.
- Urethroscopy (Fig. 14.1).

Treatment

Choice of surgical method for repair of urethral diverticula depends on the location of diverticular orifice.

- Vaginal incision.
- Exposure of entire area occupied by diverticulum.
- Diverticulum is entered and is freed from all-around.
- Connection of diverticula to urethra is established and division of urethral attachment is done.
- Urethral defect is closed, inverting the edges, and a second row of mattress sutures approximates the periurethral fascia over primary sutures.
- Vaginal flap is trimmed and approximated.

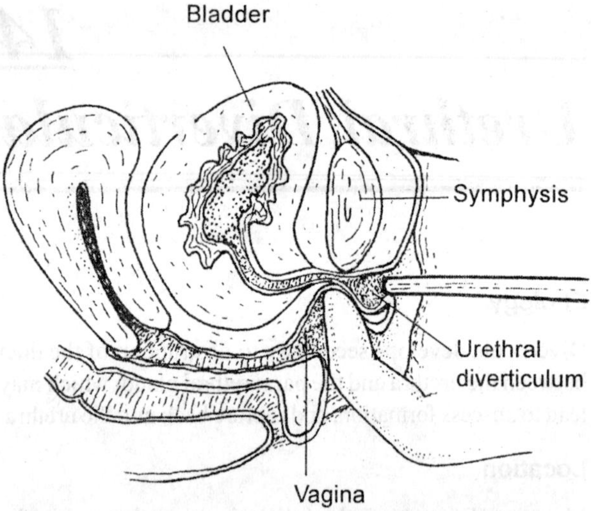

Fig. 14.1: Urethroscopy. The vesical neck is compressed against the symphysis by the surgeon's finger, allowing the urethra to distend with carbon dioxide. The urethra is then massaged to identify the opening into the diverticulum

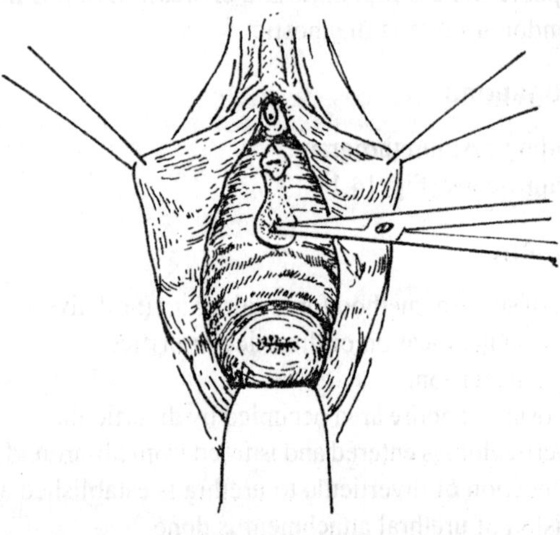

Fig. 14.2A: Spence procedure: Diverticulum distal to continence zone

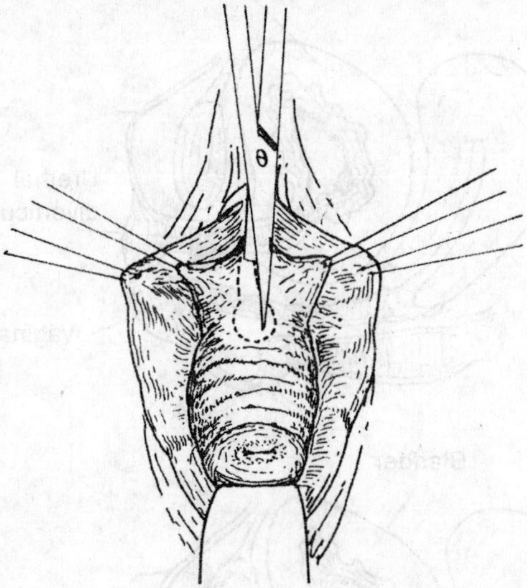

Fig. 14.2B: Spence procedure: Floor of urethra is cut

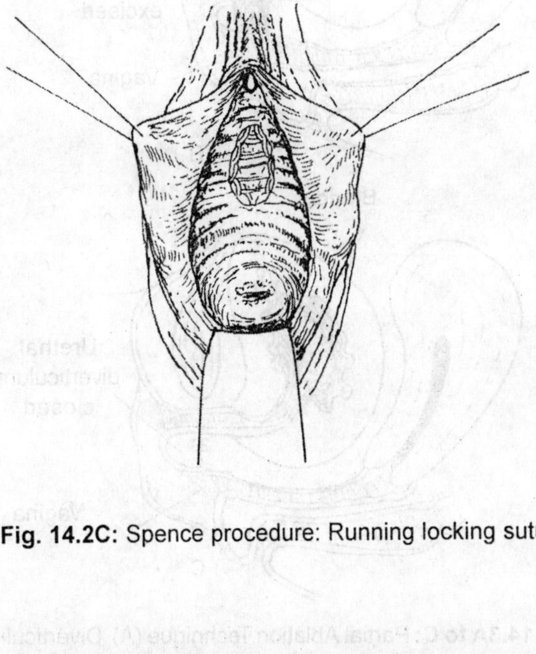

Fig. 14.2C: Spence procedure: Running locking suture

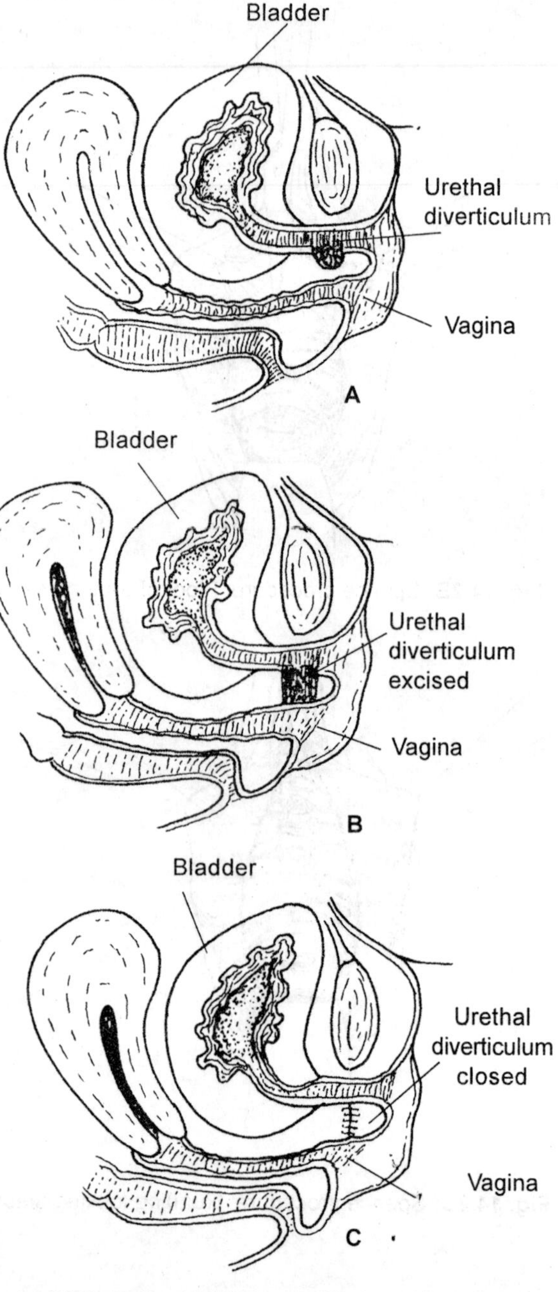

Fig. 14.3A to C: Partial Ablation Technique (A) Diverticulitis is present (B) Partial ablation (C) Urethral opening closed

Spence Procedure

It is indicated if the diverticula is located distal to continence zone.

- Diverticula is located.
- With one blade of the scissors set in the urethra and other in the vagina, the intervening septum between the floor of the urethra and the vagina is divided (Figs 14.2A to C).
- After the edges are trimmed, a running, locking suture along the edges assures hemostasis.

Partial Ablation Technique (Figs 14.3A to C)

With partial ablation technique the pathology of peridiverticulitis, the site, and the extent of lesion must be considered.

- The vaginal mucosa is dissected free, leaving the diverticulum intact.
- The sac is entered longitudinally, while the urethral opening is identified.
- The easily accessible portion of the sac is excised, attempting not to enucleate the sac at its neck.
- The opening is closed side to side with 3-0 chromic catgut.
- A second layer of sutures is placed, imbricating the previous urethral defect.

15

Miscellaneous Procedures of Reconstructive Surgery

Reconstructive surgery of the ovary, uterus, or other pelvic structures is usually performed in conjunction with tubal surgery.

UTERINE SUSPENSION

Uterine suspension is done for retroverted uterus extensively involved in the adhesive process.

The prevalent uterine attitude within the pelvis is considered to be anteflexion and anteversion. When erect, the uterine corpus is almost horizontal, resting on the bladder with the cervix pointing posteriorly.

Based on the anatomical considerations, the principle behind the numerous uterine suspension techniques is surgical shortening of the elongated utero sacral and round ligaments. Fundal ventropexy in which fundus is attached to the anterior abdominal wall is an unphysiological procedure and is therefore obsolete.

Different methods of shortening the round ligaments are as follows:

1. Abbreviation of the round ligament.
   - Plication (Figs 15.1A and B)
   - Triplication (Fig. 15.2)
   - Falope ring application
2. Ventrofixation of the round ligament.
   - Gillium suspension (Figs 15.3A and B)
   - Olhausen suspension (Figs 15.4A and B)

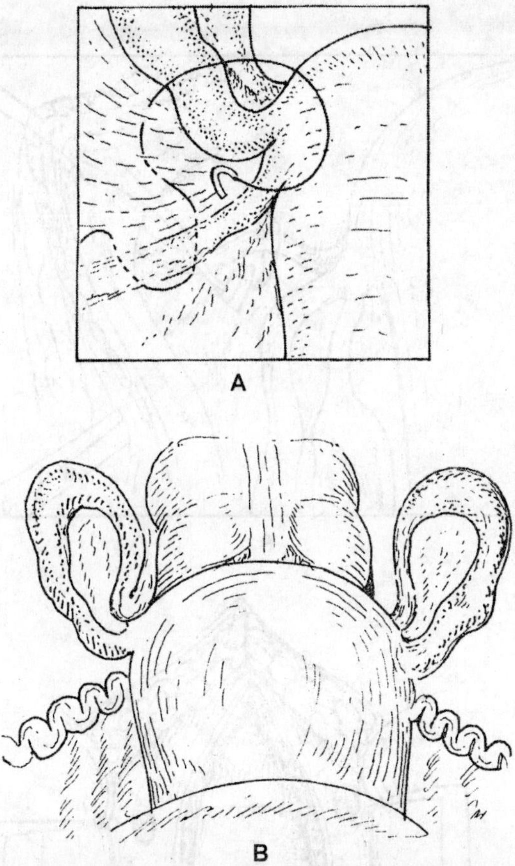

Figs 15.1 A and B: Plication of round ligament

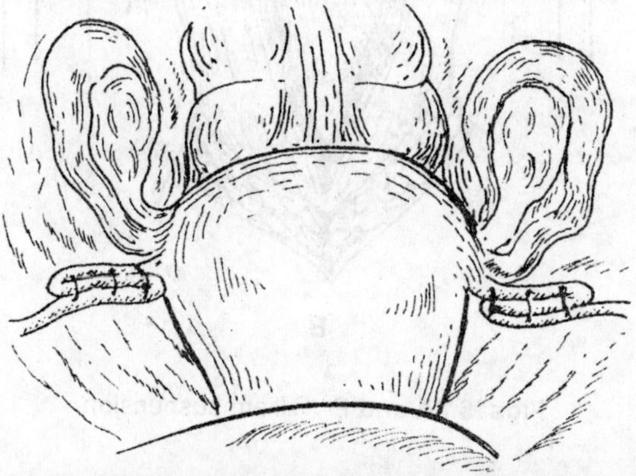

Fig.15.2: Triplication of round ligament

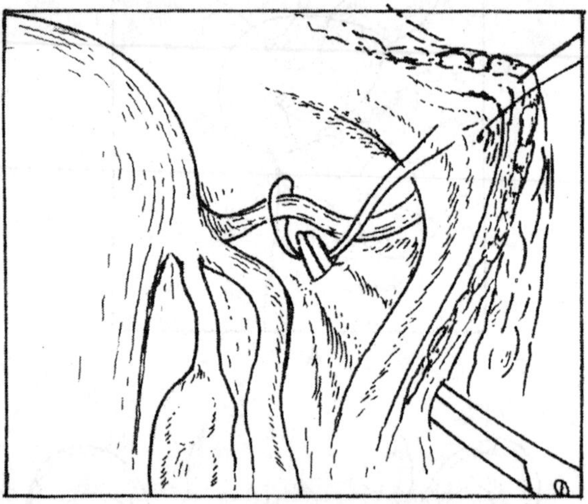

A

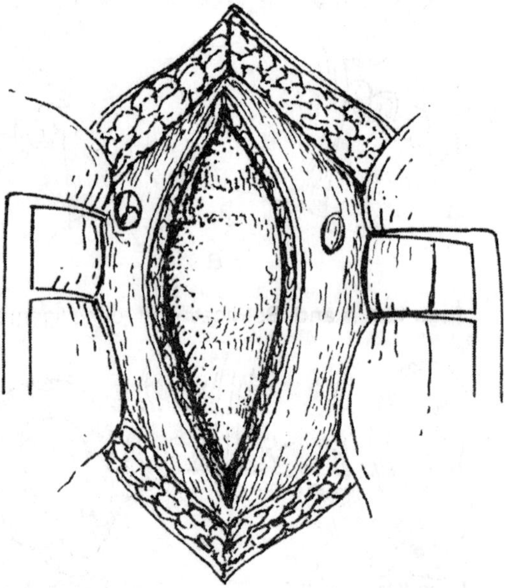

B

Figs15.3A and B: Gilliam suspension

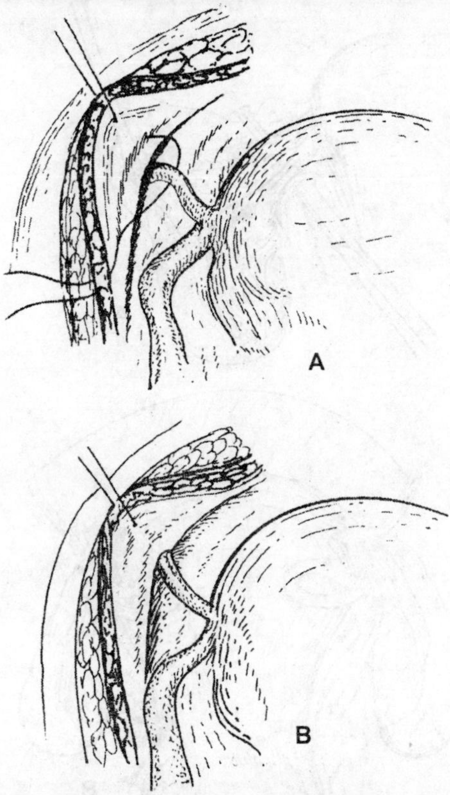

Figs 15.4A and B: Olhausen suspension

3. Uterofixation of the round ligament.
   - Baldy-Webster suspensions (Figs 15.5A and B)
   - Coffey suspension (Fig. 15.6).

In abbreviation of the round ligaments, round ligaments are shortened by folding or pleating. The anterior pull of the taut round ligament then maintains uterine anteversion.

In ventrofixation of the round ligament, the ligaments are anchored to anterior abdominal wall.

In uterofixation of the round ligament, the ligaments are shortened by affixing them to the uterus.

Revision of Tuboovarian Relationship

Tuboovarian relationship is important component of efficient fimbrial ovum pick up. Therefore, when tube is significantly shortened following a reanastomosis or tubal

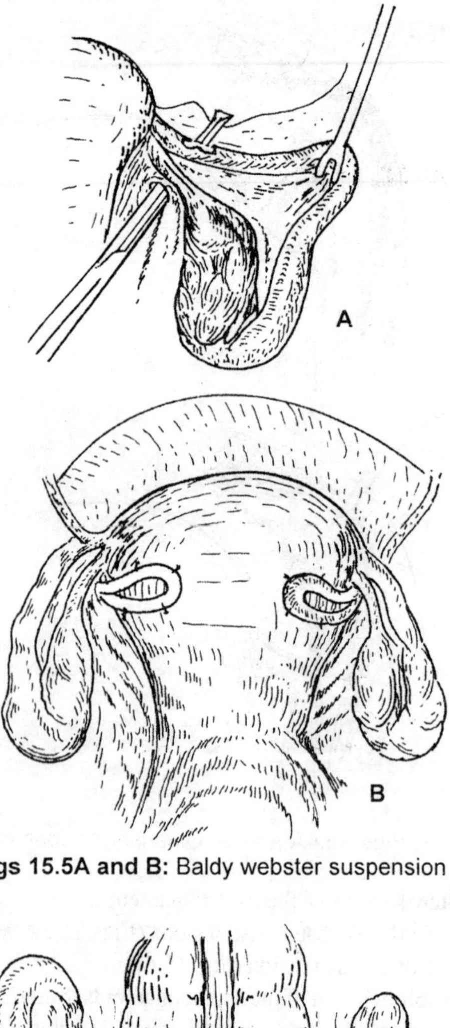

Figs 15.5A and B: Baldy webster suspension

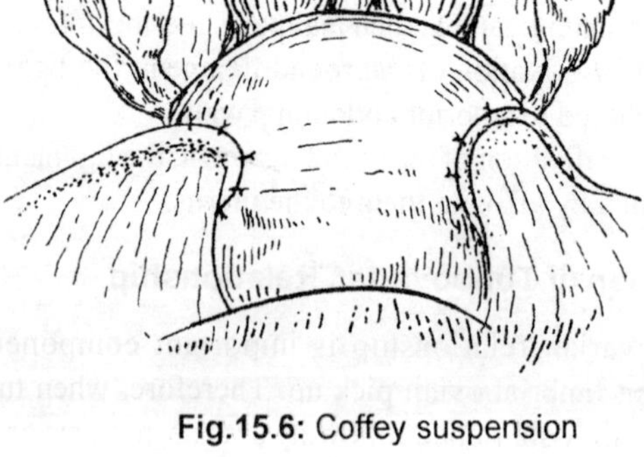

Fig.15.6: Coffey suspension

reimplantation, reapproximation of ovaries with fimbria may hasten the conception.

Shortening of the tuboovarian ligament can be accomplished by pleating or plicating the mesogastrium ovarica with fine non-absorbable suture.

Uterine Reconstructive Surgery-Metroplasty

Metroplasty is usually indicated for congenital deformities of uterus. The usual congenital deformities are given below.

Classification of Mullerian Anomalies

- Segmental Mullerian agenesis/hypoplasia
- Failure of fusion
  - Didelphys
  - Bicornate
  - Arcuate
- Failure of septum resorption
  - Single cervix
  - Double cervix
- Subseptate.

Surgical Technique

Surgical procedure of choice for bicornate uterus is the Strassman metroplasty. The principle behind this operation is to open the uterine cavity through a transverse fundal incision and unify the horns by closing the incision sagittally (Figs 15.7A to C).

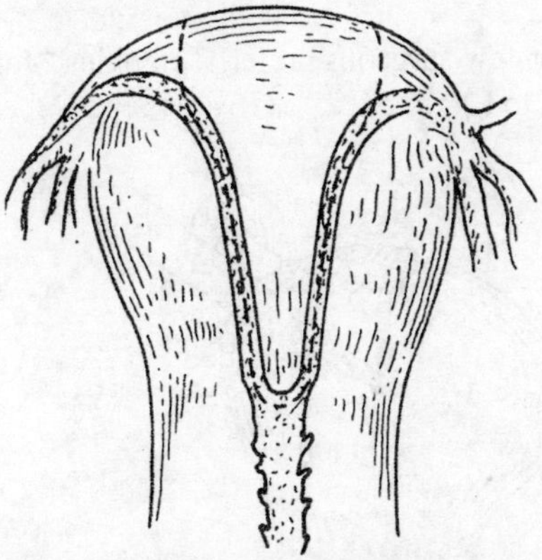

Fig. 15.7A: Strassman metroplasty

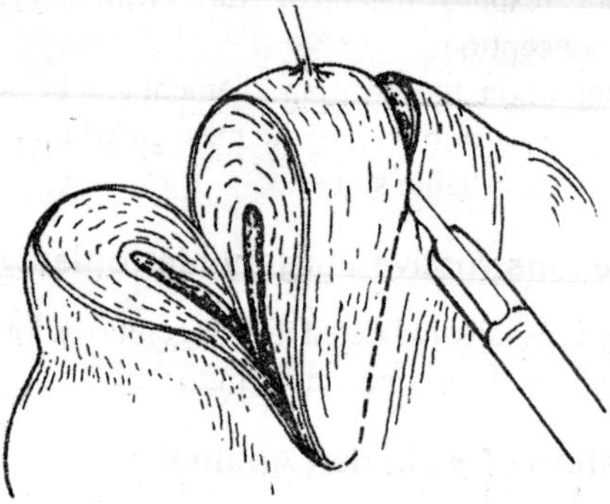

B

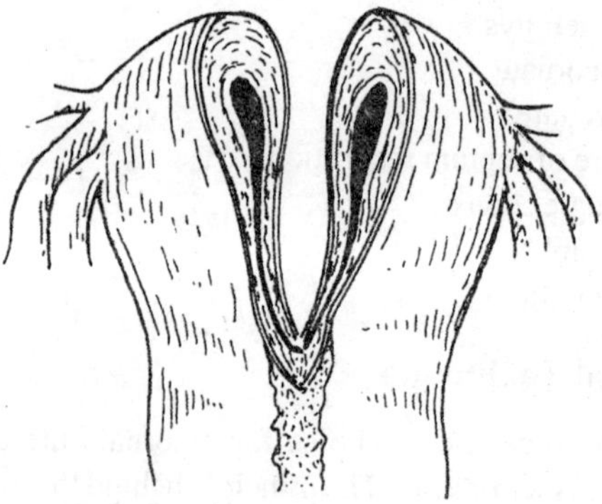

C

Figs 15.7B and C: Strassman metroplasty

However few surgeons prefer. Tompkins Metroplasty (Figs 15.8A to E).

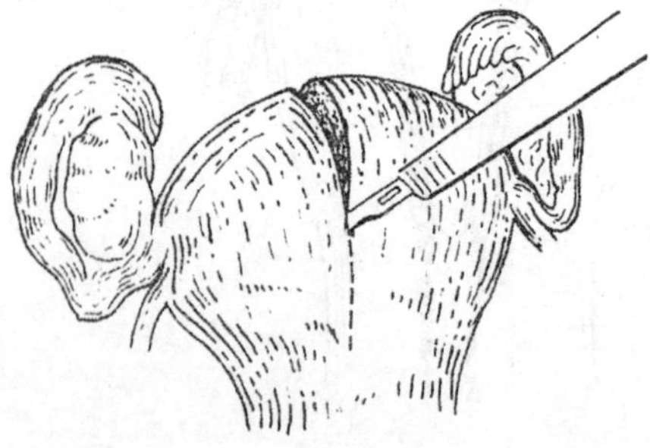

Fig. 15.8A: Tompkin metroplasty

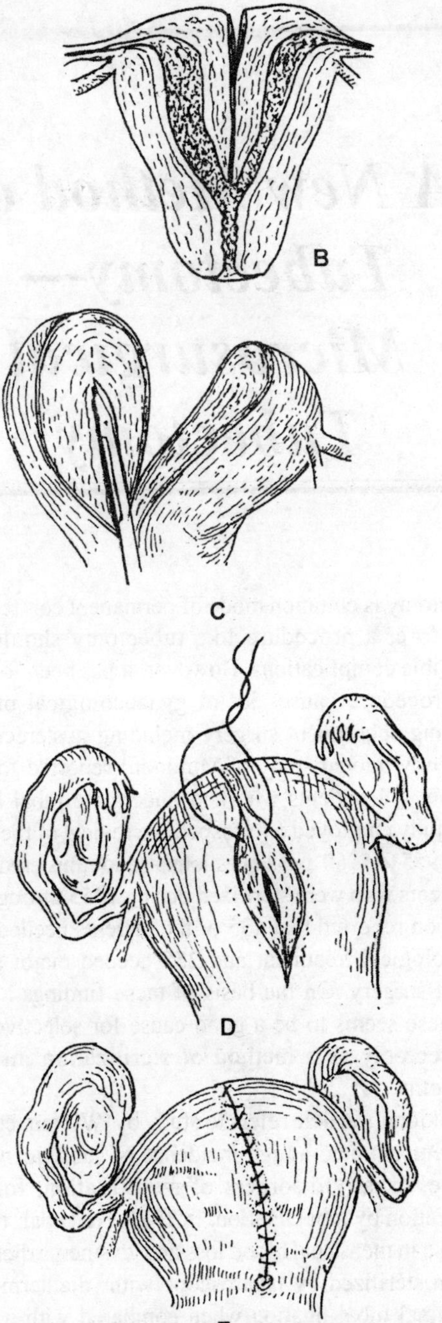

Figs 15.8B to E: Tompkin metroplasty

16

A New Method of Tubectomy—Microsurgical Tubectomy

Tubectomy is common mode of permanent contraception. Therefore, a procedure like tubectomy should have negligible complications. However, it has been found that this procedure causes lot of gynaecological problems requiring subsequent surgery including hysterectomy. A frequently quoted study of Muldoon[1] reported follow up data on 374 patients who had undergone tubal ligation. This study employed a retrospective review of the records from 1955 to 1960 and a questionnaire administered in 1972 to patients who were sterilized during 1955 through 1960. Muldoon reported that 435 of the patients needed further gynecological treatment and 255 needed major gynecological surgery. On the basis of these findings he stated that these seems to be a good cause for selective use of hysterectomy as a method of sterilization instead of tubectomy.

Muldoon's article refers to study by William et al[2] that also demonstrated a high incidence of subsequent pelvic disease, usually disorders of menstruation, following sterilization by tubal ligation. In 1975, Neil et al[3] reported increase in menstrual blood loss and dysmenorrhea in 454 women sterilized by laparoscope with diathermy or by abdominal tubal ligation when compared with a control group of 154 patients whose husbands had undergone vasectomy.

Chamberlain[4] and Foulkes found an increased incidence of dysmenorrhea in women who had undergone laparoscopic tubal sterilization.

In Stock's[5] study the overall incidence of postoperative menorrhagia was 42%.

Explanation for the causes of PTLS include impaired ovarian blood supply, altered innervation to the tube or ovary, and intermittent torsion of distal fallopian tube or ovary. So, PTLS would parallel the amount of tissue destruction that occurs in each type of the technique, producing accompanying hormonal disturbances.

Hargrove[6] and Abraham reported high serum estradiol and low serum progesterone levels in 29 patients who had PTLS consisting of pain, bleeding, and premenstrual tension.

Donnez[7] et al hypothesized that Pomeroy method alters the supplementary blood flow to the ovary by interrupting the uterovarian artery. Their proposed explanation is that the decreased blood flow might lead to deficient formation and function of corpus luteum.

Radwanska et al[8] also concluded in his study that anovulation or poor P production by the ovary may be responsible for menstrual disorders in some sterilized women and there disorders may be related to altered blood supply caused by sterilization procedure.

Despite inherent methodological problems and selection bias, all the studies suggest that some women do experience ovarian dysfunction after sterilization, and the severity may be related to the amount of disruption in blood or the nerve supply to the ovaries.

Most authors agree that PTLS is due to hormonal disturbance as during tubectomy the blood supply of the ovaries is affected, because for proper functioning of the ovaries in most of the cases the blood supply from ovarian as well as tubal artery is required.

Once a patient came to us for tubectomy. We were not interested in performing the surgery, because of various problems like PTLS syndrome. Then the senior author said, "Let us device a new and improved method to do tubectomy."

"I agreed with him. But did not know what to do."

After about three months he came to me and said, "I have devised a new method to do tubectomy. If you have any patient, let us perform the tubectomy by new method."

Soon a patient came for tubectomy and we did not microsurgical tubectomy in that patient and followed the patient for one year. The patient did not have any problem. Though nothing can be concluded by one patient, there is not doubt that this method avoids all the objections put forwards by different authors.

Technique

- The mini laparotomy is done.
- Under magnification the tubal vessels are dissected after making a longitudinal incision in serosal layer of the tubes.
- Muscular layer and mucosa are then divided. Mucosa is closed on both sides and muscles are closed over mucosa.
- Serosa is closed over (Fig. 16.1).

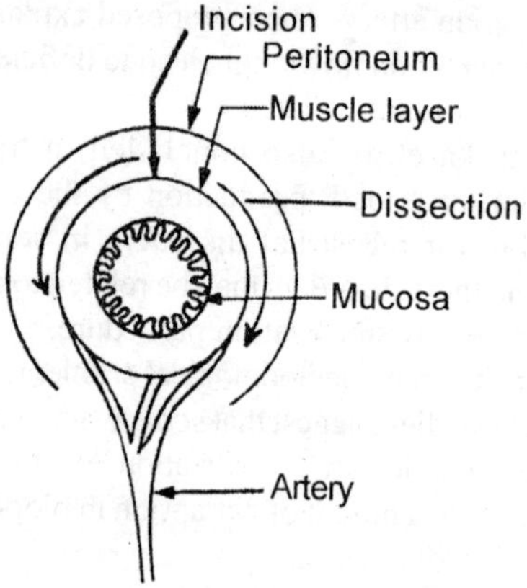

Fig. 16.1: Transverse section of fallopian tube showing incision and dissection

Advantages of the procedure are:

1. Tubal vessels and nerves are not damaged and so no alteration in blood or nerve supply.
2. Least tissue destruction.
3. Tube is in continuity so distal end cannot undergo torsion and cause pain.
4. Better chances of reversal, if required.

We have done the procedure in only one patient. However, hypothetically the procedure should be sound for tubectomy. We are planning to do a long term comparative studies of hormonal levels after out method and after other procedures of tubectomies. We will report long term results when available. But there should be no doubt that this method of microsurgical tubectomy should be the standard method of tubectomy.

REFERENCES

1. Muldoon MJ: Gynaecological illnesses after sterilization. British Medical Journal 1972;84.
2. Williams EL, Jones HE, Merril RE. The subsequent course of patients sterilized by tubal ligation: A consideration of hysterectomy for sterilization. Am J. Obstet Gynecol 51:423.
3. Neil JR, Harmond GT, Nobel AD, Rushton L. Late complications of sterilizations by laparoscopy and tubal ligation. Lancet 1975;2:699.
4. Chamberlain G, Foulkes J. Long term effects of laparoscopic sterilization on menstruation. South Medical Journal 1976;69:1474.
5. Stock RJ: Evaluation of sequelae of tubal ligation. Fertility and Sterility 1978;29:169.
6. Hargrove JT, Abraham GE. Endocrine profile of the patients with post tubal ligation syndrome. J Reproductive Medicine 1981;26:33.
7. Donnez J, Wauters M, Thomas K: Luteal function after tubal sterilization. Obstet Gynaecol 1981;57:65.
8. Radwansaka E, Headley SK, Dmowski P. Evaluation of ovarian function after tubal sterilization. J Reproductive Medicine 1982;27:376.

17

Leiomyoma and Role of Plastic Surgery

Leiomyoma which occur in one of every 4-5 women in reproductive life are the most common solid pelvic tumours in women. 20-50% of uterine leiomyomata are estimated to produce symptoms. The severity of symptoms experienced by a patient of leiomyomata will depend upon the number, size, and location of all tumours.

Treatment can be medical or surgical. However frequently both types of the approaches are combined together.

Medical Management

The following drugs are used for the medical management of fibroids:

- GnRH analogous-agonists and antagonists
- Danazol
- Progesterone
- Antiprogesterones
- Levonorgestrel releasing intrauterine devices.

Surgical treatment of the Fibroids

The textbooks of Gynecology have described two major technical concerns in the performance of myomectomy-blood loss and postoperative adhesions. Authors **have added another major technical concern—maintenance of size of uterus in very big sized fibroids.**

Maintenance of Uterine Size

In very big sized fibroids attention should be paid to maintenance of size of the uterus. However it does not mean compromising the removal of uterine tumour. It simply means replacing the lost myometrium by a skeletal muscle.

The muscles which can be used are:

- Rectus abdominis
- Latissimus Dorsi.

Rectus Abdominis Muscle

Rectus abdominis muscle is attached to pubic symphysis inferiorly and to the ribs superiorly. The muscle is supplied by inferior deep epigastric artery. While reconstructing the uterus the planning in reverse is done and then muscle is cut from superior end. This muscle is then turned down to abdominal cavity without damaging the blood supply.

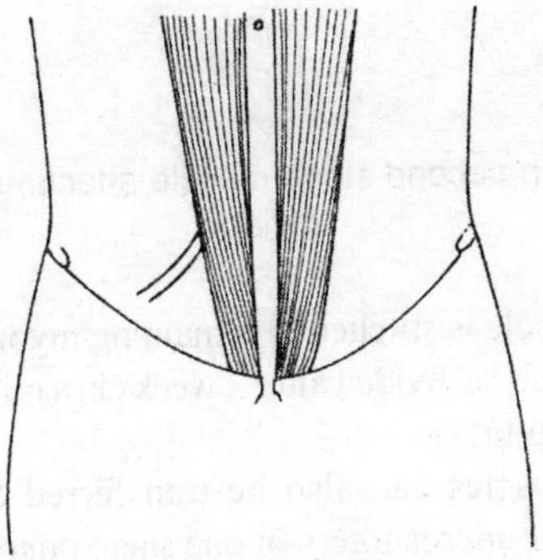

Fig. 17.1: Rectus abdominis muscles on both sides

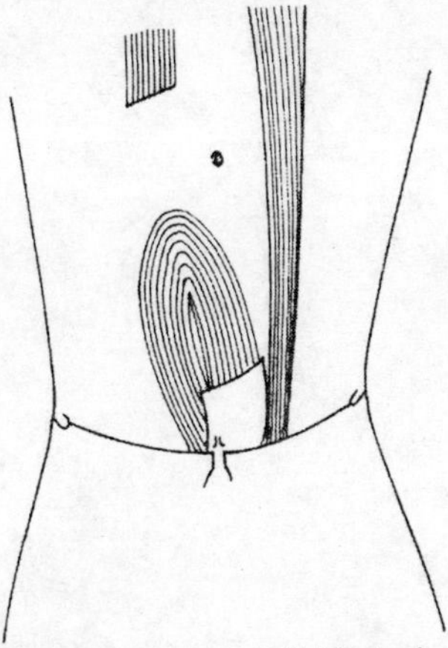

Fig. 17.2: Right rectus muscle divided above umbilicus and turned to be stitched to remaining myometrium of uterus after removal of leiomyoma

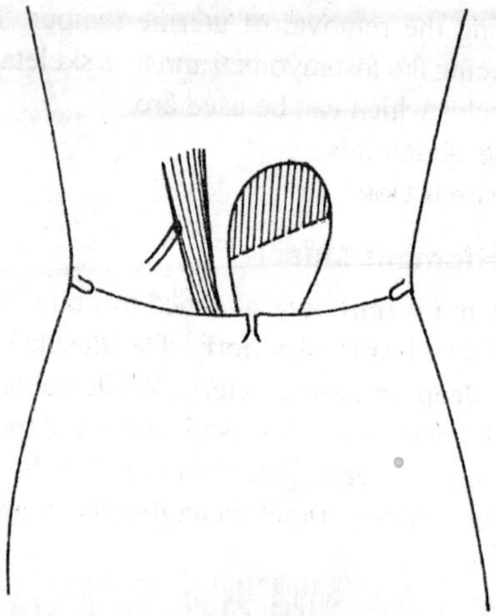

Fig. 17.3: In second stage muscle attachment to uterus divided

Turned muscle is stitched to remaining myometrium. The arterial supply is divided after 3 weeks in a minor operation (Figs 17.1 to 17.3).

Both muscles can also be transferred by using the principles of microsurgery in one stage operation.

18

Hypoplastic Uterus

Hypoplastic uterus is more commonly found than aplastic uterus. Clinically diagnosis of hypoplastic uterus is made if it is smaller with less than 5 cm of the cavity. Endometrium is less well developed and the vagina is short and narrow. The onset of the puberty is delayed and menstruation is often irregular, so that the menstrual cycle is prolonged to between 6-8 weeks. Severe dysmenorrhoea is a common symptom and there is tendency for such patients to be sterile.

There is usual medical treatment for such patients. But author is of opinion that cavity should be enlarged and muscle transfer should be done in these patients along with hormonal manipulations.

Technique

1. Patient lies in supine position.
2. Midline incision is made.
3. Rectus abdominis muscle is identified and isolated.
4. Deep inferior epigastric artery is identified and should be preserved carefully.
5. Abdoninal cavity is entered.
6. Peritoneal incision along with muscle and endometrium is made at lower level and whole part is raised as flap.
7. Rectus muscle is insetted in the defect.
8. The arterial pedicle is not divided.
9. Abdomen is closed.
10. In second sitting after three weeks, arterial pedicle is divided (See Figs 17.1 to 17.3).

19

Uterosacral Ligament Resection for Dysmenorrhea

Endometriosis is frequently associated with disabling dysmenorrhea. Conservative surgical treatment is generally satisfactory, but patients often report only partial resolution of pain or recurrence. Two uterine denervation techniques have been proposed to improve long term results—presacral neurectomy and resection of uterosacral ligaments.

In presacral neurectomy only the sympathetic nerves of the superior hypogastric plexus are sectioned; however the uterus is innervated also by the parasympathetic fibres. Both sympathetic and parasympathetic fibres run in uterosacral folds and reach the parametrium, posterolateral to the uterine cervix, where they unite to form the plexus of Franenhauser. Therefore, resection of uterosacral ligaments is better procedure for denervating the uterus in females suffering with endometriosis and midline dysmenorrhea.

The operation is done as following:

- The abdomen is opened or laparoscope inserted.
- Endometriotic lesions are excised or coagulated.
- Uterosacral ligaments are excised and coagulated.
- Check for bleeding.
- Abdomen is closed.

Vercellini et al did study of 273 women coming to clinic for dysmenorrhea. He did uterosacral ligament resection in 90 females. His most of the patients improved after surgery.

20

Immediate Plastic Surgery of Episiotomy

Episiotomy is an operation done to enlarge the introitus during delivery so as to avoid perineal tears and easy vaginal delivery. After the delivery the episiotomy is stitched back. But the author has seen the episiotomy being repaired in most callous manner without any attention to the proper repair, and the result is loss of sohincteric function of the bulbocavernous muscle. We have already described that loss of the sphincteric action is one of the important factor in development of vaginal laxity. Therefore it is important the episiotomy should be repaired with proper care and using the principles of plastic surgery

Operation

The episiotomy should be repaired in following manner:

- After delivery the mucosal margins are identified and stitched with absorbable suture.
- After that bulbocavernous muscle is identified.
- It should be separated for a distance and stitched in overlapping manner (Figs 20.1A and B).
- After repair of bulbocavernous muscle skin is repaired with non-absorbable suture after closing any dead space.

Post Operative Care

1. As the area may be infected daily dressing is required to keep the wound dry.
2. Avoid straining during stool and so stool softeners should be given.

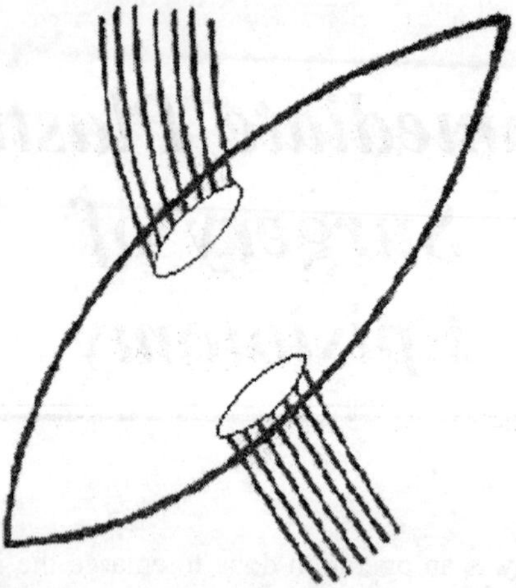

Fig. 20.1A: Episiotomy and bulbo cavernous and spongiosus muscles

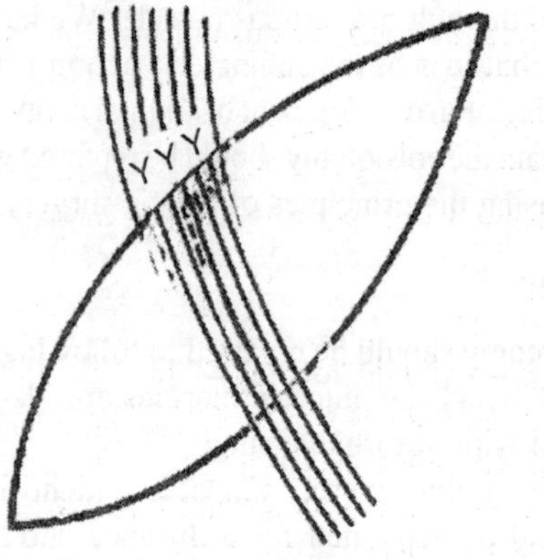

Fig. 20.1B: Muscles are to be repaired in over lapping manner

Complication

Most common complication after episiotomy is dehiscence and it is due to infection. Infection is due to lack of hygiene or small hematoma formation.

Management

- Wound should be dressed daily with Eusol.
- Repair again is done after three weeks.

Prevention of complications:

1. Avoid dead space during repair.
2. Proper attention to hygiene.

21

Different Cosmetic Surgical Procedures Related with Female Accessory Genitals

PLASTIC SURGERY OF ABDOMINAL WALL ALONG WITH CAESARIAN OR HYSTERECTOMY

With advances in management of plastic surgery of the abdominal wall females undergoing caesarean section or hysterectomy can undergo simultaneous plastic surgery of the abdominal wall, which reduces the morbidity of two operations.

With Hysterectomy

With hysterectomy any type of plastic surgery of abdomen as required can be carried out. Most common problem with females is laxity of the abdomen with deposition of fat with and without divarication of the recti.

If the age of patients is less than 40 years and her skin tone is well maintained, liposuction may be tried. But in most of the cases abdominal lipectomy is the better option as it gives proper view to recti also, which if divaricated; can be repaired at the same time. As the patient is undergoing hysterectomy it can be carried out from the same incision as made for lipectomy.

Abdominoplasty

Incision

The various incisions have been described for abdominoplasty. They are given in Fig. 21.1. All these incisions can be made and hysterectomy can be carried out through these incisions.

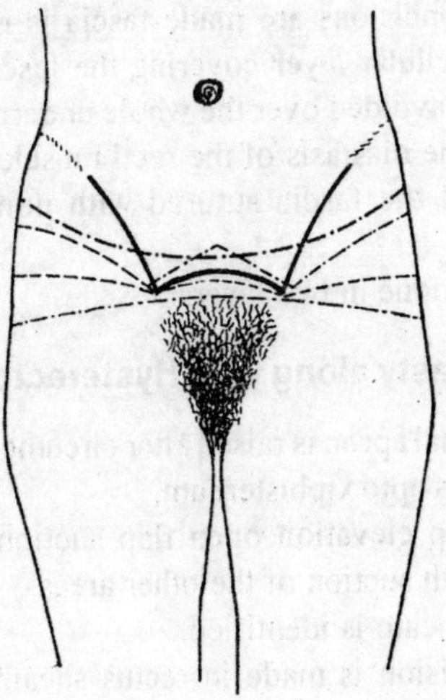

Fig. 22.1: Incisions of abdominoplasty

W Technique of Abdominoplasty

- No pattern should be used because the bodies of women are not standard and skin is more elastic than any pattern.
- W incision is located at the inguinal fold and is never on the thighs.
- The excision takes advantage of the skin's elasticity. Since skin is more supple laterally than in the midline, the basic goal of this method is to release tension in the midline and bring more tension laterally.
- The placement of the lower incision is inside the pubic hair when the tissues are very loose, or slightly above that level when skin elasticity seems only moderate.
- From mid line the incision goes downward to reach the inguinal fold either at the fold or slightly above it, depending upon the elasticity of the skin.

- The incision then goes upward and laterally, following the direction of the fold.
- Central limb of the W is usually half the length of the lateral one.
- The incision of the umbilicus is in a horizontal spindle shape.
- The upper line should never be longer than the lower ones if dog ears are to be avoided.
- After skin incisions are made fascia is reached. The very fine cellular layer covering the fascia should be completely avoided over the whole undermined area.
- Repair of the diastasis of the recti muscles is done by plication of the fascia sutured with non-absorbable material.
- Suturing is done in two layers.

Abdominoplasty along with Hysterectomy

1. Abdominal apron is raised after circumcision around umbilicus upto xiphisternum.
2. After flap elevation open flap suctioning is done along with suction of the other areas.
3. Rectus sheath is identified.
4. Now incision is made in rectus sheath in midline below umbilicus to carry out hysterectomy and rectus muscles retracted laterally.
5. Peritoneum is opened.
6. Hysterectomy is done.
7. Any divarication of the recti is corrected by plication with an interrupted non-absorbable suture no. 2.0 suture.
8. It is followed by running locking sutures of absorbable no. O chromic catgut.
9. Now marking for future site of umbilicus is done and umbilicus brought out through the incision.
10. Final closure is done with drains.
11. Adhesive dressing is done followed by abdominal binder.

Abdominoplasty with Breast Augmentation

Augmentation of the breasts without scar deformities can be carried out along with abdominoplasty and hysterectomy.

Miniabdominoplasty

This is indicated in those females in whom the laxity is more in lower abdomen. Usually it is indicated in only fewer patients as compared to full abdominoplasty.

Incisions

Incisions are same as for full abdominoplasty.

Procedure

1. Incision is made.
2. Flap is elevated.
3. If needed dissection above umbilicus is carried out but in limited fashion only in midline.
4. If needed plication of rectus is carried out.
5. Hysterectomy is carried out.
6. Closure is done with drains.

With Caesarean Section

With caesarean section excessive surgery of suctioning or dissection is not recommended. However if there is obvious divarication of the recti it should be corrected and excess skin is excised.

LIPECTOMY

Thigh Reduction

Thigh reduction is indicated when thighs are heavy and having localized deposits of fat. Overweight patients showing firm adiposity are not good candidates for surgery since the amount of tissue that can be removed safely is small. Such patients should be encouraged to reduce the weight first. The procedures for thigh reduction are:

- Semicircular
- Circular
- Vertical
- Combined circular and vertical
- Trochanteric defatting
- Correction of lower medial thigh.

Semicircular Reduction

- Planning should be done for removal with the patient standing, which helps in planning for an adequate excision.

- The upper line of the excision is marked first.
- Then by pushing upward on the thigh tissues, one can judge what width of tissue removal will give a reasonably good correction.
- The marking is continued at the back and laterally.
- One should be cautious not to plan too large a removal of the buttocks, or a flat unpleasant contour might result.
- The marking may be facilitated by having the patient wear a bikini pantie; the upper line of the marking should remain about 2-3 above the lower edge of the pantie.

Operative Technique

Semicircular excision is done in two parts anterior and posterior excision.

Anterior Excision

- Supine position.
- Legs slightly apart.
- Incision follows the markings, going through skin and fat down to superficial fascia, which is preserved along with the large veins and nerves.
- The specimen can be separated from the superficial fascia by stripping.
- Dissection is carried as far as the medial part of the thigh where the specimen is served medially and removed.
- The same procedure is done on the other thigh.
- Closure is done with absorbable suture.

Posterior Excision

- Patient is turned over.
- The arms are lifted above the head.
- The incisions follow the markings down to the musculo aponeurotic plane.
- No undermining is done medially.
- Excised tissues are removed and closure is done.
- Patient is allowed to get up the next day.
- However, sitting down is not permitted for 2-3 weeks to prevent stretching of the posterior suture line.

Circular Reduction

- Circular reduction of the thigh is indicated when a large

amount of excess skin and/or excess fat appears not only medially and laterally but also in the front of thigh.

Operative Technique

Anterior Excision

- The technique is basically the same as described in semi-circular operation.
- Anterior tissue is removed first and the specimen is divided laterally and medially as far as it is possible.
- The thigh tissues are rotated medially.

Posterior Excision

- Patient is turned over.
- Incision is marked and dissection is started laterally going progressively upward, removing skin and fat.
- Before suturing is done, the medial tissues in lower flap are rotated outward and lateral lower flap tissues are rotated inward, while upper tissue are left in position.
- Suturing is done.

Trochanteric Defatting Procedure

Correction of the trochanteric fat pad (riding breech deformity) is usually done at the same time as semicircular or circular operation.

- The area to be defatted is marked before operation with the patient standing up.
- The procedure is done with the patient prone.
- After previously described excision has been completed on the back side, undermining of the trochanteric area is done. Always leave on an average 15 mm of fat in thickness.

Lipectomy of the Lower Leg

- Lipectomy of leg is done only for functional reasons. because it leaves such visible scars.
- The excision may be posteromedially.
- If both thigh and leg need reduction, a continuous excision can be made, with a horizontal line or step placed at the level of popliteal fossa.
- Limited defatting may be done in the calf and ankle reason as long as enough subcutaneous fat is left with the skin.

Lipectomy of the Arm

Indicated in females who have lost weight and present with pendulous upper arms.

- Planning is done with the patient sitting up.
- The incision is started at the medial end of the line marked in axilla.
- Dissection is done carefully to leave the superficial fascia and the large superficial vein intact.
- Dissection is continued to the level of the posterior line of the markings and tissue elasticity is then tested.
- The resection is done according to the needs of the patient.
- Undermining is usually not done.
- Closure is done in three layers.

AUGMENTATION MAMMOPLASTY

Augmentation mammoplasty is defined as the procedure to enlarge the size of breasts. In recent years, because of improvements in breasts prosthesis and safe surgical techniques, breast augmentation has become one of the most requested cosmetic surgical procedure.

Indications

The patients presenting with micromastia is the ideal candidate for mammary augmentation.

- Postpartum involution of the breasts
- Drastic weight reduction
- Ptosis
- Larger breasts for professional reasons.

Surgical Procedures

Three basic approaches are:

- Inframammary
- Periareolar
- Transaxillary

Now another approach has also been added

- Endoscopic.

Inframammary Technique

- Most common surgical approach for breast augmentation.

- 3-4 cm incision is placed approximately 1 cm above the inframammary crease.
- The incision begins 1.5 cm medial to the reference line which is vertical line drawn from the medial aspect of the nipple inferiorly.
- The incision is made and 2 cm flap is developed inferiorly down to pectoral fascia, at which point the dissection is turned cephalad.
- Stay between pectoral fascia and the posterior capsule of the breast.
- Breast capsule is freed from the pectoral fascia by blunt dissection.
- The space is always made larger than implant.
- Dissection should not be taken too far laterally as that would cause numbness due to intercostal nerve damage.
- Meticulous haemostasis is done.
- Implant is placed.
- Stitching is done.
- A brassiere type dressing is worn (Figs 21.2 and 22.3).

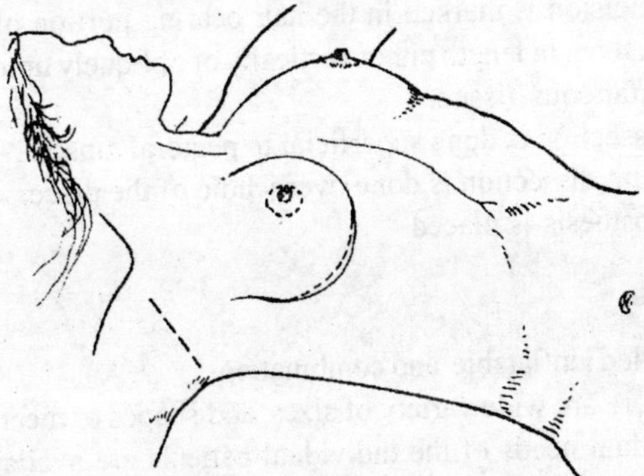

Fig. 21.2: **Broken** lines illustrate the three standard approaches to breast augmentation—the inframammary, perareolar, and transaxillary techniques

Periareolar Approach

- With the patient lying supine and the arms abducted at 90°, the incision lines are drawn circumferentially just inside the areolar border from 3 o'clock to 9 o'clock

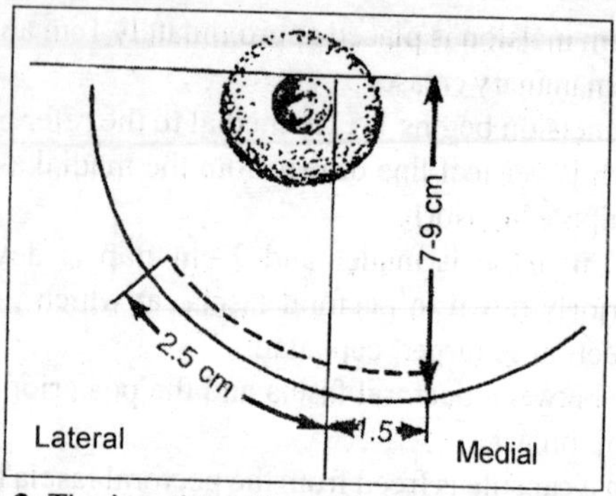

Fig. 21.3: The location of the incision for the inframammary approach. The curvillinear incision is placed 7 to 9 cm from the top of the nipple

- Subcutaneous dissection to the inferior border of the breast is done where the dissection turns cephalad and the retrommammary space is enlarged for prosthesis.

Transaxillary Approach

The incision is marked in the hair bearing portion of the axilla, 4 cm in length either vertically or obliquely upto the subcutaneous tissue.

- Dissection is done superficial to pectoral muscle.
- Blunt dissection is done over whole of the place.
- Prosthesis is placed.

Types

Gel filled , inflatable and combination.

There are wide variety of sizes and shapes to meet the individual needs of the individual patients are available. These come as contour, round, low profile and unferfill varieties.

Postoperative Care

A broad spectrum antibiotic is given.

- Two pillows cushioned behind the upper portion of the back will place the patient in a desirable semireclining position.
- As hematoma is common during the first 24 hours, patient is directed to rest for this period limiting the use of the arm to only routine acts such as eating , brushing

the teeth, and combing hair avoiding any vigorous activity involving the arms.

- May resume car driving on third day.
- During fifth day she is instructed to carry out massage.

How to do Massage

The breast is to be massaged in rotatory fashion, squeezing it and flattening it with the hand. As the breast loses the postoperative tenderness, the massage should become more vigorous.The regimen should be instituted as often as possible in the immediate postoperative period, and at least daily thereafter.

Bra

The patient should be instructed to wear a bra night and day, but she may sleep without it after 3 days. The second week she may go braless. Unlimited physical activity may resume 20 days postoperatively.

Summary of Postoperative Care

Immediate postoperative care

1. Immediate mobilization is encouraged.
2. A regular brassiere is used as the final dressing.

Three days postoperatively

1. The patient should massage her breasts twice daily for several minutes.
2. The patient may sleep without a brassiere.
3. The patient may drive an automobile.

Ten days postoperatively

The patient may go braless.

Twenty days postoperatively

The patient may resume unrestricted physical activity.

Postoperative Complications

Early complications

Early complications are:

- Changes in nipple and breasts sensations
- Hematomas
- Infection
- Wound separation
- Ptosis of prosthesis
- Leakage of prosthesis
- Mondor's disease.

Capsular Contracture

Excessive firmness of the breasts is the most common complication of the breast augmentation. It is reported to take place in about 20% of the cases.

It is noted in first six months following surgery. The firmness usually results from the contracture of the fibrous capsule, as the capsule contracts, there is a decrease in the ratio of its surface area to the volume it contains, producing an increase in the pressure within the capsule. It produces more spherical configuration of the prosthesis because the sphere is the geometric shape that has the large surface area for a given volume.

Etiology

Though various factors have been implicated. Basic problem of scar contracture is the basic aetiological factor. Following factors may aggravate the situation.

Hematoma, seroma, the type of the implant used, impurities in the silicones, fibrinogenic drugs applied locally, and overt or subclinical local infection.

Treatment

- Non-surgical
- Surgical
- Endoscopic.

Non-surgical Squeeze Capsulotomy

Closed non-surgical squeeze compression of the breasts has been found to be highly successful and is associated with small complication rate.

- The patient lies supine.
- The breast is grasped at its base with both hands and circumferential compression is administered until a popping noise is heard and the softening of the breasts is felt.
- The hands are turned 90 degrees and another squeeze is applied to complete the capsular tear-flat compression of the breasts with the palm of the hand, in a circular motion, completes the procedure.
- The patient is instructed to massage the breast vigorously and frequently for several weeks and several times a day thereafter.

Surgical Capsulotomy

- Inframammary incision.
- Subcutaneous flap is dissected.
- Capsule is splitted.
- Implant is removed.
- Capsule is incised at its base 360 degrees and the pocket is expanded to large proportion by sharp and blunt dissection.
- Implant is placed again.
- Wound is closed.

How to Measure the Volume of the Breast

Breast volume is one of the crucial measurements on preoperative planning and postoperative evaluation of the results in mammoplasty. Because symmetry is the prerequisite of beauty and normality, no matter how beautiful each of the breasts is as a result of the operation, neither the surgeon nor the patient will be satisfied with asymmetric breasts.

Erdem Tezel of Turkey had developed a device for this which consists of a container, a pliable plastic bag, and rubber stopper. The device is placed on the breasts of the patient lying in supine position. The stopper is removed and the bag is filled with warm water by using an injector. The volume of the water used is measured. The same process is applied to other breast. The difference between two measurements is the difference in volume between two breasts.

In augmentation mammoplasty, the patient wears a brassiere with a well-formed cup. This brassiere is of the size that she will prefer to wear after the operation. If needed, a sponge is placed inside the brassiere to support it. A measurement is made as described. The second measurement is made on the same breasts without bra. The difference between two measures is the volume of the prosthesis to be used. Volume can also be measured by chart as in (Figs 21.4 and 21.5).

REDUCTION MAMMOPLASTY, MASTOPEXY AND SHAPING THE BREASTS

Reduction mammoplasty is indicated in those patients in whom the breasts are hypertrophied. Excessively enlarged breasts create following problems:

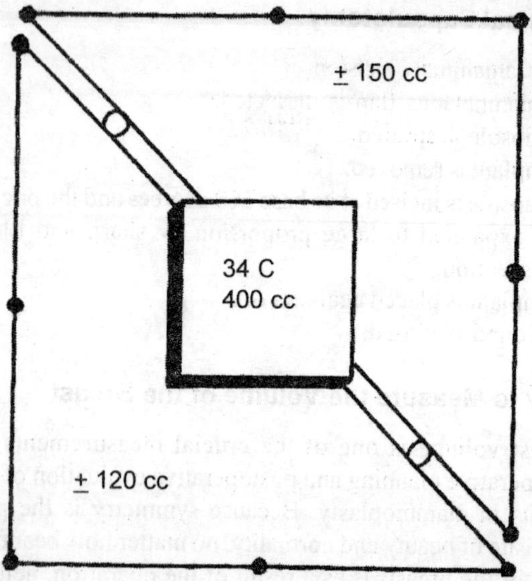

Fig. 21.4: To increase one cup size or go up one band size, add approximately 150 ml (see upper right triangle). To decrease one cup size or go down one band size, subtract approximately 120 ml (see lower left triangle)

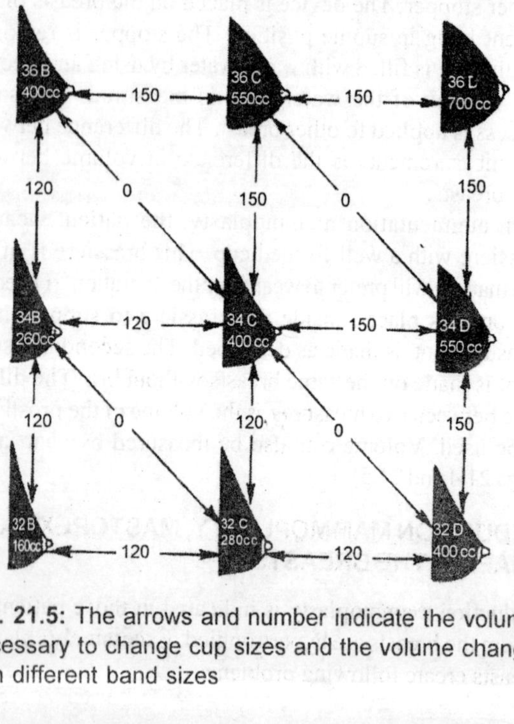

Fig. 21.5: The arrows and number indicate the volumes necessary to change cup sizes and the volume changes with different band sizes

1. Shape of the patient is distorted.
2. Shoulder pain because of heavy weight over the shoulders of the breasts.
3. Fungal infection in the inframammary fold.

Reduction mammoplasty is done by different procedures but most of them give some scar. However with advent of endoscopic surgery the problem of the scar has been minimized.

Before we proceed further let us know the aims of surgery which are:

1. A breast of ideal size elevated to a normal position on the chest wall.
2. A breast of ideal form or shape for the patient.
3. A breast with a minimal amount of scarring or visible scarring.
4. A breast with normal sensations and erectile function of the nipple.
5. A breast that can lactate and function normally for nursing, if necessary.

Etiology

1. **Endocranial hypertrophy**: This type os hypertrophy is associated with various endocrine abnormalities.
2. **Virginal hypertrophy:** This represents abnormal end organ response, but is not associated with abnormal hormonal effects any where else in the body.
3. **Obese hypertrophy:** This condition is associated with generalised obesity. However, it is not much affected by weight reduction. Histologically there is excessive fat deposition.
4. **Involutional hypertrophy:** Characterized by breast growth at middle age around the menopausal period, having the picture of lobular atrophy and fatty replacement.
5. **Gravid hypertrophy:** This condition results from the hormonal changes in pregnancy.
6. **Postgracid hypertrophy:** This condition of relative macromastia, which is characterized by larger breasts after pregnancy than existed before, results from incomplete involution and from persistence of stromal, ductal, and fatty hypertrophy of pregnancy.

Indications

1. Alleviation of the symptoms associated with weight like respiratory problem, shoulder pain.
2. Cosmetic.

Methods to do Reduction Mammoplasty

Main Features in Reduction Mammoplasty

1. Transposition of the nipple areolar segment at its best suitable position.
2. Excision of skin along with debulking procedures.

Operations are divided in three parts.

1. Lateralizing operations for breast reduction.
   This procedures are done for mild macromastia in which nipple areolar complex is shifted slightly.
2. Endoscopic
   It is also used for mild macromastia when fatty tissue is enough.
3. Pedicles operations
   Pedicled operations are the main operation for reduction mammoplasty. The pedicled operations meant that the nipple areolar is shifted on a pedicle of the breasts and skin tissue. There are various types of the pedicles described in the literature and perhaps there are not much difference in any type of the pedicle. The most commonly used pedicle is inferior pedicle. The author recently described lateral pedicle reduction mammoplasty.

Location of New Nipple Areola Complex

- All the markings should be made while the patient erect.
- Nipple should be marked at level of inframmary fold. Its position is located by placing the fingers at the infra mammary fold and thumb opposite them on new nipple line.
- The wise patter is used to mark out the skin incisions.
- The pattern is placed on the breast with its midpoint aligned on the nipple line. The nipple areolar complex is marked out with a washer of 4.5 cm diameter.
- Pedicle are created by deepithelizing the pedicle and the skin and breast tissue between the pedicle and the wise pattern are excised.
- Final closer is done.

Endoscopic Reduction Mammoplasty

Endoscopic reduction mammoplasty can be done
By periareolar incision.
By axillary incision.

PERIAREOLAR REDUCTION MAMMOPLASTY

- Marking is made in concentric circle around the nipple.
- A stab wound is made at the 6 o'clock position on the nipple, and using the long infiltration needle subcutaneous areas of the breasts are infiltrated in an area from the nipple to the sternal angle and from the nipple to the midaxillary area and upto the clavicle.
- Now sharp dissection is done subcutaneously until the upper pole of the breast is reached at which point the dissection is carried from the subcutaneous plane through the soft tissue to the fascia of the pectoralis muscle.
- The lateral quadrant of the upper hemisphere is picked up at the 12 o'clock point and advanced into or toward the sternal angle.
- With application of the full force the breast tissue is brought in the wound and the amount of the breast as determined is removed.
- If more breast tissue is to be excised, undermining of lower hemisphere is also done and desired amount of the breast is excised.
- Suture the new breast in 12 o' clock position of each upper quadrant to fascia / muscle above the second rib.

Axillary Endoscopic Reduction Mammoplasty

- Markings are made from 3-9 o'clock position on the breast and 2 cm above the chest wall, and then from 3 o'clock position to the sternal angle and from 9 o'clock position to the axilla.
- The stab wound is then made in the infra-areolar area in the 6 o'clock position and the subcutaneous tissue over the entire breasts is infiltrated.
- The incision is then made in axilla.
- Endoscope in inserted above the muscle and below the breast tissue.
- By sharp dissection the skin is dissected from breasts tissue over the area which has been marked.

Now two poles of breasts tissue are made in upper part and excision of breast tissue is done.

- Some tissue is removed from inferior segment also.
- Fat suctioning is done in lower part to remove further fat.

Reduction Mammoplasty by Open Incisions—Pedicle Operation

The usual reduction mammoplasty involves repositioning of the nipple areolar complex, reduction of larger areolar diameter, a partial resection of parenchyma, and contouring resection of excessive skin. There are various methods described for carrying out reduction mammoplasty.

Lateral Pedicle Reduction Mammoplasty (Author)

This was described with the aim to preserve nipple areola sensations as the nerve supply of the nipple and areola is from 4th intercostal nerve. This nerve is included in the pedicle.

Postoperative Care

- Suture lines are dressed with a grease impregnated gauze.
- Bulky absorbent dressings are placed over only the drain sites.
- The breasts are dressed with a wrap around dressing, providing support but not the compression.
- Within 4-6 hours surgeon should examine the patient. Hematoma and impending vascular complications should be apparent at the is point and treatment without fear of irreversible damage is possible at this time.
- Drain is removed after 48 hours.
- A well padded and fitting bra should be borne day and night for 6 weeks postoperatively.
- If hematoma is suspected it should be removed urgently otherwise there is every chance of loosing the nipple areola complex.

How to Manage Impending Vascular Complications?

- Initial treatment is directed at decompression of the breast by releasing the inframmary and vertical suture lines while retaining the general integrity of the breasts with adhesive tape and straps.

- If a responds of the treatment, breast is left in this state for several days until the resolution of edema will allow a delayed secondary closure, or until the defect is closed by skin grafting.
- On the other hand, areola fails to respond, the approach should be aborted and one should go for free nipple areolar graft.

Complications

Early

Early complications are Necrosis, hematoma, infection and wound dehiscence.

Late

Late complications are:

- Abnormal scarring, permanent sensory changes, loss of the shape, recurrent hypertrophy, and the interference with the capacity of lactation.
- Necrosis
- Nipple and areola.

Reconstruction of the breast after mastectomy

Indications

1. Localized cancers as in stage 1
2. Advanced cancers but if the patient has survived for more than three years.

Mastopexy

With aging, breasts droop. Reduction mammoplasty may not be required in every female but mastopexy is required in every female after 40 years of age or earlier. It is equivalent to drooping of perineal body with age resulting in vaginal relaxation. In a way we can say that breasts and perineal body droops with age and their reconstruction is required by every female.

Mastopexy means correcting the drooping of the breasts and give them the proptuberant shape. With age the breasts droop. However there may be following conditions.

1. Breasts are of large size and droop.
2. Breasts are of normal size and droop.
3. Breasts are of smaller size and droop.

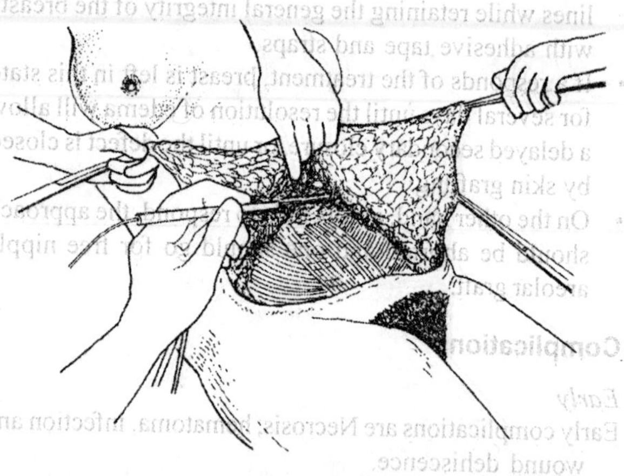

Fig. 21.6: Elevation of the panniculus utilizing electrocautery. Dissection is carried up to within a few centimeters of the umbilical stalk

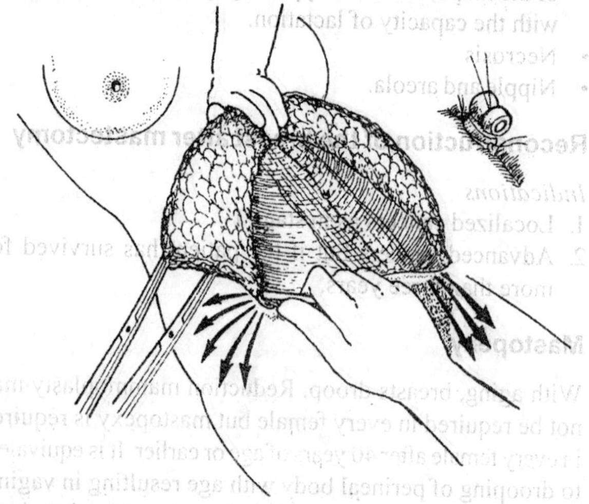

Fig. 21.7: Complete plication with the final layer closed using a running catgut suture: No. 0 general closure. Aspiration of the flank, hip and medial thigh areas is also demonstrated. (Inset) Umbilical stalk is shortened when necessary

Breasts of larger size and drooping require reduction mammoplasty either by open technique or endoscopic surgery.

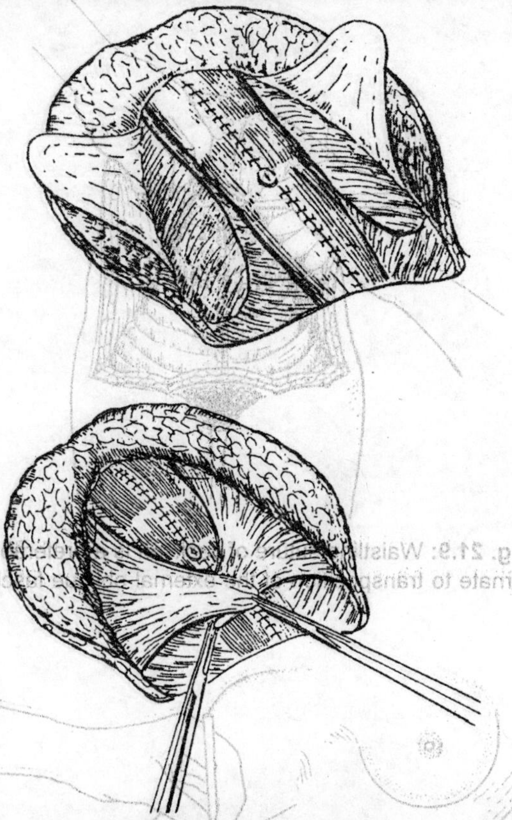

Fig. 21.8: Alternate technique of plication described by Psillakis, which we believe is needed only for extreme forms of lower abdominal deformity

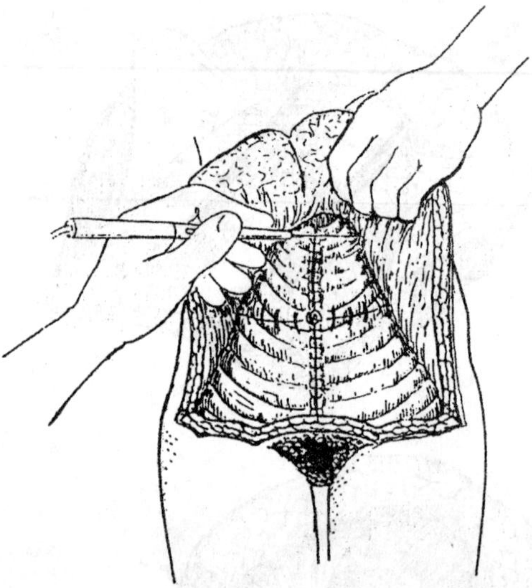

Fig. 21.9: Waistline suture of Jackson is a preferable alternate to transposition of the external oblique fascia

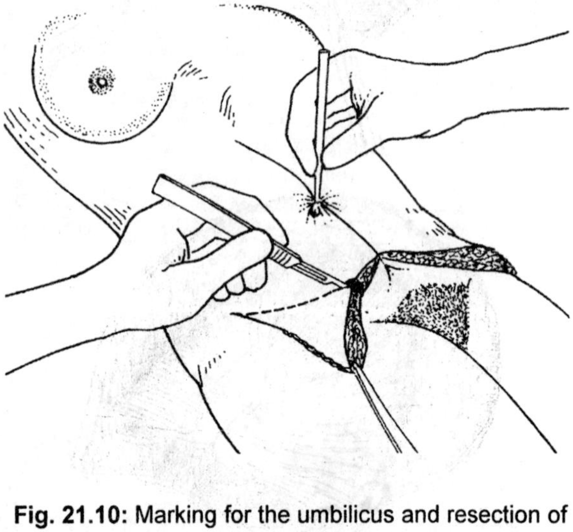

Fig. 21.10: Marking for the umbilicus and resection of excess tissue at the incision line

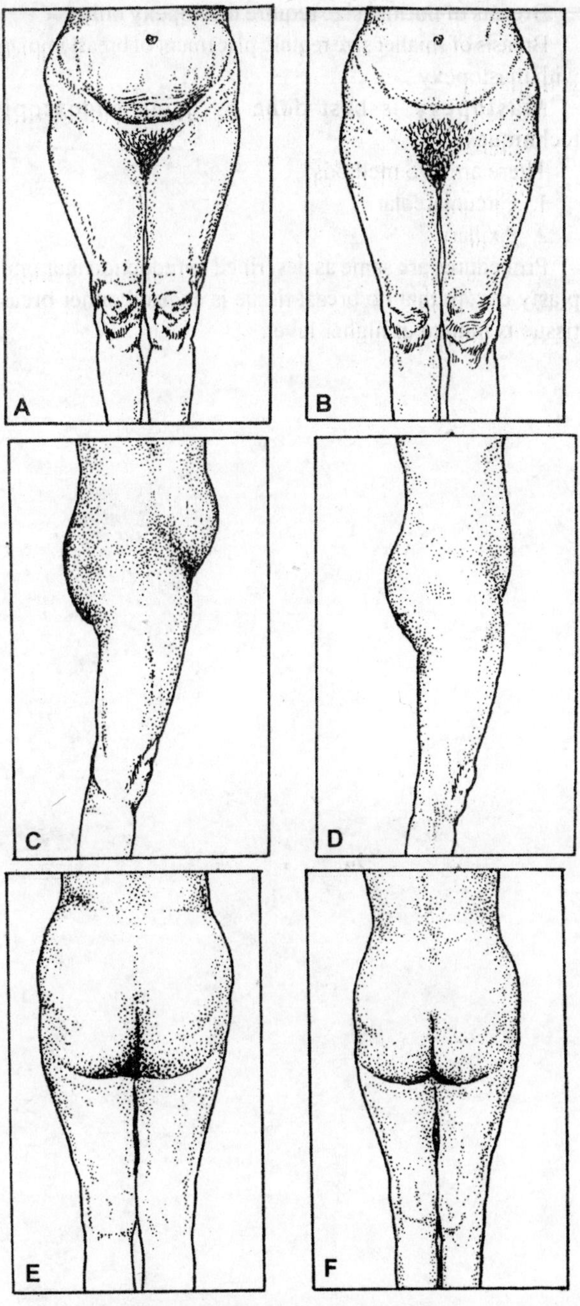

Fig. 21.11: Preoperative A C E
Postoperative B D F. Full abdominoplasty

Breasts of normal size require mastopexy only.

Breasts of smaller size require placement of breast implant with mastopexy.

Mastopexy is best done by using endoscopic techniques.

There are two methods:

1. Circumareolar
2. Axillary

Procedures are same as described in reduction mammoplasty except that no breast tissue is excised rather breast tissue is hinged at higher level.

22

Transplantation of Ovary

Recent advances in management of malignancy has changed the morbidity of the females after treatment of gynecological cancers. In most of cases irradiation is used for management of malignancy which results in premature menopause. Different treatments have been advised to protect the ovaries, including transplantation of cortical strips to the forearm.

Author has done experimental studies in animals in which he found that ovary along with the vascular pedicle can be transplanted in the forearm or abdomen using the principles of microsurgery which gives the best result.

Same principle can also be used while treating ovarian benign diseases.

Technique

- Ovary along with the vascular pedicle is dissected and taken out of abdomen.
- The recipient artery and vein are prepared over the forearm, which are radial artery and any superficial vein; or on the abdomen which are epigastric artery and vein.
- Microsurgical anastomosis is done and patient kept on anticoagulation for five days.
- As it is revascularized ovarian transfer, hormonal production is good and premature menopause is averted.

Index

ECG shows tall peaked symmetrical T waves, tent like shape with narrow base. There is lengthening of PR internal and QRS waves with decrease in R wave and decrease in height of P waves while—wave increases in depth.

Drugs Likely to Cause Hyperkalemia

Amloride, Arginine, Antineoplastic agents, Beta adrenoreceptor blockers glucose, indomethacin, potassium salts, spironolactone, suxamethonium and triamterene.

Hypokalemia is associated with clinical features such as tiredness, muscular weakness, that may result in disability in walking or climbing stairs. Neurological functions remain normal but tingling in fingers, apathy, paralips and coma may be present in extreme cases.

Long lasting hypokalemia damages renal tubular structures and results in a failure of antidiuretic response to vasopressin. These patients may present with polyurea and polydipsia.

Drugs Causing Hypokalaemia

Amphotercein B, Cardiac Glycosides Carbenoxolone, Sodium, Cadmium, Mercury, Uranium, Bismuth, Dexamethasone, Ethacrynic acid, Frusemide, Licorice, Lithium, Mercaptopurine, Neomycin, Salbutamol, Streptomycin, Sulphonamides, Triamcinolone, Tetracyclines and Vitamin D.

Serum K^+ levels must be done as symptoms of hyper as well as hypokalaemia are similar in nature.

HYPERGLYCEMIA

Drugs/Toxins Producing Hyperglycemia

Acetone, adrenalin, cadmium chloride, caffeine, clonidine, iron salts, methyl alcohol, nalidixic acid, nifedipine, phenylbutazone, phenylpropranolamine, salicylates (chronic), terbutaline, theophylline, water hemlock and few leaves.

Management

Drug induced hyperglycemia does not need active treatment as in most of the cases withdrawal of drug is sufficient to correct this problem.

RENAL TOXICITY

Poisons Causing Oliguria

Barbiturates, carbolic acid, canthridin, ethylene glycol, oxilic acid, petroleum products, salicylates and hilphonamides.

Hypernatremia indicates lack of water and hyponatremia—an excess of water in plasma.

Clinical signs associated with hypo or hypernatraemia are rare.

Hypernatreaemia is associated with thirst, mild confusion and/or disorientation severe water depletion may lead to coma and marked muscle weakness, postural hypotension, tachycardia and low jugular venous pressure.

Hyponatraemia is associated with confusional state lassitude and sleepiness that progresses to gross confusion, myoclonic jerks and generalised seizures.

Serious clinical signs occur if plasma sodium changes abruptly or if it falls below 110 mmol/L amounting to medical emergency as mortality may be as high as 40% in such patients.

Poisons Causing Volume Depletion and Hyponatraemia

Ammonium polystyrens sulfonate, acetohexamide aminoglutethemide, chlorthiazide, chlorpropamide, Demeclocyline, Ethacrynic acid frusemide. Tolazamide, glibonelamide and Lithium carbonate.

Poisons Causing Volume Excess With Hypernatraemia

Antacids (Na/K), ammonium chloride, Acetazolamide, Amitryptaline, cholestyrcemine, Carbonoxolone sodium, Chlorpromazine, Diazoxide, Dextrose, Glucocorticoids, Lequorice derwativer, mineralocortrcoids, MAO I, oxyphenbutazone, Oestrogen, Progesterone, Phenylbistazone, Sodium salts of drugs, Testosterone.

Conditions Causing Anion Gap Acidosis

Diabetic Ketoacidosis.
Renal failure.
Shock induced lactic acidosis.
Aspirin.
Methanol.

Ethyline glycol.
Isoniazid and iron.
Lactic acidosis is produced by convulsions, iron, phenformin and hypoxia.

ACID-BASE IMBALANCE

Metabolic Acidosis

Acidosis is associated with pH below 7.35.

Anion gap-($Na^+ + K^+$) – ($HCO_3^- + Cl^-$) in mEq/L
= 140 – 128 = 12 mEq/L in normal state is increased in acidosis.

Following drugs/poisons can produce acidosis.

Ammonium chloride, amiloride, anticholinesterases (neostigmine, physostigmine), barbiturates, corticosteroids, cholestyramine, chloral hydrate, ethylalcohol, Fentanyl, glutethimide, high calorie glucose nitrogen solution for neonates, I/V fructose, metformin, INH, morphine, gallamine, nitrous oxide, nalorphine, neomycin, potassium chloride, LSD, povidone, phenformin, pethidine, ritodrine, salbutamol, salicylates, sodium nitroprusside, spironolactone, strychnine and triamterene.

Anion gap is also increased by poisons that cause hypoalbuminemia, hypernatremia, hypo or hyperkalemia and hypercalcemia etc.

Management

Give sodium bicarbonate I/V at a dose of 1-2 mEq/L over 15 to 30 minutes. This dose can be repeated if required. Monitor serum Ca^{++} as hypocalcemia may develop.

Correction of acidemia helps in correcting hypotension and stopping seizures.
Disturbances in acid-base balance cause mild CNS disturbances and abnormalities of respiration.

Acidosis results in marked decline in conscious level along with confusion and irritability Kussmanl's respiration (slow, deep and sighing breathing) is classic sign of acidosis.

Following Drugs are likely to Cause Acidosis

Ammonium chloride, Arginine hydrochloride, Amiloride, Neostigmine, Physostgmine and other anticholinesterases, Barbiturates, Corticosteroids, Cholestyramine, Chloral hydrate, Iodine, Dechlorphenamide, Dimorphin, Ethanol, Fentanyl, Glycine Glutethemide, High caloric, Glucose Nitrogen solution in neonates, I/V fructose,

Metformin, Morphine, Methadone, Muscle relaxants (Gallamine), Nitrous oxide, Nalorphine, Neomycine, Potassium chloride, Povidone, Iodine (topical) Phenformin, Pethidine, Polymixin, Ritodrine, Salbutamol, Salieylic acid, Sodium nitroprusside, Streptomycin, Spironolactone, Synthetic amino acids in neonates and Triamterine.

Alkalosis is accompanied by depression of consciousness, and hypoventilation. Tetany may be present because of a low ionised calcium.

COMPLICATIONS OF POISONING

1. Hepatotoxic Agents

Many therapeutic drugs cause liver damage. In addition liver toxicity is also produced by chemicals and substances in the environment.

Paracetamol, isoniazid, iproniazid and halothane are prominent hepatotoxic agents. Genetic difference in drug metabolism have been implicated in hepatotoxicity due to isoniazid and phenytoin. Chronic use of low dose methotrexate in psoriasis results in hepatotoxicity. Chlorpromazine and androgens cause reversible toxicity.

Paracetamol is a frequent cause of death specially in individuals with induced P_{450} enzymes e.g. alcoholics, smokers, patients on rifampicin or roal contraceptives. Acetylcystein and methiomine increase GSH availability and reduce mortality in patients with severe paracetamol poisoning.

Liver damage can be produced through immunological meçhanisms e.g. halothane.

Hepatotoxic agents:

Alcohol, Isoniazid
Aminoglycoside
Anabolic steroids
Arsenic
Carbon tetrachloride
Iron
Phenothiazines
Halogenated compounds
Methyldopa
Erythromycin
Penicillin
Methyldopa
Chloroform
Paracetamol

Paraquat
Phosphorus
Naphthelene
Oral contraceptives
Sulfonamides
Indomethacin
Phenylbutazone
Tetracyclines in pregnancy.

2. Renal Failure

Paraquat, salicylate and carbon tetrachloride cause renal tubular necrosis. This coupled with hypotension and hypoxia can result in acute renal failure.

Massive destruction of skeletal muscles leads to myoglobin urea that can result in acute renal failure.

Nephrotoxic Agents

Aminoglycosides—Streptomycin, Kanamycin, Neomycin etc. Carbolic acid, EDTA, Penicillamine, Heavy metals, Methyl alcohol, Oxalic acid, Phenacetin and chronic use of Salicylates and other non-steroidal anti-inflammatory drugs.

3. Poisonous Substances Causing Rhabdomyolysis

Barbiturates, Carbon monoxide, Cocaine, Diphenhydramine, Doxepin, Heroin, Isoniazid, Isopropranolol, Methadone, Nitrazepam, Opioid analgesics (opium, morphine, codeine etc.), Oxprenolol, Paracetamol, Paraphenylene diamine pemoline, Phencyclidine, Phenelzine, Protriptyline, Pseudoephedrine, Salicylates, Strychnine, Terabutaline, Theophylline and Toluene.

Heroin reduces effective renal plasma flow and glomerular filtration rate.

Oliguria (urine volume < 500 ml/day) indicates renal failure but urinary retention must be ruled out. Therefore it is essential to maintain input-output charts in all cases of poisoning. Along with volume of urine, serum electrolytes also need constant monitoring.

POISONS WITH CHARACTERISTIC ODOUR

Smell of bitter almonds is due to cyanides while fruity smell is given by ethyl alcohol.

Smell of rotton eggs is indicative of poisoning due to hydrogen sulfide/disulfiran.

Smell of burnt rope indicates marijuana.

Smell resembling shoe polish is likely to be due to benzene.

Acrid smell is given out by patients suffering poisoning due to paraldehyde and chloral hydrate.

Garlic odour is peculiar to phosphorus, organophosphates (insecticides), arsenic, thallium etc.

Fishy or musty smell is likely to be associated with zinc phosphide.

Odours around mouth and nostrils help in reaching diagnosis, Certain drugs/agents are excreted in breath leading to characteristic odour.

Fruity smell is given by ethyl alcohol.

LIST OF RADIOOPAQUE POISONS

Arsenic.
Chloral hydrate.
Heavy metals.
Iodides.
Phenothiazines.
Enteric coated tablets.

LIST OF DRUGS IMPARTING COLOUR TO URINE

Drug	*Urine colour*
Amitriptyline, phenol, methylene blue	Green or blue
Vitamin B complex	Yellow
Quinacrine, Rifampicin, Desferroxamine, Phenytoin and Phenothiazines	Red

Brown coloured urine is produced by phenacetin, quinine, methyl dopa, metronidazole and salicylates.

Poisons Producing Metallic Taste

Heavy metals such as arsenic, lead, mercury.
Acetaldehyde.
Disulfiram.
Metoclopramide.
Metronidozole.
Tinidazole.

POISONS PRODUCING CHANGES IN NAIL

Pigmentation of nail on ingestion.

Azathioprine (pink colour).

Lithium, Tetracycline, Quinacrine—all produce yellow colour.

Methotrexate (Brown).

Phenothiazine (Grey).

Staining on contact

Copper sulfate (Blue).

Fluorescein Nitric acid (Yellow).

Formaldehyde (Gray).

Silver Nitrate (Black).

Softening and loosening of nails

5-fluorouracil

Gold, Phenothiazines, Tetracyclines and Thiazides.

Two

PROCEDURES FOR REMOVAL OF POISONS FROM THE BODY

EMESIS

Emesis should not be used in patients with compromised airway or where hydrocarbons such as petrol have been ingested. Emesis should also be avoided in poisoning due to ingestion of corrosives (strong acids and alkalies).

It is also of not much help if delayed. Mechanical induction of vomiting is unsatisfactory. **Salt water, apomorphine detergents and copper sulfate are found unsuitable** Ipecacuanha (Ipecac) is the most useful agent for this purpose.

Ipecac syrup (30 ml for adults and 15 ml for children) is given orally in 250 ml of water and can be repeated once after 15 min.

(Ipecac fluid extract should be avoided as it contains high concentration of emetine-the cardiotoxic alkaloid).

Salient Points

1. Ipecac is effective even when antiemetic medications have been taken in overdose.
2. Ipecac should not be used if patient has consumed an agent which is likely to produce convulsions (e.g. tricyclic antidepressants) as vomitus can be aspirated.
3. Apomorphine is more toxic than ipecac—especially in children.

ACTIVATED CHARCOAL

It is formed by heating coconut shell, peat and wood in an anaerobic environment till carbon is formed. This carbon is then activated by exposing it to steam at high temperatures. This leads to increase in its adsorption capacity of poisons.

It is most effective if given early in poisoning.

Poisons Absorbed by Activated Charcoal

Barbiturates, Benzodiazepines, Carbamazepine, Chloroquine, Dapsone, Digoxin, Digitoxin, Paracetamol, Paraquat, Phenytoin, Quinine, Salicylates and Theophylline.

Poisons not Removed by Activated Charcoal

Acids (hydrochloric, sulphuric and nitric acid), **alkalies** (Sodium, hydroxide and sodium bicarbonate), **Cyanide, Ethanol** (alcohol), Ethylene **glycol**, Iron preparations, **Lithium salts, Methyl alcohol and Petroleum distillates.**

Disadvantages

Patient compliance is poor and produces adverse reactions like vomiting.

Preparations

The required dose of activated charcoal is mixed with water and administered with sorbitol if required. Addition of sorbitol may cause diarrhoea that may further facilitate removal of toxins.

Repeated charcoal administration is sometimes required but the second dose should not contain purgative (sorbitol).

Adverse Reactions

1. Vomiting.
2. Is fatal if aspirated.
3. Blocks action of ipecac.
4. Repeated administration produces diarrhea.
   Systemic toxicity does not occur as it is not absorbed.

Dose: Initial dose 1 gm/kg body weight.
Or
10 times the quantity of poison ingested.

Sorbitol: Adult dose—50 ml of 70% solution.
Children—4.3 ml/kg of 35% solution.

Repeat Dose Activated Charcoal

Activated charcoal can be administered at 2 hrly or 4 hrly intervals for duration of toxicity. This helps in reducing half life of poisons and is **most useful in cases of drugs that undergo enterohepatic circulation.** The repeated doses help in keeping zero level of the poison in the gut that helps mobility of poison from blood to intestinal lumen where it gets bound to charcoal. **It is often referred to as gut dialysis. Drugs of acidic nature are easily removed by this method.**

First dose should be 1 gm/kg followed by half the dose at 2-4 hrly intervals till signs of toxicity disappear or patient cannot tolerate further administration.

Repeated doses of Charcoal is Required in Poisonings due to following:

Salicylates	Barbiturates	Nadolol
Carbamazepine	Phenytoin	
Dapsone	Quinine	
Digoxin	Theophylline	

PURGATIVES

Elimination of the unabsorbed portion of the poison is helped in the initial stages by induction of emesis and gastric lavage but in late stage (2 hours after ingestion) activated charcoal and purgatives are given for this purpose.

Saline laxatives such as **magnesium sulfate, magnesium hydroxide, magnesium citrate sodium phosphate and sodium potassium tartrate** are used to treat oral drug poisoning.

However, sorbitol and mannitol (non saline purgatives) are preferred.

Saturated solutions of these agents have high osmotic pressure that prevents absorption of water from gut and also draws water from gut wall leading to increased volume of intestinal contents with resultant increase in motility and evacuation of bowel.

Preparations and Doses

Saturated solution of magnesium sulfate containing seven molecules of water of crystallization is mixed with 45 ml of water to produce 60 ml.

30 ml of this solution is administered orally in poisoning cases.

20 ml of milk of magnesia (7-8.5% aqueous solution of magnesium hydroxide) can also be given.

Adverse effects: Dehydration and electrolyte imbalance can be produced. Hypermagnesemia can develop in patients of renal failure. **Magnesium salts should be avoided if patient is suffering from renal failure.**

Phosphate salts should be avoided as these can cause hyperphosphataemia and reduction in serum Ca^{++}.

Non saline osmotic purgatives such as **sorbitol, glycerine, lactulose and mannitol** are not absorbed and are devoid of systemic toxicity. These are preferred in treating poisoning.

Doses of Purgatives

Magnesium citrate	4 ml/kg
Magnesium sulfate (Epsom salt)	30 gm adult 250 mg child
Sodium sulfate (Glauber's salt)	30 gms adult 250 mg child
Sorbitol	1-2 gm/kg in adults **not to be given to children.**

Purgatives are contraindicated in following conditions:

1. Poisoning due to corrosive agents.
2. In presence of diarrhea.
3. Abdominal injury.
4. History of intestinal obstruction.
5. Renal failure.

GASTRIC LAVAGE

Stomach can be emptied by passing gastric lavage tube. However complete evacuation of stomach is not achieved. This procedure is indicated:

1. In unconsions patients.
2. In adults who are co-operative.
3. If vomiting does not occur after 2 doses of ipecac.

Method

Individual is kept in left lateral position with head hanging over edge of the table and face down. A single large lumen tube with multiple distal ports is necessary. A mouth gag is placed before the procedure. Catheter is passed gently to make sure that it is not in the airway.

300 ml of tap water is generally used for lavage and four or five coats are done. After fluid is instilled, it should be removed by gravity drainage or tube suction.

Catheter is pinched before it is finally withdrawn or suction is maintained during withdrawal to prevent aspiration.

Gastric lavage is contraindicated in the following.

a. If cough reflex is absent.
b. Poisoning due to corrosive agents.
c. In kerosene poisoning.
d. 2 hours after ingestion except in cases of morphine and anticholinergic agents.

In patients who are comatosed or in whom gag reflex is absent procedure can be performed after inserting endotracheal tube.

In few corrosive poisonings e.g. paraquat, danger of systemic toxicity is high therefore continuous lavage may be considered.

WHOLE BOWEL IRRIGATION

This procedure helps in evacuating the bowel rapidly and therefore is recommended for treatment of poisoning with highly toxic agents, sustained release formulations of drugs and for poisons that are not adsorbed by activated charcoal. It is also effective in cases who present late after ingestion of poison when gastric lavage is not likely to be helpful.

Patient is made to sit on a commode and a nasogastric tube is passed. Fluid is instilled through tube into stomach (in unconscious patient) or consious patient is asked to drink large volumes of fluid. Watery diarrhea develops—initially with fecal matter and 4-6 hours later without the fecal matter. **Saline is not used for this procedure** as it leads to fluid accumulation and hypokalemia. **Polyethylene glycol lavage solution with electrolytes is used.** It is instilled at the rate of 2 lt/hr in adults and 0.5 lt/hr in children.

This procedure is well tolerated even during pregnancy and childhood.

DIURETICS

Forced diuresis is often used in management of poisoning. Increasing urinary output helps in:

a. Promoting excretion of the absorbed portion of poison e.g. barbiturates.
b. Poison gets diluted in the tubule and danger from renotoxic (tubular toxic) substances is reduced.

FRUSEMIDE

It is high efficacy loop diuretic. It remains effective even at glomerular filtration rates below 10 ml/min (normal 120 ml/min). It is well absorbed when given orally. Half life is 2 hours but this rises to 10 hours in renal failure. On oral administration effect starts within one hour and diuresis lasts about 6 hours. On I/V administration effect is seen within 30 minutes.

Increase in dose matches increase in urine production.

Over treatment can result in hypovolaemia and circulatory collapse.

Dose: 20-120 mg orally/day.
20-50 mg I/M or I/V/day.

In renal failure 500 mg orally or 250 mg in 25 ml to be infused I/V at a rate not greater than 4 mg/min.

It is used to promote excretion of absorbed portion of the poison e.g. barbiturates, amphetamine etc.

Disadvantages

1. Can cause hypokalemia and hyperuricemia.
2. Indomethacin and other NSAIDs reduce its efficacy.
3. Can produce hyponatremia specially in patients who continue to take water orally. Discontinuation of diuretic and water intake corrects this imbalance.

Ethacrynic acid is not preferred as it is more prone to cause nausea and vomiting.

Mannitol

It is an osmotic diuretic, urine volume increases according to the load of osmotic diuretic. It increases volume of extracellular compartment and is not preferred in patients of congestive cardiac failure. It increases glomerular filtration rate and inhibits renin release. In addition it promotes renal blood flow. It is primarily used to maintain glomerular filtration rate and urine flow in patients with impending acute renal failure. However, **it is contraindicated if renal failure has already set in.** It is used to increase elimination of hypnotic or other poisons.

Mannitol is used to counteract low osmolality of plasma after rapid haemodialysis or peritoneal dialysis.

It is not to be used if patient has acute tubular necrosis, anuria, pulmonary oedema, cerebral haemorrhage and congestive cardiac failure.

Acidification of urine increases elimination of weak bases and reduces that of weak acids.

Ammonium Chloride acidifies urine and helps excretion of amphetamines.

Urinary alkalisation has opposite effects and bicarbonate and acetazolamide increase urinary pH and hence increase excretion of salicylates and barbiturates.

HAEMODIALYSIS

It is highly effective method for removing poisons that have small molecules (molecular weight < 350 DA) as these cross semipermeable membrane easily.

Maximum efficacy is obtained if:

a. Plasma concentration of poisons is high as in cases of **salicylates, phenobarbitone, ethylene glycol, methyl alcohol, lithium and potassium.**
b. Poison is **not** tightly bound to plasma or tissue proteins.
c. Poison is water soluble and less lipid soluble.
d. Volume of distribution of poison is small.

List of Drugs that are not Removed by Dialysis

Amphetamines, Cocaine, Benzodiazepines (Chlordiazepoxida, Diazepam, Nitrazepam, Flurazepam etc.), Chlorpromazine, Haloperidol and other antipsychotic agents, Digoxin, Glutethemide, Narcotics (morphine, heroin, codeine, etc.), Quinidine, Procainamide and Tricyclic antidepressants.

Advantages

It assists correction of fluid and electrolytes and enhances removal of poison and its metabolites e.g. formate in methanol toxicity.

Disadvantages

Complications are likely.

HAEMOPERFUSION

Arterial blood (from radial artery) is allowed to percolate through granules of activated charcoal primed with saline and then returned to patient via appropriate vein.

This technique is highly effecacious in removing **barbiturates, glutethemide, methaqualone, ethchlorvynol and meprobamates. It is not effective against tricyclic antidepressants.** It is highly effective in removing drugs with low clearance, having small volume of distribution and extensive plasma protein binding.

Haemoperfusion is indicated:

a. If poisoning is clinically servere e.g. **grade 4 coma, hypothermia, hypotension and respiratory depression or levels of the poison in blood are high.**
b. If patient's condition is worsening in spite of adequate supportive care.
c. If serious complications are present e.g. hepatic and renal insufficiency or extensive pneumonia in an unconscious patient.

Peritoneal Dialysis

It is 20% as efficacious as haemodialysis but is not a popular modality.

PLASMA EXCHANGE AND EXCHANGE TRANSFUSION

For **protein bound drugs and paraquat poisoning** this method is highly efficacious. This method is also recommended for removal of drugs that cause severe methemoglobinemia.

RESINS USED IN THERAPEUTICS

High molecular weight polymers that are insoluble in water are used as ion exchange resins. Given orally they are not affected by digestive enzymes nor absorbed into systemic circulation. These agents function by binding ions which diffuse freely or are secreted into the gut lumen.

Cationic-Exchange Resins

Sodium cellulose phosphate is given orally to reduce calcuim absorption in patients suffering from **idiopathic hypercalcemia or iotrogenic hypercalemia.**

Sodium Polystyrene Sulfonate or Calcium Polystyrene Sulfonate

These are administered orally or per rectally for management of **hyperkalemia.** The sodium and calcium changes with potassium in the gut lumen which is in equilibrium with plasma potassium.

In presence of cardiac failure calcium salt is preferred. **With all cationic exchange resins careful monitoring of serum electrolytes is essential to prevent hypokalemia, hypernatraemia or hypocalcaemia.**

Anion Exchange Resins

Extracorporeal haemoperfusion with anion-exchange resin columns has been used to treat severe barbiturate poisoning, but this procedure is no more used.

THREE

DETAILS OF DRUGS OFTEN USED IN TREATMENT OF POISONING

ANTIDOTES

FLUMEZENIL

It blocks benzodiazepine receptors and antagonises the effects of benzodiazepines. Given alone it does not produce appreciable effects on CNS.

Flumezenil can cause withdrawal syndrome in patients dependent on benzodiazepines.

Infusion of flumazenil causes reversal of consciousness within 5 minutes in patient with benzodiazepine poisoning.

It is well absorbed when given orally.

Its use is restricted to patients who are in deep coma.

ATROPINE

It is anticholinergic agent often used in poisoning associated with increased exocrine secretions (sweat, saliva, rhinorrhoea and bronchospasm).

It corrects symptoms associated with increased muscarinic but not nicotinic activity.

It is a specific antidote for **organophosphates, carbamates, physostgmine and pilocarpine.**

In addition it is highly useful in treating poisoning due to most mushrooms.

Dose: 2 mg/I.V. every 10-30 minutes till relief is obtained (absence of rales) or signs of atropinisation appear (tachycardia, dilated pupils and dry mouth). **Total dose depends on severity of symptoms and may be nearly 30 mg.**

In children: 0.02 mg/kg—0.05 mg/kg is the usual dose.

ETHYL ALCOHOL

Methyl alcohol and ethylene glycol are metabolised by the same enzyme-alcohol dehydrogenase—as ethyl alcohol. However, alcohol dehydrogenase has a much greater affinity for ethanol than the ethyleneglycol or methanol. In cases of methyl alcohol as well as ethylene glycol the symptomatology of toxicity is due to their respective metabolites. Thus use of ethyl alcohol in poisonings due to these agents slows the formation of respective metabolites.

Blood concentration of ethyl alcohol approximately 1 gm/L are optimal. It should be given as soon as possible. In early stages of poisoning ethanol can be given orally (if patient is consious and not vomiting) A loading dose of 0.6 g/kg is recommended followed by maintenance dose of 60-150 mg ethanol/kg/hr.

Ethanol can be given I/V-60 ml of absolute alcohol in 500 ml isotonic glucose in 30 min followed by 12 ml of absolute alcohol/hour.

Higher doses are recommended if patient has undergone haemodialysis or is chronic drinker.

VITAMIN K (Vitamin $K_1 + K_2 + K_3$)

A fat soluble vitamin also called coagulation vitamin.

These are of three types:

Vitamin K_1—phytomenadione is of plant origin.

Vitamin K_2—menaquinone is obtained from bacteria and is fat soluble

Vitamin K_3—is synthetically produced and has water soluble preparations e.g. menadione sodium bisulfite, menadione sodium diphosphate (Synakavite). Synthetic fat soluble preparations are—Menadione, Acetomenadione/acetomenaphthone (Kapilin).

Water soluble preparations are also available and can be absorbed even in absence of bile and can also be given parenterally.

Vitamin K preparations are used in bleeding states during salicylate or oral anticoagulant overdose.

Menadione sodium diphosphate injection—5-10 mg/ml can be given S/C, I/M or I/V.

Vitamin K tablet (10 mg) and injection (10 mg/ml)—10 mg orally or I/V.

On I/V injection vitamin K_1 may produce flushing cyanosis, breathlessness, hypotension and hypersensitivity reactions.

In large doses in neonates it can produce haemolytic anemia and jaundice.

SODIUM THIOSULFATE

It is an antidote for cyanide.

This helps in catabolizing cyanide to non toxic thiocyanate. As initial step sodium nitrite (10 ml of 3% solution) is given I/V over 3 minutes.

This generates methaemoglobin (Ferric iron), that competes with cyanide. After sodium nitrite, sodium thiosulfate (50 ml of 25% solution I/V over 10 min) should be given to eliminate cyanide by non-toxic thiocyanate formation. Oxygen administration greatly potentiaties protective effects of sodium nitrite/thiosulfate combination.

SODIUM BICARBONATE (An Alkali)

It is water soluble, acts immediately and has good neutralizing power and is capable of raising pH beyond 7.

It is often used to alkalinise urine with a view to promote acidic poisons such as barbiturates and salicylates.

It is also used to treat acidosis caused by salicylates and other poisons. It is also used to treat poisoning due to quinidine and tricyclic antidepressants.

Dose: 1-2 meq/kg I/V bolus reserves cardiotoxic effects (wide QRS, hypotension). **Avoid in congestive cardiac failures.**

GLUCAGON

It is a hormone released by pancreas. Unlike insulin it causes hyperglycemia and most actions are opposite to those of insulin.

Glucagon has **positive inotropic and chronotropic effects not blocked by beta blockers.**

It is drug of choice in treating overdose toxicity of beta blockers.

It is inactive if given orally. Half life is short.

0.5-1.0 mg is given either I/V or I/M.

It is also used to treat insulin induced hypoglycemia and cardiogenic shock.

PROTAMINE SULFATE (Heparin Antagonist)

It is commonly used heparin antagonist, has a low molecular weight and is obtained from sperms of certain fish. One mg of protamine sulfate neutralises anticoagulant effect of 80-100 units of heparin activity. If more than 30 minutes have elapsed after heparin injection only half the dose of protamine is required to neutralise it. It is used only in severe bleeding due to heparin.

Dose: 50 mg I/V slowly in 10 minutes. Maximum dose should not exceed 100 mg as it possesses anticoagulant activity.

Rapid injection can cause sudden fall in BP, bradycardia, dyspnea, flushing and feeling of warmth.

Toludine blue can be used if protamine is not available.

EPINEPHRINE (Anti Anaphylactic)

Epinephrine was used to raise blood pressure, but now it is administered to treat hypotension associated with allergic reactions. MAO inhibitors increase its hypertensive potential.

It is available as 1 ml ampoule (1 mg/ml or 1:1000) or as 10 ml ampoule (1.1 mg/ml or 1:10,000).

It is given intravenously over a period of 1-3 min. Dose can be repeated every 5 minutes during resuscitation.

As continuous I/V infusion, it is given in concentration of 4 mcg/ml in 5% dextrose or normal saline (1 mg/125 ml).

Miligrams of epinephrine to be added to 100 ml I/V solution = 0.6 × body weight in kg.

Administer epinephrine if in spite of adequate ventilation for over 30 seconds heart rate remains below 80/minute and hypotension persists.

NALOXONE

It is specific antagonist of opioids. It can antagonise all effects of all opioids **except those of buprenorphine.**

It causes pupillary dilatation, rise in respiratory rate and volume, reverses hypotension and returns consciousness in opioid poisoning. The response is specific and immediate. However **it does not produce hyperalgesia.**

In addition naloxone partly **antagonises respiratory depression produced** by non-opioids such as **alcohol** and **nitrous oxide.** It is inactive if given orally and therefore is given I/V. On I/V administration effect is seen in 2-3 minutes. Half life is short—1 hour in adults and 3 hours in children.

It is drug of choice for treatment of morphine or any other opioid poisoning and for reversing asphyxia in neonate born to a mother who is treated with opioid.

It is also given to diagnose opioid dependence as it precipitates withdrawal syndrome.

It increases BP in endotoxic or hypovolemic shock, stroke and spinal injury.

Naloxone usually reverses or partially reverses CNS toxicity of **ethanol, benzodrazepine and occassionally other drugs.**

Doses: Initial dose depends on severity of the poisoning 0.4 mg I/V reverses effects of therapeutic doses of opioids. Higher dose such as 1.2 mg I/V is required to be given in overdose toxicity.

If I/V administration is not feasible, naloxone can be instilled down an endotracheal tube or can be given intra-muscularly.

In patients with shock, naloxone can be given sublingually. Half life of naloxone being short, it needs to be repeated at frequent intervals, hence **I/V infusion is indicated. Dose of naloxone must be titrated for each case.** Reportedly 75 mg in 24 hours produces no ill effects.

***Adverse effects:* Pulmonary oedema and ventricular dysarrhythmias are reported but are rare.**

Naloxone administration in an addict precipitates withdrawal syndrome, that may be alarming, but short lived.

Failure to obtain response after adequate dose of naloxone necessitates review of diagnosis. Partial response or no response may also indicate presence of non opioid CNS depressant that may have been taken along with opioid. Patients who suffer brain damage due to severe hypoxia (late arrival of opioid patient) are not likely to respond to naloxone.

N-ACETYLCYSTEINE

It acts as glutathion precursor in early stages while after 24 hours it is advantageous because of its free radical scavanger activity. It provides nearly complete protection against liver damage by paracetamol **provided** it is **given within ten hours** of poisoning. Though it remains effective till 12 hours of poison administration, efficacy declines—late administration reduces morbidity.

It is well tolerated.

Dose: It is given I/V, 150 mg/kg of acetylcysteine in 200 ml of 5% dextrose is given over 15 minutes. This is followed by I/V infusion—50 mg/kg of acetylcysteine given over 4 hours.

Same amount of acetylcysteine (100 mg/kg in 1000 ml of 5% dextrose) is given slowly over the next 16 hours.

Alternatively acetylcysteine can be given orally: 140 mg/kg body weight followed by 17 doses of 70 mg/kg every 4 hours.

Adverse effects: About 15% of patients reportedly suffer ADRs. Anaphylactoid reaction is possible in the first hour.

Nausea, flushing, urticaria, and pruritus are among the most common adverse reactions encountered.

Angio edema, wheezing, respiratory distress, hypotension or hypertension may also occur but are rare. Skin reactions are limited to infusion site.

Most reactions are reversible and stopping drip stops symptoms. Infusion can be safely restarted but at a slower rate. Antihistamines may be given but steroids are usually not required.

METHIONINE

Like acetylcysteine this too protects liver against hepatotoxic agents such as paracetamol.

It is less expensive than acetylcysteine and can be given orally. However in patients of paracetamol poisoning who suffer from vomiting it cannot be given. Its easy availability makes it more useful in areas where acetylcysteine is not available.

CHELATORS

Dimercaprol

Also called British Anti-Lewisite and is in use since World War II to ensure protection against poisoning by arsenic. **It forms complexes with arsenic, mercury and cadmium which are non toxic and easily excretable. The complex formed however is easily dissociable. To overcome this**

dosage of dimercaprol is so adjusted as to provide a little excess of BAL.

Limitations

1. It fails to reactivate sulfhydryl enzymes if given late or when the metal is in excess.
2. It is capable of inhibiting peroxidases, catalase and carbonic anhydrase.
3. It has to be given parenterally. It is completely metabolised in 24 hours.

Doses: Ampoule of 2 ml is available and contains 50 mg/ml. It has characteristic odour. In severe poisoning due to arsenic and gold dose is 3 mg/kg given as deep I/M injection every 4 hours for first 2 days and subsequently every 6 hours on third day. This is followed by maintenance dose given twice daily for the next 10 days or till recovery is complete.

In case of eye **exposure to arsenicals,** oily solution of dimercaprol is instilled into conjunctival sac.

In case of **mercury poisoning** dimercaprol is given initially in the dose of 5 mg/kg followed by 2.5 mg/kg given 4-6 hourly till recovery.

BAL is also given to treat **copper toxicity**—including Wilson's disease in patients allergic to penicullimine. 2.5 mg/kg I/M twice daily for first two days followed by rest for next two days and repeat above dose.

D-Penicillamine

This drug forms **water soluble complex with copper, mercury and lead that are excreted in urine.** It is well absorbed when given orally and is rapidly excreted in urine. It is used to treat Wilson's disease, and is useful agent for treatment of **copper, lead and mercury toxicites.** In addition it is often used to treat rheumatoid arthritis, cystinosis, cystinuria and hemosiderosis. It is also found useful in treatment of primary biliary cirrhosis and scleroderma.

Dose: 1-2 gm base in divided doses given before meals. Dose may be increased to 4-5 gms/day and continued indefinitely for treating chronic disorders (Wilson's disease).

Clinical improvement depends upon the degree of structural damage.

Adverse effects commonly encountered are headache, nausea, lymphadenopathy, loss of sense of taste, leukopenia-thrombocytopenia and aplastic anemia. Can produce allergic reactions in patients sensitive to penicillins. **Chronic administration can produce renal damage.**

Acetyl d-penicillamine

It is less effective as well as less toxic in treating **copper** and **lead** toxicity but is more useful in managing **mercury** poisoning.

Dose: 1 gm daily in 3 or 4 divided doses for a period of 10 days can be repeated after an interval of 7 days.

Disodium Calcium Edetate and Disodium Edetate

Calcium sodium EDTA has high affinity for calcium and less affinity for Na^{+}, Mg^{++} and K^{+}. **It is employed to treat lead toxicity.** It can be given I/V or I/M but not orally.

In acute lead poisoning 40 mg/kg disodium calcium EDTA is given I/V twice daily as 0.5-3.0% solution in saline or in 5% dextrose for 5 days.

After rest of 2 days the same dose schedule can be repeated. **Smaller doses are recommended in patients with encephalopathy or with increased intracranial pressure.**

Pediatric doses: 55 mg/kg divided into two portions and given by I/V infusion.

This can also be used as diagnostic tool for detecting lead poisoning. 75 mg/kg in 3 divided doses is given as 20% solution I/M with 1.5% procaine. If excretion of lead exceeds 500 µg per 24 hours, acute lead toxicity exists.

It is also used to treat iron, cadmium and plutonium toxicities.

DITHIOCARB

It is found useful in treating poisoning due to nickel carbonyl and thallium. 200 mg I/V is followed by 2 gm/day for 7 days.

Visual disturbances produced by this drug limits its use.

DEFERIPRONE

It is orally active iron chelator used to treat iron overload in toxicity as well as diseases connected with iron overload (transfusion siderosis and thalassemia).

Chelate formed with iron is excreted in urine.

Availability—Deferiprone capsules are available (250 and 500 mg).

Dose is 50-100 mg/kg/day in 2-4 divided doses.

Triathylene Tetramine (Trientine/cuprid)

This agent chelates copper and reverses neurological changes in Wilson's disease. It can safely be used to treat copper toxicity.

Dose 400-800 mg three times a day on empty stomach. It is less toxic than penicillamine but may cause iron deficiency that can be treated by a short term administration of iron.

DOPAMINE

It is naturally occurring precursor of norepinephrine. In low doses (2-5 μg/kg/min) it stimulates dopaminergic receptors (D_1) resulting in dilatation of blood vessels in kidneys, mesentry and in brain.

5-10 μg/kg/min dopamine not only stimulates dopamenergic receptor but also stimulates β_2 receptors. This range of dose increases blood supply to kidneys, brain and in the mesenteric region. In addition it produces increase in myocardial contractility resulting in increase in cardiac output. Heart rate is only marginally increased. Peripheral resistance is either reduced or remains unchanged.

10-20 μg/kg/min produces increase in myocardial contractility and heart rate. **Arrhythmias are likely to develop in patients with history of organochlorines and halogenated drugs.**

Doses over 20 μg/kg/min stimulate alpha receptors resulting in severe vasoconstriction, decrease in renal blood flow and urinary output. This dose produces effects like norepinephrine and is not preffered.

Desirable concentration—2-10 μg/kg/min.

PLASMA EXPANDERS

These agents exert oncotic pressure and when given intravenously retain fluid and expand vascular compartment.

Human plasma is desirable and effective but is likely to transmit serum hepatitis, AIDS, malaria etc.

Substances clinically used are synthetic in nature.

Dextran, Hydroxyethylstarch (HES), Polyvinyl pyrrolidone (PVP) and degraded gelatin polymers.

Gelatin products such as **Haemacel, Gelofusine** have plasma half life of 5 hours.

Dextran

Dextran-70 is commonly used. Effect lasts for 24 hours.

Disadvantages

1. Interferes with blood grouping and cross-matching.
2. It reacts with polysaccharide reacting antibodies resulting in allergic manifestations such as **urticaria, itching, bronchospasm and fall in BP.**

Dextran 40 (Molecular weight 40,000)

Also called low molecular weight dextran.

Advantages

It reduces viscosity of blood and prevents sludging of RBCs. In addition causes improvement in microcirculation.

Disadvantages

1. Duration of action is short.
2. Gets deposited in renal tubules if there is oliguria. Total dose should not exceed 20 ml/kg/day.

Hydroxyethyl Starch (HES : Hetastarch)

It is a mixture of amylopectins of differing molecular sizes. 6% hetastarch has properties similar to human albumin. Half life is 17 days.

This may cause vomiting, mild fever, itching and flu like symptoms.

Disadvantages

It increases ESR.

Polyvinylpyrrolidone (PVP)

It is used as 3.5% solution.

Disadvantages

It interferes with blood grouping and cross matching and also releases histamine.

Management of Hypotension

1. Supine positioning with elevation of foot end of the bed raises blood pressure and should be employed as first-aid method. This technique is most useful in hypotension caused by vasodilators.
2. Correction of hypoxia may abolish hypotension.

3. Correction of acidemia (if present) helps correcting hypotension.
4. I/V fluids are necessary in patients of dehydration and hypovolumia.
5. Vasopressors such as dopamine, norepinephrine are recommended if the above fail.

MANAGEMENT OF HYPERTENSION

Labetolol and sodium nitroprusside.

LABETALOL

It is non selective beta-blocker with selective alpha, blocking action.

Given orally, labetalol reduces heart rate and myocardial contractility, slows AV conduction, decreases peripheral resistance and lowers blood pressure. Half life is 5-8 hours.

Adverse reaction: It causes GI disturbances, dryness of mouth and fluid retention and can precipitate congestive cardiac failure. Sexual dysfunctions appear.

Dose: 20-80 mg I/V bolus every 10 minutes to a maximum total dose of 300 mg or 0.5-2 mg/min till BP normalises. Intermittent I/V bolus doses are preferred to I/V infusion.

SODIUM NITROPRUSSIDE

It has immediate onset of action and is consistently effective. It can cause precipitous fall in BP. Therefore infusion rate has to be closely monitored along with BP.

It is drug of choice in patients with myocardial infarction or pulmonary edema.

0.25-10.0 mcg/kg/min I/V. Effect lasts for 1-2 minutes only.

NIFEDIPINE

Can be given sublingually and tablet thrown when BP is reduced.

TREATMENT OF CONVULSIONS

DIAZEPAM

Patients of poisoning occasionally suffer seizures.

Diazepam is the drug of choice 0.2 to 0.4 mg/kg is given I/V slowly upto a maximum of 10 mg repeat dose after 10 minutes if necessary. Diazepam can also be given per rectum (I/V dose).

Alternatively phenytoin (10 mg/kg I/V) and phenobarbitone (10 mg/kg) can also be used, but the onset is relatively slow. Diazepam is both effective and safe agent for management of acute convulsions.

Other anticonvulsants such as phenytoin and phenobarbitone can be given after diazepam as action of diazepam is short and onset of these drugs is delayed.

PHENYTOIN

It is an effective anticonvulsant and is clinically used to treat tonic-clonic seizures, and status epilepticus. In management of convulsions in poisoning it is used as second line treatment. It has long half life of 24 hours and relatively small increases in dose can produce large increases in plasma concentration resulting in drug-induced toxicity. Furthermore large genetic variations in the rate of its metabolism occur.

Phenytoin is preferred if seizures are due to acute brain injury (e.g. head injury after alcohol etc.).

Dose: 15-20 mg/kg (both for adults and children). I/V at the rate of 30-50 mg/kg/min in adults and 0.5-1.5 mg/kg/min in children.

PHENOBARBITONE: 10-20 mg/kg in both adults and children given at the rate of 25-50 mg/min. Repeat 120-240 mg every 20 minutes in adults and every 6 mg/kg in children.

PARALDEHYDE: It is still preferred as it has little respiratory depressant effect and specially if resuscitation facilities are not available.

In non-responsive cases **paraldehyde** can be given per rectum.

As a final resort if all above fails I/V lidocaine can be used.

MANAGEMENT OF RESPIRATION

Hypoxia needs to be avoided at all costs. Most importantly the airways need clearance. Outside hospital mouth to mouth breathing helps to a great extent.

In hospital setting oxygen is administered through Ambu bag via a face mask or endotracheal tube. Gas analysis should be done in arterial blood.

Mouth to Mouth Breathing

Place your mouth over the mouth of the patient. Pinch the nose and give two breaths (1 to 1.5 seconds per breath) between 2-5 rescue breaths are needed initially to ensure at least 2 effective ventilations. Correct volume for breath is assessed by adequacy of chest expansion. If rescue breathing fails to produce chest expansion despite attempts at opening of the airway, suspect foreign body or closure of airway by mucus plugs and deal accordingly.

To prevent gastric distension and aspiration, inspiratory time should be prolonged and continuous pressure applied on cricoid.

Bag and Mask Ventilation

Self inflating bags should be used to deliver adequate amount of tidal volume and this must cause visible chest rise.

Avoid excessive expansion as that compromises cardiac output and also increases risk of aspiration.

Select a mask of proper size to cover patient's nose and mouth completely without covering eyes or chin. Place the head of the patient in semiflexed position. Exert downward pressure on the mask to ensure proper air seal. After applying mask to face and sealing it, compress the ventilation bag with hand to achieve visible chest rise.

Oxygen

Is administered to all patients who are seriously ill or if there is history of consumption of an agent likely to cause hypoxia. It can be administered by face masks, nasal cannula, pharyngeal masks, laryngeal mask, tracheal tubes and ventilation.

Endotracheal Tube

If used properly this is the most effective and reliable method of ventilation as it ensures airway patency, reduces dead space, provides protection from gastric distension and aspiration and allows trachial suctioning and positive-expiratory pressure.

It is specially indicated in cases of poisoning where there is need for higher ventilation pressures (to maintain effective alveolar gas exchange) or if protective airway reflexes are absent.

Calculation of paediatric endotracheal tube size:

Age/4 + 4 = size of endotracheal tube in mm.

Following table gives size in mm and length of the endotracheal tube for paediatric population.

Age (yrs)	*Size (mm)*	*Length (cm)*
10	7	20
8	6	18
6	5.5	16
5	5	14.5
4	4.5	13
2	4	12
1	4	12
6 months	3	11

Monitoring Oxygen Therapy

Measurement of oxygen in vivo is possible using transcutaneous oxymetry or invasive oxygen electrodes. Pulse oxymetry has an important role in managing the patients. Monitoring the blood gas plays an important role in the management of patients as oxygen requirement keeps on changing during oxygen administration.

COMMON ERRORS IN MANAGEMENT OF POISONING

1. Universal antidote that contains burnt toast, magnesium oxide and tannic acid is not effective and may be harmful.
2. If ipecac syrup is used, it should be given at once and can be administered even at home. **Use of ipecac fluid extract should be avoided.**
3. Acids neutralised by alkalies, generate heat and increase tissue destruction. Therefore, dilution with milk or water (15 mg/kg) is preferred.
4. Induction of vomiting by mechanical stimulation of throat or copper sulfate can be dangerous.
5. Oil based purgatives in unconsious or semiconsious patient are likely to cause lipid pneumonia.
6. Lavage fluids containing sodium and phosphates if given in excess may cause severe electrolyte imbalance specially if kidney functions are compromised.
7. Excessive hydration worsens pulmonary functions.
8. **Large amounts of glucose lower both potassium and phosphate in serum. Hence these must be constantly monitored.**

9. Both respiratory stimulants and analeptic agents serve no purpose and may on the contrary prove harmful.
10. Hepatic and renal functioning must be monitored as many agents cause hepatic/renal toxicity.
11. **Muscle destruction may result in acute renal failure and acidification of urine in such cases increases likelihood of renal insufficiency.**
12. Catheters (I/V, bladder) increase risk from infections.
13. Large volumes of fluid (as in dialysis procedure) may reduce body temperature and worsen functioning of cardiovascular system.
14. Extreme care should be exercised in diagnosing brain death in cases of sedative hypnotic drug overdose.

CHOLINESTERASE REACTIVATORS OXIMES (Enzyme reactivators)

Anticholinesterases (organophosphorus compounds and carbamates) are commonly employed insecticides. These agents inhibit cholinesterases, resulting in excess of acetylcholine at the muscarinic receptors leading to abdominal pain vomiting, diarrhea, bradycardia etc. These effects are reversed by atropine. However the nicotinic effects of these agents (muscular fasciculations followed by muscle weakness, respiratory paralysis) are not reversed by atropine. Oximes restore neuromuscular transmission in organophosphorus poisoning by reactivation of the concerned enzymes.

Pralidoxime, however, is ineffective as antidote to carbamates (physostigmine, neostigmine, carbaryl, propoxur etc.). Indeed it may worsen the symptomatology of a carbamate poisoned individual as it has weak anti ChE activity that adds to that of a carbamate.

Efficacy of oximes depends on time of administration. These drugs must be administered before the aging of the enzyme occurs.

Pralidoxime is less toxic than obidoxime and is therefore preferred.

Pralidoxime must be administered with atropine.

Dose 30 mg/kg as slow I/V infection. Effects are observed in 30 minutes by disappearance of convulsions and fasciculations. Improvement in muscle power is observed and there is improvement in level of consiousness.

Pralidoxime is available as two salts/mesylate and chloride. Mesylate needs to be repeated 4 hourly while chloride is given 6 hourly. In severe cases of poisoning treatment with these drugs has to be given for several days. Duration of therapy is guided by clinical symptoms and estimation of serum cholinesterase activity. Though pralidoxime can be given I/M this route is not preferred in severe cases where repeated administration is required to be given. **Coadministration with atropine necessitates reduction in dose of atropine.**

A

ABRUS PRECATORIUS (Jequirty or Rosary Beads or Indian Liquorice)

Abrus belongs to family Leguminosae and is slender twine. Flowers are pea like and may be coloured. Pod is small and contains seeds 4-6 in number, less than 1 cm in size bright red in colour with a black spot on one side. Seed contains abrin (toxalbumen), Abrine (an amino acid), Abralin (a glucoside) and Abric acid as active principles. Crushed seeds were used to treat corneal opacities.

Fatal dose 1-2 seeds or
90-120 mg of abrin.

Symptoms of Toxicity

Only crushed seeds produce toxicity, produce severe gastroenteritis which may be haemorrhagic. If extract of abrus is injected it produces inflammation at the site of injection and there are symptoms associated with cardiovascular system.

Management is symptomatic.

ACETONE (Chemical Solvent)

Acetone is a volatile and inflammable organic solvent mainly used in laboratories. In houses it is used for removing nail polish. It is absorbed through the lungs, skin and alimentary tract. Poisoning in children is common but serious poisoning is rare.

Symptoms of Toxicity

CNS: Loss of consciousness, depressed rate of respiration and convulsions are the most common symptoms of the acetone toxicity. The breath smells of acetone.

Throat is inflammed, oedematous and shows presence of superficial ulcerations.

Hyperglycemia and glycosuria have been reported and oral GTT is likely to be diabetic in character.

Acetone is present in urine.

Management

Patient should be removed from the toxic atmosphere.

The skin should be washed thoroughly.

Gastric lavage is contraindicated in case of acetone poisoning as acetone is corrosive in nature.

Supportive measures like ventilator will be required if the patient is unconscious.

There is no specific treatment hence supportive measures are done.

Treatment for hyperglycemia is usually not required as it gets corrected after few weeks.

Prognosis

Recovery of consciousness occurs within a few hours. Glucose tolerance takes few months to return to normal.

ACETYL SALICYLIC ACID (Aspirin)

It is widely used as an analgesic and anti-inflammatory drug. Two distinct syndromes of intoxication may occur acute (Single large dose) or chronic (repeated large doses).

Toxic Dose

Mild intoxication: Acute ingestion of 150-200 mg/kg.

Severe intoxication: Likely after acute ingestion of 300-500 mg/kg.

Chronic intoxication: Ingestion of more than 100 mg/kg/day for 2 or more days.

Since acetyl salicyclic acid is widely used, it is a common cause of poisoning in children. Poisoning in children may not be recognized early as it produces toxic effects similar to the conditions it is used to treat e.g. fever.

Signs and Symptoms

Mild poisoning:

Pain in stomach, nausea and vomiting.

Dizziness, ringing in the ears and deafness.

Breathing is rapid and shallow.

Moderate poisoning:
Fast breathing.
Confusion and restlessness.
Fever and sweating.
Dry tongue.

Death occurs due to cardiac/respiratory failure.

Severe Poisoning

Acute ingestion: Vomiting occurs shortly after ingestion, followed by hyperpnea, tinnitus and lethargy. Mixed respiratory alkalemia and metabolic acidosis are apparent when arterial blood gases are determined. With severe intoxication, coma, seizures, hypoglycemia, hyperthermia, and pulmonary edema may occur. **Death is caused due to central nervous system depression and cardio-vascular collapse.**

Chronic intoxication: Victims are usually young children or confused elderly. The diagnosis of poisoning are usually overlooked because symptoms such as confusion, dehydration, and metabolic acidosis get attributed to sepsis, pneumonia, or gastroenteritis rather than salicylism therefore, **mortality rates are much higher than after acute overdose.** Cerebral and pulmonary edema are more common than with acute intoxication and **severe poisoning occurs at rather lower acetyl salicyclic acid blood levels.**

Management

If breathing stops, open the airway and give mouth to mouth respiration. If the patient is unconscious or drowsy, lay him or her on one side in the recovery position. Check breathing every 10 minutes.

Maintain the airway and assist ventilation, if necessary. Administer supplemental oxygen.

Specific levels: Obtain initial and serial serum acetyl salicyclic acid concentrations. Systemic acidemia increases brain acetyl salicyclic acid concentration worsening toxicity.

A level greater than 600 mg/L (60 mg/dL) accompanied by acidosis and altered mental status is considered very serious.

Treat metabolic acidosis with intravenous sodium bicarbonate. Give 0.5-1 mEq/kg IV bolus; repeat as needed to bring serum pH between 7.4-7.5. **Do not allow the serum pH to fall below 7.4.**

Other useful laboratory studies: Electrolytes (anion gap calculation), glucose, blood urea, creatinine, prothrombin time (PT), arterial blood gases, chest X-ray.

Treat hyperthermia by external cooling with sponging and fanning. Iced gastric and colonic lavage or ice-water immersion can also be performed. In case shivering occurs as a consequence of cooling, use diazepam (0.1-0.2 mg/kg IV) or midazolam (0.05-0.1 mg/kg IV) to prevent or treat it.

Replace fluid and electrolyte deficits caused by vomiting and hyperventilation with intravenous crystalloid solutions. Excessive fluid administration may contribute to pulmonary edema therefore should be avoided.

Monitor asymptomatic patients for a minimum of 6 hours (longer if an enteric-coated preparation or a massive overdose has been ingested).

There is no specific antidote for **acetyl salicyclic acid intoxication.**

Sodium bicarbonate is frequently given both to prevent acidemia and to promote elimination of acetyl salicyclic acid through the kidneys.

Decontamination is not necessary for patients with chronic intoxication.

Ipecac induced emesis may be useful for initial treatment of children at home if it can be given within 30 minutes of exposure.

Administer activated charcoal orally or by gastric tube.

Adult: 30-100 gm once and repeat without purgative every 4-6 hours in a dose of 0.5 gm/kg.

Gastric lavage is not necessary after small ingestions (< 200-300 mg/kg) provided activated charcoal has been given promptly).

Promotion of Excretion

A. Urinary alkalization:

It is very effective in enhancing urinary excretion of acetyl salicyclic acid. However, it is very difficult to acheive this in dehydrated or critically ill patients.

Sodium bicarbonate (100 meq) should be added to 1 L of 5% dextrose. To this solution, add a quarter of normal saline and potassium 30-40 meq/L (potassium depletion inhibits alkalinization). Infuse this solution at the rate of 200 ml/h (3-4 ml/kg/h). If the patient is dehydrated, start with a bolus of 10-20 ml/kg. Caution should be exercised when administering sodium bicarbonate or fluid to patients who are at a high risk of developing pulmonary edema (e.g. chronic intoxication). **Potassium should never be added if patient is in renal failure.**

B. Hemodialysis:

This procedure rapidly removes acetyl salicyclic acid and corrects acid-base and fluid abnormalities. It is indicated if:

A. **In acute poisoning:** Serum levels of acetyl salicyclic acid are more than >120 mg/dl or if there is severe acidosis or signs of severe intoxication are present.

B. In **chronic toxicity:** Serum levels of acetyl salicyclic acid are >60 mg/dl and are accompanied by acidosis, confusion or lethargy or if the patient is elderly or debilitated.

Hemoperfusion:

This procedure removes acetyl salicyclic acid but does not correct acid-base and fluid abnormalities.

Repeat-dose-activated-charcoal therapy:

Though it is effective in reducing serum acetyl salicyclic acid half-life but results in aggravating dehydration and severe electrolyte disturbances already in dehydrated patient. Therefore, dialysis is the first choice. However, if this facility is not available, consider repeat-dose-activated-charcoal therapy.

Activated charcoal Adult: 30-100 gm (orally mixed with water) as the first dose and then repeat every 4-6 hours in a dose of 0.5 gm/kg. **Not to administer purgative on the subsequent dosing.**

Child: 15-30 gm (orally mixed with water) as the first dose and then repeat every 4-6 hours in a dose of 0.25 gm/kg. **Do not to administer purgative on the subsequent dosing.**

ACIDS (Hydrochloric acid, Acetic acid, Nitric acid, Picric acid, Tannic acid, Oxalic acid, Hydrofluoric acid)

Acids are corrosive agents. Accidental poisoning occurs in children but these are sometimes used for suicidal purposes. Sometimes sulphuric/nitric acid is thrown over face of an enemy to cause injury/disfigurement. Hydrochloric acid is used to remove marks of writing on paper (forgery).

Severity of symptoms depends on concentration of acid and the chemistry of substance and therefore actual dose is not important.

Symptoms of Toxication

In case of ingestion: Severe burning pain in the mouth, throat, abdomen, dysphagia, gastritis, vomiting and diarrhoea that may contain blood/mucus.

CVS: Hypotension with cold clammy skin and rapid pulse.

Miscellaneous: Metabolic acidosis, hemolysis, massive fluid and electrolyte shifts (hyperkalemia, hyperphosphatemia, hypocalcemia, hyperchloremia).

Symptoms on inhalation: Cough, bronchospasm, dyspnea, pleuritic chest pain, pulmonary oedema, frothy sputum and hemoptysis.

Exposure of eyes to acid: Irritation, pain, lacrimation, swelling lids of eyes, chemosis, photophobia, corneal erosion and perforation due to necrosis of conjunctiva and cornea.

In case of dermal exposure: Burning pain, irritation, redness, blistering and ulceration.

Management

(A) **In case of ingestion:**
Avoid inducing vomiting.
Administer water or milk, so that acid can be diluted.
Avoid activated charcoal.
Avoid excessive amount of milk or water as they provoke vomiting.
Avoid carbonated beverages or bicarbonate for neutralization of acid.

(B) **In case of inhalation:**
Patient should be removed from site of exposure and shifted to fresh air.

(C) **In case of eye exposure:**
Irrigate eyes with large volumes of 0.9% normal saline or water for 15 minutes or more.
Eyes should not be washed with soap solution.
Remove contact lenses.

(D) **Dermal exposure:**
Wash affected skin with copious amounts of water or mild soap solution.

Avoid gastric lavage (except in acute liquid corrosive agents). However gastric lavage can be undertaken if endoscopy is required in first 24 hours to determine any perforation.

In case of airway compromise, endotracheal intubation should be done.

Administer 100% humified oxygen for inhalation. Use respirator if available and if necessary.

Gastric suction should be done using soft nasogastric tube.

Irrigate mouth frequently in patients who are cooperative and conscious.

IV fluids amount of volume should be determined by requirement of the patient.

Vasopressors (dopamine) can be used if necessary.

Perform chest X-ray to detect mediastinitis or GI perforation. Antibiotics should be given if perforation is present.

Laparotomy should be done in case endoscopy reveals necrosis of oesophagus or stomach or when signs and symptoms of GI perforation are evident at the time of admission.

ACONITE (PLANT TOXIN)

In raw state roots resemble horse radish and is used as salad in western part of the world. Dry root is conical or tapering usually archeld and shrivelled with longitudinally raised ridges. Root is twisted in its long axis, is dark brown in colour but whetish when freshly cut. It has **sweet taste.**

Roots of aconite are used for poisoning, although all parts are toxic. It is also known as Methabis and is used mainly for homicidal purposes. Powdered aconite is sprinkled in well water to poison population. Accidental poisoning may also occur as it is used in traditional systems of medicine.

Symptoms

Symptoms set in within few minutes and are due to initial stimulation followed by paralyses of sensory and secretory nerves. In addition alkaloids of aconite cause cerebro-cardiac depression.

Patient experiences sweet bitter taste and tingling sensation in mouth.

This is followed by numbness of lips, tongue, mouth and throat that spreads all over the body.

Abdominal symptoms are next to develop—nausea, vomiting and pain. Few patients may experience diarrhea, giddiness, severe muscular weakness, staggering gait, restlessness anxiety and a feeling of faintness develops that is associated with weak and slow irregular pulse. Breathing becomes slow and laboured. There are visual changes, pupils show alternate contraction and dilatation in early stages but get dilated towards the end. However, intellect remains clear. Convulsions may occur in some patients.

Death occurs due to ventricular fibrillation or asphyxia.

Fatal dose	2 gm of root 4 ml of tincture aconite 2 mg of pure aconite
Fatal period	1-5 hours.

Management

Gastric lavage with, solution of potassium iodide and iodine, tannic acid or milk. Activated charcoal is helpful. Body needs to be kept warm with help of water bottles or blankets.

Amylnitrate and atropine (0.6-1.2 mgm) I/V in 5% glucose prevents shock.

Noradrenaline can be added to the drip.

Artificial respiration will be required. Xylocaine can be given to control arrhythmia.

AEROSOL SPRAYS

Window cleaner, furniture polish, air freshner and oven cleaner are available in spray cans. Hair sprays, deodorant and insecticides are also sold in spray cans.

Aerosol abuse is habit forming and may lead to dependence and abuse of aerosols. This may cause sudden death due to the effect of the propellents on the heart.

Signs and Symptoms

Coughing and choking.

Excitement, hallucinations followed by sudden unconsciousness.

Either the patient may die suddenly or recover very quickly.

Exposure of the Eyes

Stinging and watering of eyes occurs. Eyelids become red.

Management

If the patient is unconscious or drowsy, lay him on one side. Check breathing every 10 minutes and keep the patient warm and quiet. Give symptomatic therapy.

ALDICARB (Carbamate)

It is an isecticide with anticholinesterase activity clinical picture and treatment same as other **Carbamates** *(Refer page 87).*

ALDRIN (Organochlorine insecticide)

It is widely used as pesticide in agriculture, insect control and malarial control programs. It is highly toxic among organochlorines with animal oral LD_{50} < 50 mg/kg. Estimated adult lethal dose is 3-7 gm.

Symptoms of toxicity

Nausea, vomiting, confusion, tremors, obtundation, coma, seizures and respiratory depression.

Delayed and recurrent seizure is a possibility.

Arrhythmia may occur owing to increase in myocardial senstivity to catecholamines.

Management

The clothing should be removed and the whole body sponged or washed with water and soap.

Do not give oil/milk/cream orally.

Emesis is indicated only if patient approaches within 30 minutes of ingestion of organochlorine.

Gastric lavage with lukewarm water or saline is advisable.

Activated charcoal to be given if available.

Supportive measures such as:

Ensure adequate oxygenation and undertake nasopharageal suction if necessary.

Give ventilatory support if required.

IV fluids should be given if required—the voulme should be determined by the condition of the patient.

For management of seizures:

Diazepam: Diazepam should be given in undiluted form with close monitoring of blood pressure and respiration.

Followed by either Phenytoin of Phenobarbitone:

Cholestyramine: 4 gms orally is given mixed in fruit juice every 6 hours before meals.

Do not give epinephrine or atropine as these may lead to cardiac arrhythmias.

ALKALI POISONING (Sodium bicarbonate, Potassium or Sodium hydroxide and Ammonia)

Alkalies (combination of sodium and potassium hydroxides) are used as drain, or pipe cleaners. Accidental poisoning is likely in children but is often used for suicidal purpose.

(A) **Symptoms on ingestion of an alkali:**
Local effects: Burns in lips, oral mucosa, upper airway, oesophagus.
GIT: Drooling, stridor, vomiting and gastrointestinal bleeding.

(B) **Symptoms on inhalation of alkali:**
GIT: Oedema of upper airway, dyspnea, wheezing, pulmonary oedema, pneumonitis and respiratory failure.

(C) **Exposure of eyes to alkali:**
Conjunctival irritation, corneal perforation, distortion of cellular membranes, loss of epithelium of cornea, conjunctiva and lens.

(D) **Skin exposure to alkali:**
Pain, redness, irritation, with full thickness burns.

Management

In case of inhalation: Patient should be removed from site of exposure and shifted to fresh air.

In case of eye exposure: Irrigate with large volumes of 0.9% normal saline or water for 15 minutes or more.

Remove contact lenses.

Wash affected skin with copious amounts of water for 6-8 hours.

In case of Ingestion:

Avoid inducing vomiting.

Administer water or milk so that alkali can be diluted.

Avoid Gastric Lavage

In case of airway compromise do endotracheal intubation.

Give 100% humified oxygen for inhalation. Use respirator if available and if deemed necessary.

Suction should be done using soft nasogastric tube.

Irrigate mouth frequently in patients who are cooperative and conscious.

IV fluids to be given. Volume should be determined according to the condition of the patient.

Vasopressors **(dopamine)** can be used if necessary.

Endoscopy should be performed within first 24 hours to detect absence or presence of perforation.

Perform chest X-ray for detecting mediastinitis or GI perforation. Administer antibiotics if there is perforation.

Laparotomy should be done in case endoscopy reveals necrosis of either oesophagus or stomach or when signs and symptoms of GI perforation are evident.

ALOE (Plant)

It is a small plant belonging to family Lillaceae. Aloe vera is the most common species and is used in traditional systems of medicine. It has reddish flowers.

Latex of this plant is used to treat cuts, burns and insect bites.

Symptoms

On ingestion it causes gastrointestinal irritation.

Management

Stop aloe vera and give supportive therapy.

ALPHA CHLORALOSE (Rodenticide)

Alpha chloralose is used as an anaesthetic agent in animals. It is also used to kill rodents, birds, pests and moles. Toxic dose of the L-chloralose is 1 g in adult and 20 mg/kg for an infant.

Symptoms of toxicity

The symptoms are similar to those of strychnine. Excessive salivation, increase in muscle tone, hyper-reflexia, opisthotonus and convulsions are the major symptoms. **Rhabdomyolysis is a potential complication.** Coma, generalised flaccidity and respiratory depression may occur.

Management

A clear airway and adequate ventilation must be maintained.

Convulsions are treated/suppressed with intravenous undiluted diazepam, but if not controlled, use an alternative such as phenytoin or phenobarbitone.

After control of convulsions has been achieved, repeated doses of oral activated charcoal should be given.

Gastric emptying should not be carried out as it may result in avoidable stimulation resulting in convulsions.

ALPRAZOLAM (Benzodiazepine)

Alprazolam is specially used as antianxiety drug. In addition it has some mood elevating action in mild depression, therefore is particularly useful in patients suffering from anxiety associated with depression. It also found its place in therapy of panic disorders. It has long half life (12 hrs) and also has an active meatbolite.

Clinical Features and Management

Same as with other **Benzodiazepine** *(Refer page 73)*.

ALUMINIUM PHOSPHIDE (Insecticide)

It is used to protect grains from insects.

Symptoms of Toxicity

- **GI:** Vomiting, epigastric pain, diarrhoea.
- **CNS:** Dizziness, restlessness, convulsions, CNS depression and coma.
- **Respiratory:** Dyspnea, tachypnea and pulmonary edema.
- **CVS:** Tachycardia, circulatory shock, cyanosis, cardiac arrhythmias, crepitations, congestive heart failure and acute respiratory distress syndrome.

Death in aluminum phosphide is due to shock and peripheral circulatory failure. The odour of breath is that of decaying fish.

Management

Before bringing the patient to hospital:

Patient should be shifted to fresh air.

To prevent aspiration of vomitus lay the patient on his side.

Supportive Therapy

Give activated charcoal with juice and repeat without purgative every 4-6 hours in a dose of 0.5 gm/kg.

For treating convulsions give **Diazepam** in undiluted form and closely monitor blood pressure and respiration.

Adult dose: 5-10 mg IV) Maximum dose—30 mg.

Followed by either Phenytoin or Phenobarbitone.

Dopamine is given to treat hypotension and shock: 4-6 ug/kg/min IV. Monitor blood pressure and ECG.

Ranitidine 50 mg IV three times a day.

Sodium bicarbonate is indicated if arterial bicarbonate is less than 15 mmol/L.

Intravenous fluids: 4-6 liters of saline can be given over a period of 6 hours. Closely monitor central venous pressure.

Gastric lavage is contraindicated as it releases more phosphene when it comes in contact with water in the stomach.

AMINOPHYLLINE AND THEOPHYLLINE (Bronchodilators)

These drugs are used to treat asthma, since **most of these are sustained release preparations,** it means that effects of the medicine last a long time.

Poisoning may be caused by a single overdose or by repetitive large doses.

Signs and Symptoms of Toxicity

Hypotension results in nausea and vomiting and syncope.

Arrhythmias may be present.

Restlessness, headache and sleeplessness.

Hallucinations may be present

Convulsions may occur.

Management

Put patient's head low position. If the patient is fully awake and breathing normally and is not vomiting give **activated charcoal and water.**

Treat hypotensin with fluids and **dobutamine.** Beta blockers can be used to treat arrhythmias.

AMITRIPTYLINE (Anti-depressant TCA)

It is tricyclic anti-depressant. Produces anticholinergic and cardiovascular toxicity along with convulsions.

Symptoms of Toxicity

Mild

Confusin, blurred vision, flushed dry skin and mucosa, sinus tachycardia and hypotension. Convulsions and anticholinergic activity can produce hyperthermia, rhabdomyolysis and multiple organ failure.

Moderate to Severe

1. **CNS:** Agitation, visual and auditory hallucinations, myoclonus, convulsions, ataxia, coma and death.
2. **CVS:** Hypotension, sinus tachycardia and other brady arrhythmias with prolonged PR and QRS and QT durations (>100 msec). **Prolongation of QRS complex to or over 0.12 sec is indicative of cardiotoxicity.**
3. **Respiratory:** Respiratory insufficiency or arrest, pulmonary edema, oesophageal spasm and respiratory acidosis occur in severe poisoning.
4. **Miscellaneous:** Metabolic acidosis and urinary retention occur.

   Death is due to cardiac arrest and circulatory failure.

Management

Same as with other **Anti-depressants** *(Refer page 58)*.

Special Precautions to be Taken

Do not give antiarrhythmic drugs like quinidine and procainamide as they further decrease AV nodal conduction.

Do not give phenothiazines for treatment of hyperthermia as their own anticholinergic action adds to that of the amitryptyline.

Avoid dopamine to treat hypotension as its adrenergic stimulatory effect increases arrhythmia and also increases vasodilation.

To prevent hypoxia and lactic acidosis treat convulsions immediately as these predispose to the development of life threatening ventricular arrhythmias.

After discontinuation of all supportive measures patients who suffer altered sensorium or arrhythmias should be closely monitored for the next 24 hrs.

Use of phenytoin should be avoided as it increases incidence of ventricular tachycardia.

Propranolol and verapamil should be avoided as they slow conduction velocity in heart and lower BP.

Potassium replacement during bicarbonate treatment should be done with caution as hyperkalemia may aggravate amitriptyline induced cardiac arrhythmias.

AMMONIA (Alkali)

Ammonia is released when wool, silk or nylon is burnt and can cause toxicity among bistanders.

Symptoms

In some cases of ammonia inhalation, there is formation of a pulmonary hyaline membrane producing symptoms of respiratory distress syndrome (dyspnea, tachypnea, sweating, pink frothy sputum etc.).

Ammonia poisoning can be detected by placing an open bottle of concentrated HCl near a sample of vomitus or gastric lavage. White fumes of ammonium chloride will emanate in presence of ammonia.

Management

Remove patient from contaminated area and treat symptoms. For details *Refer page 49.*

AMMONIUM NITRATE

Ammonium nitrate was widely used as diuretic and toxicological effects are primary are due to nitrate moiety.

Symptoms of Toxicity

Headache, skin flushing and orthostatic hypotension with reflex tachycardia are the most common adverse effects of nitrates and nitrites that occur commonly.

Workers or patients regularly exposed to nitrates may develop tolerance and may suffer angina or myocardial infarction due to sudden withdrawal of the drug leading to rebound coronary vasoconstriction.

Management

Maintain airway and assist ventilation if necessary. Administer supplemental oxygen.

Hypotension usually responds to supine positioning. In case no effect is seen, manage as described below:

Fluid therapy must be instituted at the rate of 10-20 ml/kg along with Dopamine 6 μg/kg/min.

Symptomatic methemoglobinemia may be treated with methylene blue if (a) patient has symptoms or (b) signs of hypoxemia (e.g. dyspnoea, confusion, chest pain) or (c) methemoglobinemia > 30%.

Methyline blue Dosage (adults and children): 1-2 mg/kg (0.1-0.2 ml/kg of 1% solution) IV slowly over 5 minutes. May be repeated in 30-60 minutes. If no response occurs, do not repeat dosing.

On ingestion: Administer activated charcoal without purgative. Ipecac induced emesis may be useful for initial treatment. Gastric emptying is not necessary for small ingestion if activated charcoal can be given promptly.

Hemodialysis and hemoperfusion are not effective. Severe methemoglobinemia in infants not responsive to methylene blue therapy may require exchange transfusion.

AMOXAPINE (Tricyclic Anti-depressant)

Amoxapine is moderately toxic anti-depressant. Rhabdomyolysis with resultant acute renal failure is often associated with amoxapine.

Symptoms

(A) Mild toxicity: Confusion, blurred vision, flushed dry skin and mucosa, vasodilatation sinus tachycardia and hypotension.

(B) Moderate to severe:

CNS: Agitation, visual and auditory hallucinations, myoclonus, convulsions, ataxia and coma Grade 2 or 3 with strabismus.

CVS: Hypotension, sinus tachycardia and other brady arrhythmias both are possible. QRS interval may not change.

Respiratory: Respiratory insufficiency or arrest, pulmonary edema, oesophageal spasm and respiratory acidosis.

Miscellaneous: Urinary retention.

Death is due to cardiac arrest and circulatory failure.

Management

Same as of other anticholinergics. However, renal dialysis is advocated if renal failure occurs along with other appropriate measures.

Maintain proper airway. Adequate oxygenation to be given. Give assisted respiration if indicated.

In case of seizures, prevent injury to the tongue by placing a spoon in the mouth of the patient.

Nasopharyngeal suction to be done if required.

Induce emesis by mechanical stimulation of the back of the tongue.

Gastric lavage:

Adult: 150-200 ml of lukewarm water or normal saline per wash.

Child: 50 to 100 ml of normal saline in children below 5 years. This can be repeated every 6 hrs, if necessary.

Laboratory tests to be advised are:

- ECG monitoring.
- Blood-gases, bicarbonate and pH.
- Serum electrolytes.
- Quantitative test for amoxapine (if available).

Activated charcoal:

Adult: 30-100 gm once and repeat without purgative every 4-6 hours in a dose of 0.5 gm/kg.

Children: 15-30 gm orally mixed with water (single dose) and repeat 0.25 gm/kg every 4-6 hours.

For treating convulsions:

Diazepam:

Adult: 5-10 mg, intravenously slowly over 2-3 min (maximum rate 5 mg/min). Repeat if necessary every 10-15 min. Maximum dose not to exceed 30 mg/day.

Children: 0.25-0.4 mg/kg IV slowly over 2-3 min. Repeat if necessary every 2-5 min (maximum dose is 5 mg in children below 5 years of age and 10 mg in those above 5 years).

Or

Lorazepam: 1-2 mg IV over several minutes.

IV fluids: Given if there is dehydration and hypotension.

Adult: 100 ml of 50% dextrose.

Child: 0.5-1gm/kg of 25% dextrose.

Sodium bicarbonate: 500-800 ml IV by slow infusion (7.5% v/v). Maintain blood pH of 7.5.

Dobutamine: 2.5-1.5 ug/kg/min infusion if hypotension is due to loss of inotropy.
Potassium chloride: If indicated along with monitoring.

Special Precautions to be Taken

Same as with other **Amitriptyline** *(Refer page 53)*.

AMPHETAMINES (Sympathomimetic Agent)

Special Risk Groups

Drug smugglers who swallow large amounts of amphetamine/cocaine in sealed bags get severe poisoning if the bags burst inside the body.

Symptoms of Toxicity

CNS: Euphoria, restlessness, confusion, delirium, hallucinations and paranoia are prominent.

CVS: Tachycardia, peripheral vasoconstriction, tachypnea, tremors and dilated pupils may occur.

Miscellaneous: Nausea, vomiting, facial flushing and sweating are also common.

Hypertension produced by amphetamines can precipitate dissection of the aorta, myocarditis, myocardial infarction, dilated cardiomyopathy, subarachnoid haemorrhage, and cerebral infarction. Chronic use produces cerebral vasculitis, transient cerebral ischaemic attacks, hyperpyrexia, convulsions, metabolic acidosis, impaired consciousness, impaired respiration and paranoid psychosis.

Management

Activated charcoal:

Adult: 30-100 gm once and repeat without purgative every 4-6 hours in a dose of 0.5 gm/kg.

Child: 15-30 gm orally mixed with water (single dose) and repeat 0.25 gm/kg every 4-6 hours.

Maintain proper airway.

Adequate ventilation is necessary if conscious is impaired.

Arterial blood gas tension should be measured.

Correct hypoxia and metabolic acidosis if these are present.

For treatment of convulsions and agitation: Convulsions should be managed by administering diazepam in undiluted form with closely monitor of blood pressure and respiration to be followed by either phenytoin or phenobarbitone.

Hypertension is controlled immediately using **labetalol** given IV at a rate of 2 mg/min and further dose should be adjusted according to response. Total dose should not exceed more than 200 mg.

Propranolol or any non-specific beta blockers should be avoided because they can cause paradoxical increase in blood pressure. Beta-adrenoceptor blocker is contraindicated if ECG shows signs of ischaemia as these drugs potentiate coronary vasoconstriction.

For treating arrhythmias or severe tachycardia give beta adrenoreceptor blocker.

Forced diuresis should be avoided as it can lead to serious disturbances specially in patients of arrhythmias.

ANTI-DEPRESSANTS (Tricyclic and Tetracyclic Compounds) Amitryptyline, Amoxapine, Dothiepin, Doxepin Imipramine, Nortptyline, Protriptyline, Lofepramine, Loxapine, Propriphyline and trimipramine, Maprotiline is tetracyclic compound

---

Tricyclic Anti-depressants Available in India

Amitryptidine	Amiline, Amitone, Limbicon, Sarotena
Amoxapine	Demolox
Imipramine	Antitep, Depsol, Depsonil, Impramine
Nortryptyline	Primox, Senswal
Trazodone	Depryl, Sedodep, Trazolin, Trazalon, Traze, Trazolin, Trittico.

Clinically amtriptyline, doxepin and dothiepin are most commonly used preparations. Amitriptyline is more toxic maprotline, amoxapine and oxapine are moderately toxic while lofepramine is relatively safer.

Symptoms

(A) Mild Toxicity

Confusion, blurred vision, flushed dry skin and mucosae, vasodilatation, sinus tachycardia and hypotension.

(B) Moderate to Severe Toxicity

CNS: Agitation, hallucinations, impaired consiousness, respiratory depression, myoclonus, hyperreflexia and extensor plantar responses followed by coma of grade 2 or 3 with strabismus.

Convulsions occur in early phase and are of short duration but are more frequently encountered in toxicity due to **maprotiline.**

Cardiovascular system: Hypotension (specially orthostatic type) occurs during early part of. Degree of hypotension is less as compared to barbiturates with comparable degree of consciousness and may result from tachy/brady-arrhythmias, vasodilatation and depression of myocardial contractibility.

ECG shows prolongation of PR and QRS intervals and P wave may be lost in preceding T wave. AV nodal blocks may be seen.

Due to anticholinergic activity sinus tachycardia may also occur. In small number of patients Torsade de pointes occurs resulting in sudden death in these patients.

Delirium and hallucinations may be present initially. Anticholinergic activity contributes to retention of urine. Rhabdomyolysis with renal failure is reported with **Amoxapine and Loxapine.**

Respiratory system: Pneumonine, adult respiratory distress syndrome.

Plasma concentrations do not often correlate with symptomatology and severity of toxicity.

Most of these drugs have active metabolites and late toxicity is a possibility.

Alcohol, benzodiazepines and antipsychotics increase toxicity. If given with MAO inhibitors there is danger of hypertensive criseis accompanied with hallucinations and excitement. Similarly aspirin and phenylbutazone can precipitate toxicity.

Management

1. Ensure adequate oxygenation and maintain proper airway. Give assisted respiration if indicated.
2. Laboratory tests advised are:
   ECG monitoring.
   Blood gases, bicarbonate and pH.
   Serum electrolytes.
3. Nasopharyngeal suction should be done whenever needed.
4. Induce emesis by mechanical stimulation of the back of the tongue.
5. To prevent injury to tongue put a spoon in patient's mouth in case of seizures.

6. **Gastric lavage:**

   Adult: 150-200 ml of lukewarm water or normal saline per wash.

   Child: 50 to 100 ml of normal saline in children above 5 years. This can be repeated every 6 hrs if necessary.

   Give activated charcoal:

   Adult: 30-100 gm once and repeat without purgative every 4-6 hours in a dose of 0.5 gm/kg.

   Child: 15-30 gm orally mixed with water (single dose) and repeat 0.25 gm/kg every 4-6 hours.

   IV fluids: IV fluids are given if there is dehydration or hypotension.

Physostigminee salicylate (2 mg I/V given over 2 minutes in adults and 0.5 mg for a child) reverses anticholinergic effects of tricyclic anti-depressants. It reverses tachycardia and improves clinical picture.

It has short half life and needs to be repeated every 30 minutes. **Infusion is not desirable as it increases bronchial secretions and reportedly causes ventricular tachycardia. However its use is restricted.**

For treating convulsions: Diazepam: In adult—5-10 mg, intravenously slowly and repeat if necessary every 10-15 min. Half the dose is to be given to children. Or give **Lorazepam:** 1-2 mg IV over several minutes.

Sodium bicarbonate: 50-80 ml IV by slow infusion (7.5% v/v). Maintain blood pH at 7.5.

Thiamine hydrochloride: 100 mg IV to be given only if altered sensorium.

Dobutamine: 0.5-1.5 ug/kg/min infusion if hypotension is due to loss of ionotropy.

Potassium chloride: (If indicated) is given with constant monitoring.

ANTI-DIABETIC AGENTS OR ORAL HYPOGLYCEMICS (Sulfonylureas, Meglitinides, Glitazones)

Sulphonylureas are used to treat NIDDM.

Trade Names of Anti-Diabetic Agents

Chlorpropamide	Chlorformin, Diabinase
Glipizide	Glibetic, Glynase
Tolbutamide	Rastinon

Phenformin	Chlorformin, DBI
Metformin	Diaphage, Glyciphage
Insulins	Human insulatard Human mixtard Human monosulin Insulatard Human Nordizulin Mixtard, Monosulin Nordisulin

Symptoms

Hypoglycemia is most common event in these patients and can be precipitated by excessive dose, fasting, vomiting or by associated liver and kidney disease. It is also precipitated by co-administration of beta blockers (nonspecific), anticoagulants and salicylates. Allergic reactions are common.

Chlorpropamide can cause cholestatic jaundice and occasionally pulmonary eosinophilia.

Management

Stop offending drug. Administer glucose I.V. Monitor blood sugar constantly.

ANTIHISTAMINICS (CARBINOXAMINE, DIMENHYDRINATE, DIPHENHYDRAMINE, DOXYLAMINE, PYRILAMINE, TRIPETENNAMINE, BROMPHENIRAMINE, CHLORPHENIRAMINE, CYCLIZINE, MECLIZINE, HYDROXYZINE, ASTEMIZOLE, TERFENADINE)

Antihistaminics (H_1 blockers) are used to treat allergy, travel sickness and cough. They are also used in ointments for treating stings, sunburns and skin rashes. (H_2 receptor blockers such as cimetidine, ranitidine, famotidine inhibit gastric acid secretion but otherwise share no effects with H_1 agents. They do not produce significant intoxication).

Accidental poisoning in children is common.

Common Anti-Histaminic Preparations

Astemizole	Acctinol, Alespl, Cortomine, LA histalog, Minastem
Azatidine	Zadine
Buclizine	Longifene

Chlorpheniramine	Corex, Corecidin F, Ephedrex, Febrex plus, Grilinctes, Hystalin, Pruton, Polaramine, Zeel
Cinnarizine	Cinzan, Dizeron, Stugeron
Cyclizine	Marzine, Megril
Cyproheptadine	Cyslactin, Cydine Practin
Diphenhydramine	Benodryl, Bronolax, Daslin, Mucosal, Lupihist
Mebhydrolin	Incidal
Orphenadrine	Desipal, Orphamol, Orphelgin
Phenuramine	Avil, Cosavil
Promethazine	Phenergan, Phensedyl, Promasun, Tixylex
Terfenadrine	Terdane, Terf, Terfed, Tofril, Trexyl, Zoter.
Trimeprazine	Vellergan
Tripelennamine	Bradex-vcoform
Triprolidine	Actidil, Actifed, Actilex, Deletus D

Signs and Symptoms

Acute intoxication results in symptoms very similiar to those of anticholinergic poisoning.

The usual effects are:

CNS: Drowsiness, Headache, Nausea, Drowsiness and Confusion, Hallucinations, Unconsciousness, Tremors, Excitement and Convulsions.
Tachycardia.
Retention of urine.
Dry mouth.
Shallow breathing mydriasis.
Hyperpyrexia.

Massive diphenhydramine overdose has been reported to cause QRS widening and myocardial depression similiar to cyclic anti-depressants.

QT interval prolongation and torsades-type atypical ventricular tachycardia is associated with elevated serum levels of **terfenadine or astemizole.** These usually occur after overdose or excessive daily dosing or use of an interacting drug (e.g. erythromycin, ketaconazole, itraconazole). **For details see terfenadine or astemizole.**

If there is urinary retention it may be necessary to catheterize the patient.

Maintain the airway and assist ventilation if necessary.

Treat hyperthermia by external cooling with ice packs—it is most efficient. Alternatively gastric lavage with iced water or ice water immersion can be done. In case shivering occurs as a consequence of cooling, use diazepam (0.1-0.2 mg/kg IV) or midazolam (0.05-0.1 mg/kg IV) to prevent it.

Administer **activated charcoal** or **Ipecac-induced emesis may be useful** for initial treatment of children at home if it can be given within 30 minutes of exposure.

For treatment of convulsions:

Diazepam: IV undiluted form with close monitoring of blood pressure and respiration.

Adult dose: 5-10 mg IV given slowly over a period of 2 to 3 minutes. (Maximum rate of administer 5 mg/min). Repeat diazepam dose every 10-15 min if necessary. Maximum dose—30 mg.

Children: 0.25-0.4 mg/kg IV slowly over 2-3 min. Repeat every 2-5 minutes. Maximum dose 5 mg in children below 5 years of age and 10 mg for children above 5 years.

Followed by:

Phenytoin:

Adult: 10-15 mg/kg given slowly IV. Maximum rate of administration 50 mg/min 100 mg orally or IV every 6-8 hours. Patient's blood pressure and ECG should be closely monitored.

Children: 15-20 mg/kg IV slowly. The rate of administration is 1mg/kg/min or 1.5 mg/kg at every 30 min. Do not exceed the maximum dose of 20 mg/kg/day.

or

Phenobarbitone:

Adult: 600-1200 mg or 10-12 mg/kg IV diluted in 60 ml of normal saline. The rate of administration is 25-50 mg/min 120-240 mg every 20 min. Maximum dose should not exceed 2 gm.

Children: 15-20 mg/kg IV the rate of administration is 25-50 mg/min 5-10 mg/kg every 20 min. Maximum dose should not exceed 40 mg/kg.

For atypical ventricular tachycardia (in case of terfenadine or astemizole poisoning); use overdrive pacing or isoproterenol 1-10 µg/minute IV to increase the heart rate (this makes repolarization more homogenous and abolishes the arrhythmia).

Monitor the patient for at least 6-8 hours after ingestion.

For terfenadine or astemizole, monitor patients for minimum of 18-24 hours after recovery.

ANTISEPTICS (Benzalkonium cetrimide, Cetylpyridinium, Chlorhexidine, Hydrogen peroxide, Phenol, Cresol, Chlorocresol, Chloroxylenol or Tar acids, Pine oil and Soap)

They are widely used in households, food industry and hospitals and include cationic detergents.

Signs and Symptoms

Cationic detergents may cause unconsciousness and affect breathing because of their surfactant action.

Strong solutions of potassium permangnate may cause burns in mouth, throat and muscles of this region.

Hydrogen peroxide is a strong oxidizing agent and rapidly breaks into oxygen and water. Generation of oxygen gas in closed body cavities causes mechanical distension resulting in gastric/intestinal perforation.

Management

Exposure of eyes:
Wash the eyes for at least 15-20 minutes with water.

On the skin:
Immediately remove contaminated clothes.

Upon Ingestion:
In case of ingestion of concentrated solution, the airway should be monitored for evidence of swelling and intubated if considered necessary.

In cases of potassium permangnate poisoning, methylene blue should be used to counteract methemoglobinemia.

Dose (adults and children): 1-2 mg/kg (0.1-0.2 ml/kg of 1% solution) IV slowly over 5 minutes

Copious amounts of water or milk should be offered to the patients to dilute the ingested chemical.

Gastric lavage should be performed cautiously. **Forced emesis should not be done because of risk of corrosion.**

Activated charcoal/cathartics are not effective.

ANTS

Most ants grasp skin with their jaws and sting or spray locally irritating venom. Fire ants have well developed abdominal stingers and inflict multiple stings.

Ant venom contains alkeloids sprotens.

Symptoms and Management

Same as with other **Bees.**

ARSENIC AND ARSENIC CONTAINING CHEMICALS

They are used in farming and forestry to kill weeds, ants, termites, insects, rats and mice, to protect wood from decaying, in electronic industry. In veterinary medicine these are used to deworm. It is also used in herbal and traditional remedies.

Arsenic oxide, arsenious trioxide or white arsenic is often used for homicidal purposes in India. It is colourless, tasteless and odourless. 0.2 gm is sufficient to kill an adult. It is cheap and readily available. Symptoms mimic cholera or gastroenteritis and therefore easily misdiagnosed. However arsenic can be easily detected in hair and nails years after death.

Coloured salts of arsenic are also available such as acid cupric arsenite (Scheele's freen), oceto-arsenite of copper (Paris green), Arsenic bisulphide is red sulphide of arsenic while arsenic trisulfide is yellow in colour.

Arsenic salts are used in arts, calico printing, in artificial flowers as fly paper and in preservation of timber against white ants.

It is irritating to the skin, lungs and gut. If swallowed or it comes in contact with skin it can be problematic. Chronic poisoning occurs from repeated doses of small amounts as **it is cumulative.**

People exposed to arsenic fumes or dust are at risk of chronic arsenic poisoning. They need to wear protective clothing.

Signs and Symptoms of Toxicity

These salts exert irritant effect locally and dilate capillaries but also exert effect on CNS.

If swallowed:

Sudden pain in abdomen along with vomiting occurs that is followed by severe diarrhoea.

Sore throat, dry mouth and thirst.

The breath may smell of garlic.

Signs of shock may be present, pulse is weak and rapid cold clammy skin, low blood pressure and even blue skin.

These symptoms may be followed by delirium and sudden unconsciousness.

Convulsions.

Differences between arsenic poisoning and cholera (gastroenteritis)

Features	*Arsenic poisoning*	*Cholera*
Pain	Pain in throat and abdomen	None
Vomiting	Uncontrollable vomiting. Vomitus contains bile and streaks of blood	Watery and is not blood stained
Diarrhea	Diarrhea follows vomiting. Rice water stools initially followed by mucus and blood. Burning sensation in rectum.	Diarrhea is initial symptom followed by vomiting. No burning pain in rectum
Voice	Hoarse and husky in later stages	Husky from the beginning
Conjunctival	Inflammed margins of eye lids are red	Normal
Circumstantial evidence	Sudden onset in an individual or a family simultaneously in locality	Usually many patients suffer

Arsenic neuropathy differs from lead neuropathy as it is usually more painful and is associated with sensory manifestations. **Arsenic is teratogenic in nature and chronic exposure can result in lung and skin cancer, leukemia etc.**

Arsenic gas is highly toxic and differs from arsenic as it causes severe hemolysis and renal failure. BAL is not effective and haemodialysis need to be done.

Management

Gastric lavage is recommended supportive treatment is given.

Chronic Poisoning

Is usually seen as occupational hazard.

Chronic generalised weakness.

Loss of appetite, nausea and vomiting.

Diarrhoea as well as constipation are possible.

Skin rashes.

Thickening of skin on the palms.

Hoarse voice and sore throat.

Management

On Ingestion

Gastric lavage

Activated charcoal in usual doses.

Adult: 30-100 gm once and **repeat without purgative** every 4-6 hours in a dose of 0.5 gm/kg.

Child: 15-30 gm orally mixed with water (single dose) and repeat 0.25 gm/kg every 4-6 hours.

For treatment of convulsions:

Diazepam:

Followed by:

Phenytoin (To treat seizures if diazepam fails)

Correct hypovolumia and electrolyte imbalance.

Chelation therapy: Chelation therapy should be started as soon as possible. Administer 2-3 dimercaprol in dose of 3-5 mg/kg IM every 4-6 hourly for 24 hours or till serum arsenic levels become less than 50 μg/L.

ASTEMIZOLE (Antihistaminic—H_1 Blocker)

Information on the effects of overdosage is limited.

Symptoms

According to case reports with ingestion of 200 mg astemizole the following symptoms were seen:

Drowsiness, Prolongation of QTC interval and Ventricular tachycardia.

In some cases Torsade de pointes with or without giant U waves had been seen.

Management

Put the patient under observation for atleast 12 hours.

If QT interval is prolonged, cardiac monitoring is required.

Intravenous magnesium sulphate appeared to abolish ventricular ectopic beats and tachycardia in one man.

ATROPA BELLADONA (Plant Containing Atropine)

Atropa belladona has shiny black berries and is accidentally ingested by children in India. It is used by practitioners of traditional systems of medicine. Overdose toxicity can result in patients consuming these drugs.

Pharmacologically—the active principle—atropine has strong anti-cholinergic activity.

Symptoms of Toxicity

Initially: Blurred vision, mydriasis, dry flushed skin, hallucinations, agitation, disorientation and delirium.

Later: Hyperthermia, tachycardia, decreased bowel sounds, urinary retention and seizures.

Death occurs due to respiratory failure and cardiovascular collapse.

Management

For treating hypertherima body should be sponged with cold water.

Ice bags and alcohol sponges should be given.

Induce emesis or do gastric lavage.

Give gastric lavage

Activated charcoal in usual dose with purgative

IV dextrose (50%) and multivitamin.

Specific antidote: Physostigmine.

Trial dose: 2 mg IV given slowly over 5 min. A second dose of 1-2 mg may be attempted if no reversal has occurred.

Therapeutic dose: 1-4 mg IV slowly over 5-10 min. should be repeated if anticholinergic symptoms recur.

(Do not give physostigmine as a continuous drip. Monitor anticholinergic toxidrome i.e. hyperthermia, mydriasis, dry flushed skin and hallucinations).

Diazepam: 5-10 mg IV slowly over 2-3 min (maximum rate 5 mg/min). Repeat every 10-15 min, if required. Maximum dose 30 mg.

Propranolol:

Adult: 10 mg/dose IV infusion at the rate less than 1 mg/min.

ATROPINE (Anticholinergic Agent)

Atropine drops are put into the eyes, as drops or as ointment during eye examination or to treat some eye conditions. It may be given sometimes to treat some stomach problems like ulcers. Atropine affects heart, eyes, gut and bladder.

Clinical Picture and Management

Same as with other **Atropa Belladona** *(Refer page 67)*.

AZINPHOS (Organophosphorus Insecticides)

It belongs to organophosphorus group of widely used pesticides that may cause acute or chronic poisoning. It is a highly toxic organophosphorus compound with a LD_{50} of 10 mg/kg.

Signs, Symptoms and Management

Same as of any other **Organophosphorus compound** *(Refer page 219)*.

B

BARBITURATES (Sedatives, Hypnotics, Anti-convulsant)

Classification

Ultra short acting (theopentone, hexa barbitone, methohexitone). These are used as anaesthetic agents.

Short acting barbiturates such as butobarbitone, secobarbitone and pentobarbitone were used as hypnotics.

Long acting barbiturates are phenobarbitone and mephobarbitone. These are used as antiepileptic agents.

From toxicological point of view classification into short long is not useful (except phenobarbitone) as CNS depression is comparable for all barbiturates.

Signs and Symptoms

CNS: Drowsiness and ataxia are early features. These are followed by coma, hypotension and respiratory depression. Deepening of coma is indicated by loss of gag and cough reflexes. Respiration becomes shallow though rate is not reduced. Skeletal muscle tone is reduced, but there is no change in size of pupils.

Hypothermia develops in 6% of patients may develop blisters on skin. Blood levels correlate with symptoms except in chronic users and in patients who may consume these drugs with other CNS depressants such as alcohol or benzodiazepines.

During recovery plasma levels in initial phases fall gradually and then decline rapidly as enzyme induction occurs.

Management

Repeated doses of activated charcoal to be given.

Gastric emptying is advocated if patient presents within 2 hours of ingestion or patient is unconscious. Supportive therapy can save lives. Forced alkaline diuresis helps to promote excretion.

Haemodialyses is indicated if barbiturate levels are over 6 mg.

Charcoal haemoperfusion gives good results.

BARIUM CARBONATE

Symptoms

Nausea, vomiting, diarrhoea, paresthesias, hypokalemia resulting in profound skeletal muscle weakness. Respiratory failure results in death.

Management

Gastric lavage: 150-200 ml of lukewarm water/saline with magnesium sulphate.

Furosemide: Administer (40 mg) IV furosemide to increase barium elimination.

Potassium chloride: Administer IV potassium chloride according to serum K^+ levels.

BENDIOCARB (Carbamate)

It is used as insecticide. It acts by reversibly inhibiting cholinesterase.

Clinical Picture and Management

Same as of other **Carbamates** *(Refer page 87)*.

Oximes are Contraindicated.

BENFURACARB (Carbamate type Insecticide)

Symptoms and Management

Same as of other **Carbamates** *(Refer page 87)*.

BENZALKONIUM CETRIMIDE (Detergent)

It is a cationic detergent and is widely used as antiseptic in households, food industry and hospitals. **It is highly toxic.**

Symptoms

Local effects—Irritant

On ingestion:

Nausea, vomiting and diarrhoea are common. 10% solution or solutions of higher concentrations cause corrosive lesions of upper GI.

B Systemic toxicity includes CNS manifestations in the form of coma, convulsions, muscle weakness, respiratory failure, metabolic acidosis and renal failure.

Management

In the eyes:

Wash the eyes for at least 15-20 minutes with water.

On the skin:

Immediately remove contaminated clothes and wash skin with water.

Upon ingestion:

In case of ingestion of concentrated solution, the airway should be monitored for evidence of swelling and intubated if considered necessary.

Copious amounts of water or milk should be offered to the patient to dilute the ingested chemical.

Gastric lavage should be performed cautiously.

Forced emesis should not be done because of risk of corrosion.

Activated charcoal/cathartics are not effective.

BENZENE

It is present in automobile fuel and is used in many industrial processes. If workers do not use proper protection or safety measures, working with this chemical can prove dangerous.

Chronic exposure: Seen in industrial workers because it is used in many industrial processes and is also present in automobile fuel. It is not usually a household product.

Signs and Symptoms of Toxicity

Acute exposure of benzene:

Brain and heart get affected. The kidneys and liver may also be affected during acute exposure.

Euphoria, weakness, headache, nausea, blurred vision, irritation to nose and eyes, incoordination of movements, tight chest and shallow breathing, signs of pulmonary oedema, irregular pulse, unconsciousness and convulsions. Acute exposure may cause sudden death.

If skin is exposed: Redness, dry skin and blisters.

If eyes are exposed: Pain, redness, watering and photophobia.

B

Management

Move the patient away from poisonous gases or liquid spills. Protect workers by making them wear breathing equipment and protective clothing. If the patient is unconscious or drowsy, lay him or her on one side in the recovery position.

Treatment is Symptomatic

Give fluids if needed. Maintain patency of airway and administer oxygen. Give diazepam if patient has convulsions.

BENZODIAZEPINES (Alprazolam, Diazepam etc.)

List of Benzodiazepines

Alprazolam
Bromazepam
Chlorazepate
Chlordiazepoxide
Clobazam
Clonazepam
Diazepam
Flumitrazepam
Flurazepam
Ketazolam
Loprazolam
Lorazolam
Lormetazepam
Medazepam
Nitrazepam
Oxazepam
Temazepam
Triazolam

Benzodiazepines used as hypnotics: Diazepam, flurazepam, nitrazepam, flunitrazepam, temazepam, triazolam and midazolam.

Used for antianxiety effect: Chlordiazepoxide, oxazepam, lorazepam and alprazolam.

Anticonvulsant: Diazepam, clonazepam and clobazam.

Elderly population as well as patients with asthma are likely to be more seriously affected.

Flurazepam, flunitrazepam and triazolam are relatively more toxic. Triazolam and flunitrazepam are short acting and produce rebound insomnia leading to increase in demand as well as dose. Flurazepam and quazepam

B are slowly eliminated (t½ = 85 hours) and frequent dosing can lead to toxicity.

Benzodiazepines potentiate toxicity of all CNS depressants e.g. alcohol, barbiturates etc. All produce psychological dependence. Many of these drugs have active metabolites that are responsible for hangover and impairment in machine handling.

Drugs	*Therapeutic dose in adults*	*Dose in children*
Alprazolam	0.25-1 mg upto 4 times a day	
Bromazepam	6-30 mg/day in divided doses	
Clorazepate	7.5-15 mg 2 to 4 times a day Maximum = 90 mg/day	
Chlordiazepexide	4-50 mg/3-4 times a day Maximum = 300 mg/day	Over 6 years-10 mg/6 hourly
Chlorazepate-dizodium	7.5-60 mg/day Maximum = 90 mg/day Maximum = 60 mg/day	Between 9-12 7.5 mg/twice a years day
Diazepam	2-10 mg/day orally-3-4 times Maximum = 30 mg/day I/V	0.1-0.3 mg/kg every 2-4 hours For status-0.2-0.4 mg/kg I/V
Istazolam	1-12 mg orally at bed time 0.5-1.0 mg in elderly	Not approved forchildren
Flurazepam	15-30 mg orally at bed time	
Corazepam	15 mg/day orally 0.05 mg/kg I/M to a maximum of 4 mg 2 mg or 0.044 mg/kg I/V	
Lormetazepam	1 mg at bed time 2 mg preoperatively	
Medazepam	10-12 mg/day in divided doses	
Midazolam	1 mg I/V maximum 2.5 mg	
Nitrazepam	2.5-10 mg/day	
Oxazepam	10-30 mg TDA or QID	
Pinazepam	5-20 mg/day	
Prazepam	10-60 mg/day in divided doses	
Quazepam	7.5 to 15 mg/day	
Temazepam	15-30 mg/day	
Triazolam	0.125 to 0.5 mg/day orally	

MAXIMUM TOLERATED EXPOSURE

Specific Substance

Alprazolam: Patients with 20-60 mg presented with mild lethargy and combativeness.

Chlordiazepoxide: Concomitant ethanol and chlordiazepoxide (levels 2-25 mg/l) ingestion produce more CNS depression than chlordiazepoxide (levels 2-15 mg/l) alone.

Diazepam: Ingestion of 500-2000 mg of this drug produced only minor toxicity.

Estazolam: Recovery from overdose (as high as 40 gm) of estazolam has been reported.

Flunitrazepam: 40 mg and above are toxic.

Flurazepam: 2.4 gms are toxic.

Lorazepam: 2.5-25 mg is associated with mild to moderate toxicity.

Oxazepam: 900 mgms produce grade I coma.

Triazolam: 2-20 mg produce toxic symptoms.

THERAPEUTIC CONCENTRATIONS

Diazepam

For anti-anxiety effect: 300-400 nanograms/milliliter.

For anticonvulsant effect: Greater than 600 nanograms/milliliter.

Flunitrazepam

In adult: 10 nanograms/milliliter is the minimal sedative concentration.

TOXIC CONCENTRATIONS

Bromazepam: 7.7 mg/L.
Chlorazepate: 0.7 and 5.1 micrograms/milliliter.
Chlordiazepoxide: 10 micrograms/milliliter.

Diazepam:

a. **Postmortem concentrations:** Diazepam concentrations ranged 0.004 to 64.0 micrograms/milliliter.
b. **Overdose concentrations:** N-Desmethyl diazepam concentrations ranged 0.10-13, 40 micrograms/milliliter.

Flurazepam:

a. Postmortem blood concentrations of Flurazepam: 5.5 micrograms/liter.

B b. N-1-desalkyl flurazepam: 0.73 micrograms/milliliter serum concentration.

Flunitrazepam:
In children: 0.1 milligram/kilogram.
In adult: Plasma concentration of 650 nanomoles/liter.

Midazolam: 2.4 micrograms/milliliter.

Nitrazepam: 200 nanograms/milliliter.

Temazepam: 885 to 14,000 micrograms/liter in fatal cases.

Symptoms of Toxicity

Mild: Drowsiness, ataxia and generalised weakness. Intensity of toxicity increases with age.

Moderate to Severe

CNS: Apathy, dizziness, lethargy, headache, vertigo, slurred speech, partial ptosis, nystagmus, response to verbal stimuli may remain intact. Hypotension and respiratory depression.

GIT: Nausea, vomiting, epigastric discomfort. In case of epileptic patients, excess dose may produce convulsions.

Management

These are generally less toxic compounds unless associated with other CNS depressants e.g. alcohol or barbiturates or narcotics.

For suicidal purposes often these are taken in combination. Gastric emptying is not indicated except if large doses are consumed.

Repeated doses of activated charcoal are advocated.

Hypotension is treated conventionally.

Assisted ventilation may be required in deeply comatosed patients.

Specific antidose: Flumazenil is benzodeazepine antagonist capable of reversing even serious toxicity due to these drugs. It is reserved for serious cases only (deep coma).

Half life of flumazenil is shorter than most benzodiazepines. I/V infusion (2 mg/hour) is indicated in toxicity due to long acting benzodiazepines **(Flurazepam** and **quazepam).**

Dose: 0.2 mg I/V given over 30 seconds. If consiousness is not regained in 60 seconds administer 0.3 mg I/V of flunazemil followed by another dose of 0.5 mg I/V given after 60 seconds of second dose.

Except in profound coma maximum total dose should not exceed 3.0 mg in one hour.

If abolishes hypnotic, psychomotor, cognitive and EEG effects of benzodinazepines 1-3 mg is sufficient to reverse coma due to benzodiazepines. In patients who partially respond to 3 mg dose a total dose of 5 mg is justified.

But failure to respond to 5 mg of flumazenil over 5 minutes excludes possibility of toxicity due to benzodiazepines.

Half life of flumazenil being short, the dosage needs to be repeated in the responders and patients must be observed for next 12 hours.

Flumazenil has anxiogenic activity and can precipitate convulsions in patients on chronic treatment with benzodiazepines, therefore patient should be monitored closely.

Adverse effects of flumazenil can be minimised by correcting hypoxia, severe hypotension and arrhythmias before its administration.

Caution must be exercised in using flumazenil in patients of epilepsy, or those suffering from cardiac toxicity or toxicity of tricyclic anti-depressants.

Flumazenil has short half life, so should be given for 24 hours even after patient has recovered.

Forced diuresis, hemoperfusion and dialysis not helpful.

Toxicity of benzodiazepines increases if taken with alcohol or other CNS depressants. Haemodialysis may be undertaken in mixed toxicity provided the second drug is dialysable.

BETA-BLOCKERS IN INDIA

Beta-blockers in India (Trade Names)

	Trade names
Atenolol	Aloten, Altol, Atcardil, Atelol, Aten, Atenoera, Beta-card, Beten, Catenol, Hipres, Lonol, Presolar
Labetalol	Normadate
Metoprolol	Betaloc, Lopressor, Metocard, Metrozide
Oxprenolol	Trasicor
Sotalol	Sotagard
Timolol (for glaucoma)	Glaucare, Glucomol, Iotium

B These drugs are often used to treat hypertension, angina pectoris and cardiac arrhythmias. Toxicity occurs due to accidental/intentional overdose.

Symptoms

Congestive cardiac failure is precipitated. Most of these drugs cause AV block and arrhythmias. In asthmatics, these drugs will worsen bronchospasm.

Chronic use produces fatigue and muscle cramps. These drugs prevent correction of hypoglycemia by adrenergic and cause hypoglycemia that is symptomless. Cold extremities and absent pulses may be observed in a few patients.

Management

Stop the drug. Manage symptomatically. For correction of arrhythmia glucagon can be given.

BHANGBALL STALKS OF PLANT BHANG IS TAKEN AS SHARBAT OR IN SWEETS. IT CONTAINS 15% CANNABIS

Fatal dose is 10 gm/kg body weight.

Symptoms of Toxicity and Management

Same as with other **Cannabis** *(Refer page 90)*.

BHC (Organochlorine)

It is widely used as a pesticide in agriculture, insect control and malarial control programs. It is moderately toxic among organochlorines with animal oral $LD_{50} > 50$ mg/kg. Estimated adult lethal dose is 10-30 gm and as little as 1 gm can produce seizures in a child.

Symptoms of Toxicity

Nausea, vomiting, confusion, tremors, obtundation, coma convulsions and respiratory depression.

Sudden onset of convulsions is a possibility but delayed and recurrent seizures can also occur.

Arrhythmias may occur due to myocardial sensitivity to catecholamines.

Management

The clothing should be removed and the whole body should either be sponged or washed with water and soap.

B

If seizures are present, place a spoon in the mouth of the patient to prevent injury to tongue.

Do not give oil/milk/cream orally.

Emesis is indicated only if patient approaches within 30 minutes of ingestion of organochlorine.

Gastric lavage is advisable.

Activated charcoal is indicated and can be repeated without purgative every 4-6 hours.

Ensure adequate oxygenation and undertake naso-phageal suction if necessary.

Give ventilatory support if required.

IV fluids should be given if required—the voulme should be determined by the condition of the patient.

For management of seizures:

Diazepam should be given in undiluted form and closely monitor blood pressure and respiration.

Maximum dose - 30 mg in adults and 10 mg for children above 5 years, 5 mg for under 5 years.

Followed by either Phenytoin (in usual doses).

or

Phenobarbitone.

Patient's blood pressure and ECG should be closely monitored.

Cholestyramine: 4 gms orally is given mixed in fruit juice every 6 hours. before meals.

Do not give epinephrine or atropine as these may lead to cardiac arrhythmias.

BISMUTH SUBNITRATE

Bismuth subnitrate is used as antidiarrhoeal and toxico-logical effects are primarly due to nitrate moiety.

Symptoms

Headache, skin flushing and orthostatic hypotension with reflex tachycardia.

Workers or patients regularly exposed to nitrates may develop tolerance and may suffer angina or myocardial infarction owing to rebound coronary vasoconstriction upon sudden withdrawal of the drug.

Treatment

If the patient is unconscious or drowsy, lay him or her on one side in the recovery position. Check breathing every 10 minutes and keep the patient warm.

B Maintain airway and assist ventilation if necessary. Administer supplemental oxygen.

Vasodilator overdose induced hypotension usually responds to supine positioning and rewarming of the patient. In case no effect is seen, manage as described below:

Fluid therapy must be instituted at the rate of 10-20 ml/kg.

Dopamine: Infuse 10-20 μg/kg/min.

On Ingestion: Administer activated charcoal if available. Ipecac induced emesis may be useful for initial treatment at the scene. Gastric emptying is not necessary for small ingestion if activated charcoal can be given promptly.

Symptomatic methemoglobinemia may be treated with methylene blue. It is indicated if patient has symptoms or signs of hypoxemia (e.g. dyspnea, confusion, chest pain) or methemoglobinemia > 30%.

Dosage of methylene blue (adults and children): 1-2 mg/kg (0.1-0.2 ml/kg of 1% solution) IV slowly over 5 minutes. May be repeated within 30-60 minutes. If no response occurs, do not repeat dosing.

Hemodialysis and hemoperfusion are not effective. Severe methemoglobinemia in infants not responsive to methylene blue therapy may require exchange transfusion.

BITTER ALMONDS (Plant Toxicity)

Bitter almond is seed of Prunus amygalis varamara belonging to family Rosaceae. Like sweet almonds it also grows in Kashmir. The volatile oil of bitter almonds is toxic as it contains hydrocyanic acid. It contains amygdalin—a toxic alkaloid. The oil is used in traditional systems of medicine.

Symptoms

Vertigo, vomiting, confusion, tachypnea followed by bradycardia, hypotension and CVS collapse.

Breath smells of bitter almonds.

Management

Activated charcoal is not effective. Stomach wash can be done after antidotal therapy. 100% oxygen is given through assisted ventilation.

Hyperbaric oxygen not recommended. Nitrites are given.

Amylnitrite (0.2 ml inhalation) every minute until I/V sodium nitrite is begun (10 ml of 3% solution). Gastric lavage with 158 gm of ferrous sulphate and 3 gms of citric acid dissolved in 1 liter of cold distilled water along with 60 gms of anhydrous sodium bicarbonate dissolved in 1 liter of distilled water is recommended.

Metabolic acidosis and electrolyte imbalance to be corrected.

BORAX, BORIC ACID AND SODIUM PERBORATE

Borax is used in some ant killers, wood preservatives, water softeners, eye drops, mouth washes and skin creams. Boric acid is also used in talcum powder. Sodium perborate is used as a bleach, cleaner for dentures and a water softener.

These are very poisonous chemicals but the amount in most household products such as detergents and ant killers is small. Individual may not be poisoned if these products are ingested in small amounts.

Chronic poisoning may occur from using mouthwash or boric acid over period of weeks, months or years.

However, skin creams or talcum powders containing boric acid may cause serious poisoning in infants and young children. Elderly people may suffer toxicity due to accidental swallowing of denture cleaning tablets.

Signs and Symptoms of Toxicity

Acute poisoning.

If swallowed:

Nausea, severe vomiting and diarrhoea.

Restlessness, agitation and convulsions.

Unconsciousness.

Signs of kidney failure may appear.

If eyes are exposed:

Stinging and a burning feeling may manifest.

Watery eyes.

Red swollen eyelids.

On the skin:

Itching and redness.

When the skin is exposed or there are cuts or scratches, the patient may also have signs and symptoms similar to those reported under ingestion.

Chronic poisoning:

Repeated swallowing or skin contact with these chemicals may result in:

Loss of appetite and loss of weight.

Vomiting and mild diarrhoea.

B A red skin rash, with peeling skin, particularly on the buttocks, palms and soles.
Hair loss.
Signs of kidney failure.
Convulsions.

Management

In case of ingestion:
Avoid inducing vomiting.
Administer water or milk orally.

In case of inhalation:
Patient should be shifted to fresh air.

In case of eye exposure:
Wash with large volumes of 0.9% normal saline or water repeatedly.

Avoid soap solution to wash eyes.

Wash affected skin with copious amounts of water or mild soap solution.

Do not give gastric lavage. Gastric suction should be done using soft nasogastric tube.

In case of airway compromise-endotracheal intubation should be done.

Give 100% humified oxygen with assisted ventilation.

IV fluids to be given if necessary.

Give vasopressors as and when required.

Administer appropriate antibiotics if chances of infection are there e.g. GI perforation.

Endoscopy should be done within first 24 hours to detect perforation and chest X-ray for detecting mediastinitis or GI perforation.

Laparotomy should be done (a) in case endoscopy reveals grade B burns, (b) if there is necrosis of oesophagus or stomach or (c) when clinical picture of GI perforation is evident.

BROMOPHOS (Organophosphorus compound)

It is widely used pesticide that may cause acute as well as chronic poisoning. It is relatively less toxic organophosphorus compound with an LD_{50} of 3750-8000 mg/kg.

Symptoms

Same as with other **Organophosphorus compounds** *(Refer page 219)*.

B

Treatment

Same as other **Orgenophosphorus compounds** *(Refer page 219)*.

BROMPHENIRAMINE (Anti histaminic)

It is an H_1 blocker used to treat allergy, travel sickness and cough. Its toxicity is common among children.

Symptoms of toxicity: Acute intoxication results in symptoms very similar to those of anticholinergic poisoning.

The usual effects are:

Drowsiness.

Dry mouth.

Headache.

Nausea.

Rapid pulse.

Retention of urine.

Confusion.

Hallucinations.

Unconsciousness.

Shallow breathing.

Some children may suffer from:

Wide pupils.

Tremors.

Excitement.

High temperature and warm skin.

Convulsions.

Management

If breathing stops, open the airway and give mouth to mouth respiration.

If the patient is unconscious or drowsy lay him or her on side in the recovery position and check breathing every 10 minutes.

If a patient is anxious, confused, very restless or aggressive or who has hallucinations he should be kept in a quiet dark place and protected from injury.

If there is urinary retention it may be necessary to catheterize the patient.

Ipecac-induced emesis is useful. Administer activated charcoal without purgative if it can be given within 30 minutes of exposure.

Maintain the airway and assist ventilation if necessary.

B Treat hyperthermia by external cooling with cold. This method is most effective. In case shivering occurs as a consequence of cooling, use diazepam (0.1-0.2 mg/kg IV) or midazolam (0.05-0.1 mg/kg IV) to prevent/treat it.

For treatment of convulsions:

Diazepam should be given in undiluted form and closely monitor blood pressure and respiration.
Maximum dose—30 mg/day in adults and 5 mg in children below 5 years of age and 10 mg for children above 5 years.

Followed by:
Phenytoin:
(10-15 mg/kg) slowly IV. Repeat 100 mg orally or IV every 6-8 hours. Patient's blood pressure and ECG should be closely monitored in adults and 15-20 mg/kg IV slowly in children. The rate of administration is 1mg/kg/min 1.5 mg/kg at every 30 minutes interval. Do not exceed the maximum dose of 20 mg/kg/day.
Or
Phenobarbitone in usual doses:
Monitor asymptomatic patient for at least 6-8 hours after ingestion.

BUTANE (Organic solvent)

It is a volatilate and inflammable organic solvent mainly used in laboratories. In house it is used as nail polish remover. It can be absorbed through the lungs, skin, GI tract. Poisoning in children is common.

Symptoms of Toxicity

Loss of consciousness, depressed rate of respiration and convulsions are the most common symptoms of toxicity.

Management

Patient should be evacuated from the toxic atmosphere (If butane is present in the air).

Clothes must be removed and the skin thoroughly washed.

Supportive measures like ventilator will be required if the patient is unconscious but there is no specific treatment. **Give symptomatic therapy.**

Prognosis

Recovery of consciousness may occur within a few hours but glucose tolerance may take few months to return to normal.

C

CALOTROPIS GIGANTEA (Madar, Akanda) AND CALOTROPIS PROCERA (Plant Toxicity)

It is a shrub that grows wild in all parts of India. There are two varieties. Caltropis gigantea with purple flowers and calotropis procera bearing white flowers.

C. gigantea and C. procera have purple and white flowers respectively. Leaves and stalk yield milky juice that contains active principles—**Calotoxin, calotropin, calactin, gingantin and escharin.** Juice when applied on skin produces bruises and blisters. If introduced into vagina it causes abortion.

Madar juice is used by tanners to remove hair from the hide. Application of juice in addition destroys offensive odour and imparts yellow colour to the hide.

In villages in India it is used for infanticidal purposes.

Symptoms

Symptoms are due to irritation of gastrointestinal tract. Causes acrid bitter taste and burning pain in throat and stomach. This is followed by salivation, stomatitis, diarrhea and dilated pupils.

In later stages it may produce convulsions, coma and death. Time between ingestion and death is usually 12 hours.

Management

Perform gastric lavage and administer activated charcoal without a purgative.

Administer milk and other demulcent drinks.

Morphine is given to treat excruciating pain.

Hypotension and shock are managed by I/V fluids, dopamine and assisted respiration.

CALOTROPIS (Plant Toxicity)

In folklore medicine juice is used to treat certain skin conditions and as a depilatory. Poultice prepared from leaves is used to treat pain—Root extract is used as emetic.

CAPSECUM (Chilly) PLANT

It belongs to family Solanaceae, has long tapering fruits which become red when ripe. Fruit has pungent odour, taste and contains number of seeds.

Capsicum annuum and capsicum fruitescers are too most common varietes in India. Fruits of capsicum annuum are larger than the other variety.

Capsicum is an alkaloid that is the active principle of the seeds.

Seeds are used in India as spice.

Symptoms

Contact produces irritation—lacrymation results if eyes get exposed. Ingestion of large quantities of chillies cause burning in mouth, abdominal pain, vomiting and diarrhea. Profuse salivation and sweating may result.

Management

On skin exposure—wash the area with 5% acetic acid (vinegar) or with cold water. In case of massive ingestion make the patient drink large volumes of cold water or ice cubes for relief of burning sensation in mouth.

Ranitidine can be given to reduce acidity in stomach.

Convulsions

Certain clinical conditions such as hypoglycemia and hypoxia produce convulsions. Drugs/agents producing hypoglycemia (insulin and oral hypoglycemia) therefore produce convulsions in toxic doses.

CNS agents such as **anticholinerfics sympathomimetics, MAOIs, opioid analgesics, mefenamic acid atenolol, antidepressants, phenothiazines, flupenthixol, Halothane, Lignocaine, Isoniazid, Indomethacin, Katamine, Maprotiline, Oxacillin, Penicillin, Propandid, Ticarcillin and Vincristine C** also produce convulsions.

Noise and painful stimili can precipitate convulsions in these individuals. Therefore, nursing care should be accordingly convulsions are treated by administering diazepam 5-10 mg I/V is given and repeated, if needed.

C

CARBAMATES (Physostigmine, Neostigmine, Pyridostigmine, Edrophonium, Donepezil, Carbaryl, Propoxur)

Aldicarb	Bendiocarb Benfuracarb	Carbaryl Carbofuran Carbosulfan
Ethiofencarb	Methiocarb Methomyl	Oxamyl
Pirimicarb Propoxur	Thiofanox	

Insecticides with Carbamates as active agent

Trade name/Brand name	Active principle
BPMC 5 DEC	Fenobycarb 50 EC Febicarv
Tagwin 50% WDP	Carbaryl 50%

Classification according to degree of toxicity

Highly toxic	*Trade names*
Aldicarb	
Aprocarb	Baygon
Carbufuran	
Moderately toxic	
Carbaryl	Sevin
Primicarb	
Propoxicr	Hit spray
Organochlorines	
Highly toxic	
Endrin	
Moderately toxic	
Aldrin	
Chlordane	
Dieldrine	
Endosulfan	
Luidane	Gammaxane
Aldicarb	
Bendiocarb	
Benfuracarb	
Carbaryl	
Carbofuran	
Carbosulfan	
Ethiofencarb	

Contd...

Contd...

C

Methiocarb
Methomyl
Oxamyl
Pirimicarb
Propoxur
Thiofanox

Symptoms are due to excess of acetylcholine in system. Carbamylated enzyme is much slower to hydrolyse as compared to acetylcholine cholinesterase, but the reaction is relatively faster than the phosphorylated enzyme (organophosphorus compounds).

Thus effects are reversible and half life of reactivation of carbamylated enzyme is about 30 minutes and is far less than that of synthesis of fresh enzyme.

Autonomic effects include bradycardia hypotension, excessive secretions (lacrymation, salivation and awea-ting) along with severe bronchoconstriction.

There is hypermotility of gastrointestinal tract and decrease in intraocular tension.

Muscle fasciculation is followed by muscle paralysis.

Management

Gastric lavage with 5% sodium bicarbonate or potassium permagnate is given.

Remove individual from the contaminated area and wash skin thoroughly as these agents are absorbed from the skin and lumps.

Shock is treated with I/V drip and dopamine. Atropine sulphate 2 mg I/M and is repeated every 20 minutes till symptoms of atropinisation appear or rales disappear. Dehydration needs correcting with I/V fluids.

Enzyme reactivators—P_2AM or DAM other oximes are contraindicated.

CARBINOXAMINE (Antihistaminic)

It is H_1 blocker used to treat allergy, travel sickness and cough. It is often kept in home and children can easily get hold of it, as a result, its toxicity is common among children.

Clinical Picture and Management

Same as with other **Antihistaminics** *(Refer page 61)*.

CENTEPEDS

Belong to family Myriopoda class of arthropods. These have long segmented bodies with numerous pairs of legs. These can inflict painful bites associated with erythema, edema and sometimes regional lymphangitis.

Management

Wash the bite site with soap. To relieve pain analgesics (NSAIDS) can be adminstered.

CERBERA ODOLLAM (Ordeal tree or Tangena nut) Plant Toxicity

It is small tree found in Kerala which bears fruits resembling unripe mangoes-accidental poisoning therefore occurs.

Kernel stone of the fruit contains toxic glycoside-cerebrin—which produces symptoms like oleander.

Suicidal cases are often reported with this plant in Kerala.

Symptoms and Management

Gastric lavage followed by symptomatic treatment.

CALCIUM CHANNEL BLOCKERS

Trade Names of Calcium Channel Blockers

	Brand names
Diltiazem	Angizem, Cardem, Dicard, Dilcardia, Dilgard, Dilgina, Dilzem, Masdil, Nengil etc.
Nifedipine	Angibloc, Beta-mcardia, Calcigard, Cardules, Depicor, Depin, Myogard, Nicardia, Nifedin, Niflat, Nilol.
Verapamil	Calaptin, Cordilox, Harteze, Isoptin, Vasopten.

These drugs are given for treating angina, hypertension and cardiac arrhythmias.

Verapamil produces constipation, vertigo, bradycardia, heart block, congestive heart failure and hypotension. Rarely it may cause cardiac asystole.

C

Diltiazem: It can precipitate congestive cardiac failure and causes AV block if given with either beta blockers or digitates.

Amlodipine and felodipine are less likely to cause bradycardia and AV block. These drugs produce vasodilation and hypotension.

Management

Stop the offending drug and treat symptomatically.

CETYLPYRIDINIUM (Detergent)

It is a cationic detergent and is widely used as antiseptic in house holds, food industry and hospitals. It causes unconsciousness and affects breathing because of its surfactant action.

Symptoms and Management

There is irritation:

In the eyes:
Wash the eyes for at least 15-20 minutes with water.

On the skin:
Immediately remove contaminated clothes.

Upon Ingestion:
In case of ingestion of concentrated solution, the airway should be monitored for evidence of swelling and intubated if considered necessary.

Copious amounts of water or milk should be offered to the patients to dilute the ingested chemical.

Gastric lavage should be performed cautiously. **Forced emesis should not be done because of risk of corrosion.**

Activated charcoal/cathartics are not effective.

CHARAS AND CANNABIS INDICA

It is the resinous exudate from the leaves, branches and stalks of Cannabis India. It is also known as **Hashish.** It is usually smoked and is the most potent amongst agents of cannabis. Fatal dose 2 gm/kg body weight.

Clinical Picture and Management

Symptomatic treatment given.

CHLORHEXIDINE

Symptoms and Management

Same as with other **Cetylpyridinium** *(Refer page 90)*.

CHLOROCRESOL (Disinfectant)

It is a phenolic compound and is widely used as a disinfectant in households, food industry and hospitals.

It is a strong irritant and may cause damage to mucus membranes if ingested.

Management

Same as with other **Cresol** *(Refer page 94)*.

CHLORPHENIRAMINE (Anti histaminic)

It is H_1 blocker used to treat allergy, travel sickness and cough. It is often accessible to children, as a result, its toxicity is common among children.

Clinical Picture and Management

Same as wtih other **Antihistaminics** *(Refer page 61)*.

CLAVICEPS PURPUREA (Ergot, mother of rye)

Claviceps purpurea is fungus that infests cereals particularly rye and barley. It invades interior of cereal resulting in black mass called sclerotium. Ergot is an important alkaloid of this fungus which produces toxicity when the contaminated rye is ingested. Ergotamine, ergotoxine and ergometrine are three important alkaloids of ergot. All of these alkaloids cause severe contraction of uterus resulting in abortfacient effect. Clinically ergotoxine is used to treat migraine, senile dementia and ergometrine is used to prevent/treat post partum haemorrhage.

Symptoms

Chronic use causes gangrene, abortions and certain neurological disorders such as hallucinations, ataxia and convulsions.

Management

Withdrawal of ergot consumption. I/V nitroprusside for treatment of gargrene with low dose heparin.

C

COAL GAS AND CARBON MONOXIDE

Clinical Symptoms of Carbon Monoxide-poisoning at Different Levels of Blood Carboxyhaemoglobin

Carboxyhaemoglobin level	*Symptoms*
10-20%	Dyspnea on exertion, mild frontal headache
20-30%	Increase in dyspnea, severe headache
30-40%	Vertigo, blurred vision, confusion and nausea
40-50%	Weakness trismus, muscle spasms, vomiting and tachypnea
50-60%	Convulsions, respiratory failure, coma and death.

Leaking of coal gas from pipes specially if the rooms are also ill ventilated. Carbon monoxide is the main constituent of coal gas responsible for poisoning coal gas contains 0.46% of carbon dioxide.

COCAINE

It is obtained from a plant called Erythroxylon cocca. It was used as local anaesthetic, but because of its abuse liability, now it is not used clinically.

Symptoms

CNS: Insomnia, euphoria, talkativeness, restlessness, confusion, delirium, hallucinations, paranoia are prominent symptoms. Headache, convulsions, transient ischemic attacks are also reported. Patient has dilated pupils giving rise to photophobia.

CVS: Tachycardia, peripheral vasoconstriction, myocarditis, arrhythmias and MI can occur. ECG shows sinus tachycardia with impaired cardiac conduction (due to local anaesthetic activity), tachypnea, facial flushing, sweating and tremors.

GI: Nausea and vomiting.

Serious vascular, cardiac and neurological complications are known to be associated with cocaine and related products.

Miscellaneous: Rhabdomyolysis myoglobin urea and coagulopathies have been reported.

Cocaine body packer syndrome: It is a condition that occurs in individuals who swallow condoms, balloons filled with cocaine with a view to smuggle this agent. The rupture of these agents, in individuals can lead to cocaine intoxication. These objects can be detected on X-rays.

Differential diagnosis: Clinical picture due to amphetamines, anticholinergic and phencylidine toxication is similar to that produced by cocaine. However, this can be differentiated by the following features—Amphetamine lacks local anaesthetic activity and its actions last longer than cocaine. Phencylidine, though produces sympathomimetic activity, does not produce dilation of pupils. On the contrary pupils are small sized and there is multidirectional nystagmus with encephalopathy. Anticholinergic drugs produce dry skin whereas patient of cocaine intoxication has clammy skin.

Management

Maintain proper airway.

If consciousness is impaired adequate ventilation is clearly imperative.

Activated charcoal in usual doses is found to be helpful.

Hypoxia and metabolic acidosis to be corrected if required.

Convulsions and agitation: Convulsions are managed by diazepam.

Hypertension is controlled by labetalol 10-20 mg IV given at a rate of 2 mg/min. Further dose is adjusted according to response but maximum dose should not exceed 200 mg/day.

Labetalol should be avoided because betablockers can cause paradoxical increase in blood pressure. ECG shows signs of ischaemia as beta blockers potentiate coronary vasoconstriction.

Arrhythmias: Extreme tachycardia responds to beta adrenoreceptor blockers. Other cardiac arrhythmias may not be treated unless life threatening.

Forced diuresis should not be produced because diuresis can lead to serious trouble in patients with dysarrhythmias.

C

CORROSIVES (Strong Acids and Alkalies)

In case of doubt whether a patient has ingested acid or an alkali, pH of saliva can be checked with litmus paper (red for acids and blue for alkalies).

Symptoms and Management

Same as with other **Acids and Alkalies** *(Refer page 44, 49)*.

CRESOL (Antiseptic/Disinfectant)

It is a phenolic compound and is widely used as a disinfectant in households, food industry and hospitals.

Symptoms of Toxicity

It is a strong irritant and may damage mucus membranes. If ingested, it results in blood in stools and vomiting.

Management

In the eyes:
Wash the eyes for at least 15-20 minutes with water.

On the skin:
Immediately remove contaminated clothes and wash skin.

Upon Ingestion

Copious amounts of water or milk should be offered to the patient to dilute the ingested chemical.
In case of ingestion of concentrated solution, the airway should be monitored for evidence of swelling and intubated if considered necessary.
Gastric lavage should be performed cautiously. **Forced emesis should not be done because of risk of corrosion.**
Activated charcoal/cathartics are not effective.
Symptomatic treatment given.

CYCLIZINE (Antihistaminic)

It is H_1 blocker used to treat allergy, travel sickness and cough. It is often kept in home in places where children can easily get hold of it. As a result, its toxicity is common among children.

Clinical Picture and Management

Same as with other **Antihistaminics** *(Refer page 61)*.

D

DDT POWDER AND ITS ANALOGUES (Aldrin, Dieldrin) (Organochlorines)

It is widely used as a pesticide in agriculture, insect control and malarial control programs. It is moderately toxic among organochlorines with animal oral $LD_{50} > 50$ mg/kg.

Fatal dose is 20 gms.

Fatal period = 6 hrs.

Symptoms of Toxicity

Nausea, vomiting, confusion, tremors, obtundation, coma seizures and respiratory depression.

There can be sudden onset of convulsions.

Arrhythmia may occur owing to increased myocardial sensitivity to catecholamines.

In severe poisoning: Myoclonic jerking movements, generalised tonic clonic convulsions followed by coma, respiratory depression and death.

Management

If the chemical has been swallowed **do not give oil/milk/ cream orally.**

Wash the skin and the eyes and remove contaminated clothes.

Ensure adequate oxygenation and undertake naso-pharyngeal suction if necessary. Give ventilatory support if required.

Emesis is indicated only if patient approaches hospital within 30 minutes of ingestion of organochlorine.

Gastric lavage is advisable between 30 minutes to 3 hours.

Activated Charcoal needs to be given

IV fluids should be given if required—the voulme to be determined by the condition of the patient.

For management of seizures:

Diazepam followed by either phenytoin or phenobarbitone in usual doses.

D **Cholestyramine:** 4 gms orally is given mixed in fruit juice every 6 hours before meals.

Do not give epinephrine or atropine as these may lead to cardiac arrhythmias.

DEMETON-S-METHYL (Organophosphorus Compound)

It is an organophosphorus compound used as insecticide.

Symptoms and Management

Same as with other **Organophosphates compounds** *(Refer page 219)*.

DESIPRAMINE (Antidepressant)

It is **tricyclic antidepressant** but has lesser sedative, anticholinergic and adrenergic blocking actions and is better tolerated than imipramine.

Thus compared to other compounds in this group patient is likely to have less marked tachycardia and hypotension.

Clinical Features and Management

Same as of other **Tricyclic antidepressants** *(Refer page 58)*.

DETERGENTS (Soaps etc.)

Soaps contain sodium and potassium salts of fatty acids.

Di-alkyl, dimethyl ammonium chloride is present is fabric conditioners used to make clothes soft and fluffy.

Sodium silicate or sodium triphosphate are present in washing powders.

Sodium hypochlorite or sodium perborate act as bleaching agents.

Benzalkonium chloride—a toxic compound—is a detergent.

Accidental poisoning due to detergents is often reported in children.

Symptoms of Toxicity

Poisoning due to ingestion of detergent:

Local effects on ingestion: Burns on lips, oral mucosa, upper airway and oesophagus.

GIT: Drooling strider vomiting and gastrointestinal bleeding.

Oedema of upper airway, dyspnoea, wheezing, pulmonary oedema, pneumonitis and respiratory failure.

Exposure of eyes: Conjunctival irritation, corneal perforation, distortion of cellular membranes, loss of epithelium of cornea, conjunctiva and even lens may occur.

Skin exposure to detergents: Pain, redness, irritation and full thickness burns may occur.

Management

In case of ingestion:

Avoid inducing vomiting: Administer water or milk so that acid. as well as alkali can be diluted.

In case of inhalation: Patient should be removed from site of exposure and shifted to fresh air.

In case of eye exposure: Depending upon severity, irrigate with large volumes of 0.9% normal saline or water for 15 minutes or more.

Remove contact lenses.

Wash skin with water for atleast 6-8 hours.

Avoid Gastric Lavage

In case of airway compromise do endotracheal intubation. Give 100% humified oxygen for inhalation. Use respirator if available and if necessary.

Suction should be done using soft nasogastric tube.

Irrigate mouth frequently in patients who are cooperative and conscious.

IV fluids—The volume to be given should be determined according to the condition of the patient.

Vasopressors can be used if necessary.

Endoscopy should be performed within first 24 hours to detect absence or presence of perforation and chest X-ray for diagonsis of mediastinitis or GI perforation. Administer antibiotics if there is perforation.

Laparotomy should be done in case endoscopy reveals necrosis of oesophagus or stomach or when signs and symptoms of GI perforation are evident at the time of initial presentation.

DEXAMPHETAMINE (Amphetamine)

D Same as with other **Amphetamine** *(Refer page 57).*

DEXTROMETHORPHAN AND DEXTROPROPOXYPHENE (Opioids)

These drugs are used to treat pain, cough and diarrhoea. These drugs are opioids and therefore abused because of their euphoric activity.

People may become dependent on them. People taking opiates for a long time may need to take larger doses to get the same effects, and may take a fatal dose by mistake.

Symptoms of Toxicity

Sign and symptoms of acute poisoning usually begin within 20-30 min after oral ingestion and within minutes following parenteral administration.

Poisonous amounts can cause death within an hour particularly if taken with alcohol or other substances causing sedation. The patient becomes deeply unconscious, breathing becomes slower and may stop suddenly.

Shallow breathing with depressed respiratory rate, coma, pinpoint pupils, bradycardia, hypotension, hypothermia, convulsions, decreased urinary output and gastrointestinal motility are the likely symptoms. Respiratory depression may lead to hypoxia cyanosis, bronchospasm, pulmonary edema and respiratory arrest. Deaths in opioid poisonings are due to respiratory depression and cardiorespiratory arrest.

Management

Maintain proper ventilation and put the patient on artificial respiration.

Perform chemical analysis of urine, blood and a gastric output for presence of opioids.

Give IV fluids to maintain life line for drug administration.

Dopamine: 4-6 μg/kg/min IV for maintaining BP.

Perform gastric lavage to reduce absorption of opiates. This is useful even in cases where opioids have been taken parenterally.

Give **activated charcoal** in the form of slurry or mixed with sorbitol.

Diazepam to be administered only if convulsions develop.

D

In adults: 5-10 mg IV initially. Maximum rate of infusion—5 mg/min.

Repeat every 10-15 min. Maximum dose 30 mg/day.

Specific Antidote

Naloxone:

Adult and children dose: 0.4 to 2.0 mg IV bolus injection. Repeat as needed to reverse signs and symptoms of toxicity.

Neonates: Initial dose 10-30 μg/kg IV.

Alternatively continuous IV infusion of naloxone can be given—2/3 of initial as bolus and remaining amount as infusion. **Infusion is also indicated in poisoning with long acting opioids.** Monitor respiratory rate and CVP carefully during infusion.

Naloxone has short half life and needs to be repeated. Dose of naloxone needs to be titrated depending on clinical response.

If no response is observed after 10 mg of naloxone has been administered diagnosis of opioid induced poisoning is questionable.

DATURA ARBOREA, CANDIDA, METAL, ROSEL, STRAMONIUM, SUAVEOLENS (Plants with Anti Cholinergic Activity)

Poisoning due to this plant is common in India. All parts of the plant are poisonous but leaves and seeds are mostly used. **Hyoscine, hyosciamine and traces of atropine** are present in this plant. Both hyoscine and atropine block muscarinic receptors in the body. Hyoscine has sedative activity while atropine causes mild CNS stimulation. Seeds/leaves are used to stupify individuals.

Datura seeds resemble seeds of capsicum.

Differences between Datura and Capsicum (chilly) seeds

Features	*Datura*	*Capsicum*
1. Shape	Kidney shaped	Rounded and smooth
2. Colour and size	Brownish red in colour Size is bigger than capsicum seeds	Yellowish in colour
3. Odour	Odourless	Pungent
4. Taste	Slightly bitter	Pungent
5. Appearance	Double ridge of convex border	Single ridge

Contd...

Contd...

Features	*Datura*	*Capsicum*
6. Effect of heating	Seeds on burning do not yield irritant vapours	Seeds on burning yield irritant vapours
7. Instillation of watery decoction in eyes	Causes dilatation of pupils	Causes painful irritation with watering of eyes

D

Symptoms

There is stage of delirium followed by stage of coma. Initially voice becomes husky and later there is aphonia. Vomiting occurs immediately if crushed seeds have been consumed. There is dryness of mouth, dilatation of pupils, diplopia and photophobia. Light reflex is lost. Skin is hot and dry with rise in body temperature.

Burning and itching appear all over the body.

Swallowing becomes difficult due to dryness of throat and spasm of laryngeal muscles. **There is difficulty in urination.** Patient talks incoherently, grasps imaginary objects, pulls imaginary threads. Initially respiration is slow but then there is tachypnea.

Initially there is tachycardia but later pulse becomes weak and irregular.

Drowsiness and coma develops.

Death occurs due to cardiorespiratory failure.

100-125 seeds (1.2 to 1.23 gm) is fatal dose.

Management

Same as for **Atropine.** Strong solution of tannic acid or strong tea is a useful household antidote.

These plants have strong anti-cholinergic activity. Datura stromonium is employed by practitioners of traditional system of medicine for treating parkinsonism.

Symptoms of Toxicity and Treatment

Same as of **Atropa belladona** or **Atropine** *(Refer page 67).*

DIAZEPAM (Benzodiazepine)

It is a benzodiazepine that is often used to treat status epilepticus. It is also used as day time sedatives. It has an active metabolite, therefore with regular use accumulation of oxazepam (active metabolite) occurs. It is easily available and is often used for committing suicide. However safety margin is large.

D

Clinical Picture and Management

Same as with other **Benzodiazepines** *(Refer page 73)*.

Symptoms

Mild: Drowsiness, ataxia, weakness.

Moderate to severe: Apathy, dizziness, lethargy, slurred speech, partial ptosis, nystagmus, response to verbal stimuli may be intact. Hypotension and respiratory depression.

Management

Maintenance of patent airway and respiratory support are the mainstay of treatment.

If the patient is unconscious or drowsy, lay him or her on one side in the recovery position. Check breathing every 10 minutes and keep the patient warm.

DIAZINON (Organophosphorus Compound)

It belongs to organophosphorus group, widely used pesticide—that may cause acute or chronic poisoning. It is a moderately toxic with LD_{50} of 300-400 mg/kg.

Signs, Symptoms and Treatment

Same as of other **Organophosphorus compounds** *(Refer page 219)*.

DIAZOXIDE (Vasodilators)

It is a peripheral vasodilator and serious acute overdose toxicity seldom occurs.

Toxic levels: Minimum toxic levels have not been established.

Signs and Symptoms of Toxicity

CNS: Headache, Nausea, Dizziness, Weakness, Syncope, Ataxia.

CVS: Orthostatic hypotension, Warm flushed skin, Palpitation.

General Lethargy

Severe hypotension may result in cerebral and myocardial ischemia and acute renal failure.

There is skeletal muscle relaxation.

D

Management

If the patient is unconscious or drowsy lay him or her on one side in the recovery position raise food end of the bed. Check breathing every 10 minutes and keep the patient warm.

Administer assisted ventilation with oxygen supplementation if it is necessary.

Hypotension due to this drug usually responds to supine positioning. In case no effect is seen, manage as follows:

1. **Fluid therapy**—at the rate of 10-20 ml/kg.
2. **Dopamine**—Infuse 5-10 μg/kg/min.

Activated charcoal is effective. Gastric emptying is not necessary if activated charcoal is given promptly.

DICHLORVOS (Organophosphate)

It is an organophosphorus compound used as insecticide.

Symptoms and Management

Same as of other **Organophosphorus compounds** *(Refer page 219).*

DIEFFENBACTRIA (Plant)

Diffenbactria belongs to the P Araceae family of plants that are commonly grown for decorative value. Poisoning with this plant is most common in children.

Symptoms of Toxicity

Burning pain in lips and mouth, hypersalivation inflammation of buccal mucosa, swollen lips, tongue and palate. Respiratory obstruction, retrosternal pain and oesophageal necrosis.

Management

Symptomatic treatment is required.
Advise patient to suck ice and milk.

For immediate relief give antacid followed by Ranitidine:

Adult: 50 mg IV 6-8 hourly.

Children: 1.25-2 mg/kg/day. Maximum dose should not exceed 300 mg/day.

Endotracheal intubation (if possible) is advised but in serious respiratory obstruction tracheostomy can be done.

Corticosteroids: May be given but their value has not been assessed.

DIELDRIN (Organochlorine)

It is widely used as a pesticide in agriculture, insect control and malarial control programs. It is highly toxic among organochlorines with animal oral LD_{50} < 50 mg/kg. Estimated adult lethal dose is 2-5 gm.

Symptoms of Toxicity

Nausea, vomiting, confusion, tremors, coma, seizures and respiratory depression.

Sudden onset of convulsions not preceded by premonitory manifestations is possible.

Arrhythmias may occur owing to myocardial sensitivity to catecholamines.

Management

The clothing should be removed and the whole body should either be sponged or washed with water and soap.

Do not give oil/milk/cream orally.

Emesis is indicated only if patient approaches within 30 minutes of ingestion of organochlorine.

Activated charcoal is advocated. Gastric lavage is advisable if activated charcoal is not available.

Ensure adequate oxygenation and undertake nasopharageal suction if necessary.

Give ventilatory support if required.

IV fluids should be given if required—the volume to be determined by the condition of the patient.

For management of seizures: Give diazepam I/V followed by either Phenytoin I/V or Phenobarbitone IV.

Cholestyramine: 4 gms orally is given mixed in fruit juice every 6 hours before meals.

Do not give epinephrine or atropine as these may lead to cardiac arrhythmias.

DIESEL FUEL, NAPTHA, PETROL, TURPENTINE etc.

Poisoning due to these substances is common among children as these are easily available at home. Absorption through inhalational route is also possible. **Repeated hand washing with diesel has reportedly caused toxicity.**

D

Symptoms of Toxicity

Vomiting is common but not necessary. Diarrhoea is uncommon.

There may be excitement, but in severe poisoning drowsiness is seen which may lead to coma.

The most common complication of this poisoning is pulmonary troubles which occurs in almost 60% of the cases and results from aspiration of the poison into the bronchial tree. This results into cough, choking, wheezing and breathlessness.

Respiratory involvement is usually evident within few minutes after poisoning but in some cases it may be delayed for hours but never more than a day. Severe poisoning can cause hemorrhagic pulmonary oedema which is fatal within 24 hours. Pneumonitis mostly involves two or more lobes and is peripheral in distribution. **Fever and polymorph leukocytosis are common.**

Rare complications include pneumatocele formation, intravascular hemolysis and renal failure.

Diagnosis of hydrocarbon ingestion may be confirmed by finding a double gastric level on the X-ray of the abdomen taken in the erect position.

Management

Gastric emptying is advocated if sufficiently large amount of the poison has been ingested, but the patient should be sufficiently alert and be able to cough effectively and second the airway should be protected by cuffed endotracheal tube.

Indications for gastric emptying:

a. If the amount of ingested poison is more than 1 ml/kg of body weight. Or

b. If the solution contains another toxin (such as pesticide). Or

c. If signs of serious poisoning are evident.

Antibiotics should be given in patients who develop secondary bacterial infections.

If cyanosis is present, oxygen may be necessary. Intermittent positive pressure is indicated for patients with pulmonary oedema.

No specific antidote available.

DIETHYL TOLUAMIDE (Insect Repellent)

Diethyl toluamide is used on skin as an insect repellent to prevent bites from mosquitos and flies.

This agent can damage the brain due to acute poisoning.
Repeated use on the skin may cause rashes and dermatitis.
Children are mostly at risk if sprayed chronically on their skin or on bed.

Signs and Symptoms

If swallowed (small amounts):

Nausea and vomiting, abdominal pain, diarrhoea

Large amounts:

Unconsciousness and convulsions.
Signs of liver damage.
Tachypnea and tachycardia.
Bright yellow urine followed by oliguria.
Pulmonary oedema.

Management

Move the patient to fresh air and wash chemical off the lips.

Give lots of water to drink.

Wash skin.

Symptomatic treatment is given as no specific antidote is available.

DIETHYLPROPION (CNS Stimulant)

Causes sympathetic stimulation.

Symptoms

Euphoria, talkativeness, restlessness, tachycardia, peripheral vasoconstriction, tachypnea, tremors and dilated pupils may occur. Nausea, vomiting, facial flushing and generalised sweating are other features.
Confusion, delirium, hallucinations, paranoia are prominent.
Serious vascular, cardiac and neurological complications associated with cocaine and related products are also seen with this compound.
Hypertension produced by this drug may precipitate dissection of the arota , myocarditis, myocardial infarction, dilated cardiomyopathy, subarchnoid hemorrhage, cerebral infarction and transient cerebral ischaemic attacks. Hyperxia, convulsions, metabolic acidosis, impaired consciousness, impaired respiration, paranoid psychosis are often seen.

Management

Maintain proper airway, adequate ventilation is necessary specially if consciousness is impaired.

D

Arterial blood gas tension should be measured.

Hypoxia and metabolic acidosis need correction as and when required.

Activated charcoal: 30-100 gm orally in repeated doses should be given.

For treatment of convulsions: Diazepam should be given in undiluted form with close monitoring of blood pressure and respiration.

Followed by either phenytoin or phenobarbitone.

Hypertension should be controlled immediately with **labetol** given IV at a rate of 2 mg/min and further doses adjusted according to response. Maximum dose should not exceed more than 200 mg.

Propranolol as well as other beta blockers should be avoided because it can cause paradoxical hypertension and ECG show signs of myocardial ischaemia because beta blockers potentiate coronary vasoconstriction.

Arrhythmias: For extreme tachycardia beta adreno-receptor blockers. Can be given continously.

Note: Forced diuresis should not be produced because forced diuresis can lead to serious troubles in patient with arrhythmias.

DIFENCOUM (Rodenticide with anti-coagulant activity)

These chemicals are used to kill rats and mice. Warfarin is also used as a medicine to stop blood clotting. Swallowing a small amount does not lead to poisoning. Children can accidentally consume this poison.

Signs and Symptoms of Toxicity

If swallowed:

Bleeding from cuts.
Bruising and skin rashes.
Haematuria.
Haemophysis.
Blood in stools, showing that there is bleeding inside the gut.
Back or abdominal pain.

Management

Cholestyramine 4 gms orally in fruit juice every 6 hours before meals (cholestyramine orally enhances the elimination of this drug).

Administer vitamin K_1 (60 mg/day) along with infusion of fresh frozen plasma.

DIGOXIN (Cardiotonic Agent)

Digoxin is a cardiac glycoside and has narrow therapeutic range therefore therapeutic intoxication is common. Acute massive overdosage is relatively rare. However acute digoxin and digitoxin poisoning occurs occasionally in children and adults with normal hearts. Over dosage results due to ingestion but poisoning by the IV route has also been reported (due to wrong calculations of dose). **Digoxin is cumulative in nature.**

Ingestion of certain plants such as oleanders also produces same toxicity.

Symptoms

Nausea, vomiting, diarrhoea and extreme degree of uneasiness. Drowsiness, confusion and delirium are commonly reported. Pale cold extremities and hypotension indicate decreased cardiac output occurring due to arrhythmias.

Hypokalemia, sinus bradycardia, sinus arrest, sinoatrial block with PR prolongation, AV block, and AV dissociation, disturbances of ventricular rhythm-bygemini trigeminy and ventricular fibrillation, hypoxia and metabolic acidosis are usual features of digitalis toxicity.

Management

Supportive:

Oral activated charcoal: Should be given to interrupt entro-hepatic circulation of the drug and given until signs of serious toxicity disappear.

Cholestyramine is given to reduce further absorption of digoxin-4 gm orally four times daily.

Colestipol: 5 gm orally four times daily.

Atropine: 1-2 mg IV or as required.

ECG should be monitored and sinus bradycardia, ventricular ectopics, AV block and SA standstill are often reduced or even abolished by atropine.

Specific Antidote

D

Digoxin specific antibodies: Severe intoxication is an indication for treatment with **Fab fragments** of digoxin antibodies. However these antibodies also cross react with digitoxin and lanatoside C. The dose requirement is based on total body load of glycoside.

Total body load of cardiac glycoside can also be calculated by the use of either of the two methods described below:

1. If dose that is ingested is known multiply the amount ingested by 0.8 (bioavailibility factor).
2. If amount of digoxin ingested is unknown:

Determine plasma concentration of digoxin and calculate digoxin body load using following formula.

$$\frac{\text{Plasma conc. in ng/ml} \times 5.6 \times \text{body weight}}{1000}$$

$$\text{Fab dose} = \text{digoxin body load} \times 64$$

DIMENHYDRINATE, DIPHENHYDRAMINE, DOXYLAMINE (H_1 Receptor Blockers)

These are H_1 blockers used to treat allergy, travel sickness and cough. It is often kept in home in places where children can easily get hold of it. As a result, its toxicity is common among children.

Signs and symptoms: Acute intoxication results in symptoms very similar to those of anticholinergic poisoning.

The usual effects are:

Drowsiness.
Dry mouth.
Headache.
Nausea.
Rapid pulse.
Retention of urine.
Drowsiness and confusion.
Hallucinations.
Unconsciousness.
Shallow breathing.

In addition some children may suffer from:
Mydriasis, tremors, hyperpyrexia and convulsions.

Management

If the patient is unconscious or drowsy lay him or her on one side in the recovery position, and check breathing every 10 minutes.

If a patient is anxious, confused, very restless or aggressive or who has hallucinations keep patient in a quiet dark place protected from light, noise and injury.

If there is urinary retention it is necessary to catheterize the patient.

Maintain patency of airway and assist ventilation if necessary.

Treat hyperthermia by external cooling. This evaporative method is most efficient. Other methods include iced gastric/colonic lavage or total body immersion in ice-water. In case shivering occurs as a consequence of cooling, use diazepam (0.1-0.2 mg/kg IV) or midazolam (0.05-0.1 mg/kg IV) to treat it.

Administer activated charcoal in usual doses.

For management of convulsions:

Diazepam 5-10 mg I/V given in undiluted form with close monitoring of blood pressure and respiration.

Followed by Phenytoin (10-15 mg/kg IV) or Phenobarbitone 600-1200 mg or 10 mg/kg.

Monitor the patient for atleast 6-8 hours after ingestion.

DIMETHOATE (Organophosphorus Compound)

It belongs to organophosphorus group. It is widely used pesticide—may cause acute as well as chronic poisoning. It is a moderately severe toxic organophosphorus compound with an LD_{50} of 50 mg/kg.

Signs, Symptoms and Treatment

Same as of other **Organophosphorus compounds** *(Refer page 219).*

DIMETON (Organophosphorus Compound)

It belongs to organophosphorus group of pesticides that can cause acute as well as chronic poisoning. It is a **highly toxic** organophosphorus compound with an LD_{50} of 2.5-6 mg/kg.

Signs, Symptoms and Treatment

Same as of other **Organophosphorus compounds** *(Refer page 219).*

D

DIPHENOXYLATE (An Opioid)

It is an opioid with anti-diarrhoeal activity.

Symptoms

Shallow breathing with depressed respiratory rate, coma, pin point pupils, bradycardia, cardiac arrhythmias, hypotension, hypothermia, convulsions, decreased urinary output and gastrointestinal motility. Respiratory depression may lead to hypoxia, cyanosis, bronchospasm, pulmonary edema and respiratory arrest.

Management

Perform laboratory analysis for presence of altaloid of opium in urine, blood and a gastric lavage.

Maintain proper ventilation. Put the patient on artificial respiration if needed.

Administer IV fluids and **Dopamine:** 4-6 μg/kg/min IV.

Gastric Lavage

Activated charcoal: Slurry aqueous or mixed with sorbitol.

Adults dose: 30 to 100 gms.

Children: 10 to 30 gms.

Infant: 1-2 g/kg.

Specific antidote: Naloxone 1-2 mg IV. Repeat doses of naloxone as half life of naloxone is shorter than diphenoxylate.

DISOPYRAMIDE (Antiarrhythmic and Anticholinergic Agent)

It is a type 1a antiarrhythmic agent and in high doses reduces myocardial contractility and excitability with severe depression of cardiac conduction velocity. Repolarization is delayed resulting in a prolonged QT interval associated with polymorphic ventricular tachycardia. Disopyramide also has anticholinergic activity.

Toxic dose is 1 gm and serum disopyramide levels >2-4 mg/L are considered toxic.

Diagnosis: It is based on history, positive ECG abnormalities and specific signs and symptoms.

Signs and Symptoms of Toxicity

Cardiac toxicity Sinus bradycardia, SA arrest, prolongation of PR, QRS and QT intervals , Polymorphous ventricular tachycardia, Sinus tachycardia, Depressed myocardial contractility.

CNS Toxicity Seizures, Coma.

Dry mouth dilated pupils, delirium.

Respiratory arrest.

Management

Do not induce emesis as it may precipitate seizures.

Administer activated charcoal, if available.

Maintain patent airway. Assisted ventilation with oxygen supplementation may be necessary in some cases.

Treat hypotension on the folloowing guidelines:

a. Fluid therapy must be instituted at the rate of 10-20 ml/kg.
b. Dopamine. Infuse 6 µg/kg/min.

For treatment of convulsions

Give diazepam in undiluted form followed by either phenytoin or phenbarbitone.

Ventricular tachycardia should be managed by **Lidocaine/ Phenytoin.**

Dose (adults and children): 1 mg/kg IV bolus over 1 minute duration. This is followed by continuous intravenous infusion of 1-4 mg/min (20-50 µg/kg/min). A repeat dose (0.5 mg/kg IV) can be given if after the initial dose significant ectopy persists. **Do not use lidocaine if third-degree atrioventricular or intraventricular block is present.**

Or

Phenytoin

Loading dose: 15-20 mg/kg IV for adults and 1 mg/kg in children diluted in 50-150 ml of normal saline and given at the rate of 50 mg/min.

Maintenance dose: 5 mg/kg/day/as a single oral dose

Treat "atypical" or polymorphic ventricular tachycardia using overdrive pacing or **isoproterenol,** 1-10 mcg/min IV.

Monitor ECG and other vital signs for a minium period of 6 hours after normalisation.

Specific therapy: Hypertonic sodium bicarbonate:

Dose: 1-2 meq/kg rapid IV bolus and repeat injection every 5-10 minutes. If no response occurs on conduction or high degree atrioventricular block, insertion of cardiac pacemaker is the only other option.

Disopyramide can be removed by hemoperfusion as well as dialysis.

D

DIURETICS

Diuretics are used to rid body of extra fluid and are often used for treatment of oedema, hypertension, congestive cardiac failure and pulmonary oedema.

Loop diuretics (frusemide), is the most popular diuretic.

Osmotic diuretics: Mannotol is used to treat barbiturate poisoning, and to reduce intracerebral and intraocular tensions.

Glycerol can be used in dehydration as well as cardiac failure. It causes hyperglycemia.

Thiazides: Chlorthalidone, chloroxozone and clopamide are used as diuretics. These are ineffective if GFR is below 30 ml/minute.

Trade Names of Diuretics available in India

Thiazides	
Indapamide	Lorvas, Natrilixina
Chlorthalidone	Catapres, Diu
Hydroflumethlazide	Aldactide
Loop diuretics	
Freesemide	Lasix
Amiloride	
Speronolactose	Aldactide, Aldactone, Lactone
Triamunolone	Dytole

Symptoms of Toxicity

Mannitol can cause dehydration and can precipitate congestive cardiac failure.

Glycerol causes hyperglycemia.

Thiaznpides are likely to cause hyperglycemia, hyperuricemia, hypercalcemia and thyperlipidemia.

Loop diuretic—Frusemide: Can cause serious electrolyte and water disturbances as it causes excessive loss of water, sodium and potassium.

Patient may complain of weakness, fatigue, dizziness and cramps, orthostatic hypotension. In elderly it may precipitate urinary retention. I.V. and I.M. administration can cause sudden death due to cardiac arrest.

Frusemide can precipitate hepatic coma in presence of liver disease.

Rarely it can cause nausea, diarrhea and pancreatitis and acute hypoglycemia.

Very large doses cause transieent/peroxanent hearing loss without tinnitus.

Ethacrynic acid resembles frusemide in adverse reactions.

Potassium sparing diuretics—spironolactone: In presence of renal disease it can cause K^+ retention, drowsiness, increase in blood urea nitrogen and serum uric acid.

Management

Stop the offending drug. Correct water and electrolyte balance.

DISULFOTON (Organophosphorus Compound)

It belongs to organophosphorus group of pesticides that may cause acute or chronic poisoning. It is a highly toxic organophosphorus compound with an LD_{50} of 4 mg/kg.

Signs, Symptoms and Treatment

Same as of other **Organophosphorus compounds** *(Refer page 219).*

DOXAZOSIN (Vasodilator)

It is a peripheral vasodilator and serious acute overdose toxicity seldom occurs, but unlike diazoxide muscle relaxant activity is less.

Signs, Symptoms and Treatment

Same as with other **Diazoxide** *(Refer page 101).*

DOXEPIN (Antidepressant)

It is a tricyclic antidepressant. It has prominent sedative effect. Produces anticholinergic and cardiovascular toxicity along with convulsions.

Symptoms

Mild: Confusion, blurred vision, flushed dry skin and mucosa, sinus tachycardia and hypotension. Convulsions and anticholinergic activity can produce hyperthermia, rhabdomyolysis and multiple organ failure.

D

Moderate to Severe Poisoning

CNS: Agitation, visual and auditory hallucinations, myoclonus convulsions, ataxia, coma and death.

CVS: Hypotension, sinus tachycardia and other brady arrhythmias with prolonged PR and QRS and QT durations (>100 msec). Prolongation of QRS complex to or over 0.12 sec is indicative of cardiotoxicity.

Respiratory system: Respiratory insufficiency or arrest. Pulmonary edema occurs in severe poisoning, oesophageal spasm and respiratory acidosis can also occur.

Miscellaneous: Metabolic and urinary retention.

Death is due to cardiac arrest and circulatory failure.

Management

Ensure adequate oxygenation and maintain proper airway. Give assisted respiration if indicated. Nasophageal suction should be done whenever needed.

Induce emesis by mechanical stimulation of the back of the tongue.

To prevent injury to tongue put a spoon in patients mouth during seizures.

Perform gastric lavage with warm water or saline.

Activated charcoal is advisable.

For treating convulsions normal doses of diazepam and lorazepam are administered.

IV fluids: IV fluids are given if there is dehydration or hypotension.

Adult: 100 ml of 50% dextrose.

Child: 0.5-1 gm/kg of 25% dextrose.

Sodium bicarbonate: 500-800 ml IV by slow infusion (7.5% v.v.). Maintain blood pH at 7.5.

Thiamine: 100 mg IV to be given only if there is altered sensorium.

Dobutamine: 2.5-1.5 μg/kg/min infusion if hypotension is due to loss of ionotropy.

Potassium chloride: (If hypokalemia) is given with constant monitoring.

Special precautions to be taken:

Do not give antiarrhythmic drugs like quinidine and procainamide as they further decrease AV nodal conduction.

Do not give phenothiazines for treating hyperthermia and fever as their own anticholinergic action potentiates that of amitryptyline.

Avoid dopamine to treat hypotension as its adrenergic stimulatory effect increases arrhythmia and exacerbate peripheral beta adrenergic mediated vasodilation.

To prevent hypoxia and lactic acidosis treat convulsions immediately as these predispose to the development of life threatening ventricular arrhythmias.

After discontinuation of treatment patients on therapeutic support suffering from altered sensorium or arrhythmias should be closely monitored for the next 24 hours.

Use of phenytoin should be avoided as it increases the incidence of ventricular tachycardia.

Propranolol and verapamil should be avoided as they slow conduction velocity in heart and lower BP.

Potassium replacement during bicarbonate treatment should be done with caution as hyperkalemia may aggravate dopamine induced cardiac arrhythmias.

Clinical Picture and Management

Same as of other **Tricyclic antidepressants** *(Refer page 58)*.

E

ENDOSULFAN (An Organochlorine)

It is widely used as a pesticide in agriculture for insect and malarial control programs. It is highly toxic among organochlorines with animal oral $LD_{50} < 50$ mg/kg.

Symptoms

Nausea, vomiting, confusion, tremors, obtundation, coma seizures and respiratory depression.

Arrhythmia may occur owing to myocardial sensitivity to catecholamines.

Management

Same as with other **Dieldrin or Organochlorine** *(Refer page 218).*

ELDRIN (Organochlorine insecticide)

It is widely used as a pesticide in agriculture, insect control and malarial control programs. It is **highly toxic** among organochlorines with animal oral $LD_{50} < 50$ mg/kg.

Signs, Symptoms and Management

Same as with other **Organochlorines** *(Refer page 218).*

ETHANOL (Ethylalcohol, Alcohol, Beverages)

Varying amounts of ethanol are present in beer, wine and liquor. It is also found in a variety of colognes, perfumes, after-shaves, mouthwashes, food flavorings (e.g., vanilla, almond, and lemon extracts), pharmaceutical preparations (e.g., elixirs), and many other products. It is used for recreation and is usually taken along with other drugs in suicide attempts. **CNS depression is the main symptom of ethanol ingestion that is exacerbated by concurrent ingestion of other CNS depressants (barbiturates, benzodiazepines, anti-depressants and antipsychotics).**

E

Approximate Percentages of Alcohol in Beverages

Whiskey	40-50%
Brandy	40-50% (fatal dose 5-10)
Gin	40%
Sherry	18-22%
Beer	2-6%
Winé	10-15%

Ethyl Alcohol

Signs and symptoms of alcohol withdrawal:

1. Abstinence syndrome occurs in chronic alcoholic 6 to 8 hours after sudden withdrawal. There is nausea, agitation, tremors, headache and insomnia.
2. Alcoholic hallucinations are seen 24-36 hours after alcohol withdrawal. There can be both auditory and visual hallucinations.
3. Seizurs occur after 48 hours. These are clonic tonic in nature with or without unconsciousness.
4. Delirium tremens-usually develops 4-5 days after withdrawal and is characterised by confusion, delusions hallucinations, agitation, fever, sweating and hypertension. Death can also occur.
5. Wernicke-Korsakoff syndrome and beri-beri occur in **chronic alcoholics** and are due to deficiency of thiamine. Main features include mental confusion, nystagmus, ophthalmoplegie and unsteady gait. Pellagra may also manifest. Psychotic personality, polyneurity insomnia, illusions and hallucinations may be experienced by the patient.

Clinical picture of a drunk patient closely resembles a patient suffered concussion (head injury) therefore the two conditions need to be identified.

Features	*Drunkenness*	*Head injury*
1. Behaviour	Uncooperative and somewhat aggressive	Cooperative but dazed
2. Face	Flushed and warm, conjunctiva are congested	Pale and clammy face
3. Pulse	Rapid and bounding	Slow
4. Pupils	Are contracted during coma sluggish response to light	Contracted or unequal
5. Respiration	Smell of alcohol	Shallow, slow or irregular
6. Memory	Confused	Retrograde amnesia

E

Toxic Levels

According to the American Medical Association, ethanol concentration 100 mg/dl indicates a drunken state while less that 50 mg/dl is not considered legally drunk. Blood levels between 50 and 100 mg/dl do not indicate impairment of mental facilities. The level sufficient to cause deep coma or respiratory depression is highly variable and depends on the degree of tolerance of the individual. In novice drinkers, levels >300 mg/dl usually cause coma while chronic alcoholics may be awake with levels of 500-600 mg/dl or higher. The average serum ethanol concentration in fatal cases is about 400 mg/dl.

Symptoms

Mild-Moderate Intoxication:
Euphoria.
Mild incoordination.
Ataxia.
Nystagmus.
Impaired judgments and reflexes.
Boisterous/aggressive behaviour is common.

Signs and Symptoms of Severe Intoxication

Coma.
Respiration depression.
Pulmonary aspiration.
Small pupils.
Hypothermia, hypotension and decreased pulse.
Rhabdomyolysis (rare).

Chronic Alcohol Abusers Suffer from

GIT bleeding because of ulcers.
Esophageal varices.
Mallory-Weiss tears.
Pancreatitis.
Hepatitis, Cirrhosis, Hepatic encephalopathy.

Metabolic disorders such as Hypokalemia, Hypophosphatemia.

Hypomagnesema and Thiamine deficiency (Wernicke's encephalopathy, alcoholic ketoacidosis).

Alcohol withdrawal in chronic users is characterized by tremulousness, anxiety due to sympathetic nervous system overactivity and convulsions. Occasionally, this may progress to **delirium tremens**, which is a life threatening syndrome constituting severe autonomic hyperactivity, hyperthermia and delirium and has significant morbidity and mortality if untreated.

Diagnosis

Care is needed in making diagnosis as different diseases mimic clinical picture e.g., diabetic coma may be mistaken for severe alcoholic intoxication. Other conditions include hypoglycemia, head injury, hypothermia, meningitis or intoxication with other drugs or poisons.

Breath test is an unreliable guide. Therefore, concentration of ethanol in the blood, exhaled air or urine should be determined, especially for MLC purposes.

Ethanol abusers or alcoholics are likely to ingest ethanol substitutes such as isopropyl alcohol, methanol or ethylene glycol. Therefore poisoning due to methanol alcohol is common.

Specific Blood Levels

Ethanol levels should be determined in blood, urine or expired air. The concentration in expired air and urine is about 0.05% and 130% respectively of the concentration in the blood. An ethanol levels <300 mg/dl in a comatosed patient indicates that coma is of non alcoholic origin.

In case, facilities for ethanol levels are not available, it may be estimated by calculating the **OSMOLAR GAP**. To obtain serum ethanol levels (in mg/dL), multiply osmolar gap by 4.6, which can be calculated in following manner:

Osmolar gap = Measured – Calculated osmolality.

Calculated osmolality = 2[Na] + [Glucose]/18 + [BUN]/2.8

Na (serum sodium) in meq/L.

Glucose and BUN (urea nitrogen) in mg/dL.

Management

Prevent aspiration of fluid. Intubate and give assisted ventilation, if necessary.

Administer glucose.

Adults: 50%, dextrose, 50 ml (25 gm) IV.

Children: 25% dextrose, 2 ml/kg IV.

Administer **thiamine** to prevent abrupt precipitation of Wernicke's syndrome, especially in a chronic alcoholic. It should not be given routinely to children.

Dose of thiamine: 100 mg in the IV bottle (slow) or IM. Repeat every 6 hours. Doses as high as 1 gm over the first 12 hours have been given safely to patients with acute Wernicke's syndrome.

Correct hypothermia with rewarming.

Precautions

No specific antidote exists. However a few case reports of alcohol reversal with **naloxone** are available (2-5 mg IV), but **its use is not generally recommended.**

E

Emesis or gastric lavage is not indicated except if high volume has been ingested and the patient is conscious and cough reflex is present. It should be done in the following manner:

a. Ipecac induced emesis is helpful if given within few minutes of ingestion (e.g. accidental ingestion by children at home).
b. Gastric lavage is beneficial if performed within 30-35 minutes of ingestion.

Activated charcoal does not efficiently remove ethanol but should be given when there is a doubt of concurrent ingestion of other toxins.

Forced diuresis is not effective.

Hemodialysis efficiently removes ethanol but is generally not needed, as supportive care is sufficient in majority of cases.

ETHER (Solvent and Anaesthetic)

It is a volatilate and inflammable organic solvent mainly used in laboratories and in house (nail polish removal). It can be absorbed through the lungs, skin and alimentary tract. Poisoning in children is common though serious poisoning is rare.

Symptoms

Loss of consciousness, depressed rate of respiration, hyperglycemia and convulsions are the most common symptoms of toxicity.

Management

Patient should be evacuated from the atmosphere of ether vapours.

Clothes must be removed if soaked in ether and the skin thoroughly washed.

Supportive measures like ventilator will be required if the patient is unconscious. **There is no specific treatment.**

Treatment for hyperglycemia will not usually be required.

Recovery of consciousness may be within a few hours (if respiration is in order) though glucose tolerance may take few months to return to normal.

ETHIOFENCARB (Carbamates)

It is highly toxic carbamate compound used as pesticide. **It is not listed for sale in India.**

Clinical Picture and Management

Same as with other **Carbamates management** *(Refer page 87)*.

ETHION (Organophosphorus Compound)

It belongs to organophosphorus group of widely used pesticides that may cause acute or chronic poisoning. It is a moderately toxic organophosphorus compound with LD_{50} of 21-208 mg/kg.

Signs, Symptoms and Management

Same as with other **Organophosphorus compounds** *(Refer page 219)*.

ETHOPROPHOS (Oganophosphorus compound)

Is an organophosphorus compound used as insecticide.

Signs, Symptoms and Management

Same as with other **Organophosphorus compounds** *(Refer page 219)*.

ETHYLENE DIBROMIDE (Insecticide/Pesticide)

Used as insecticide, pesticide and as fumigant for grains.

Symptoms of Toxicity

In case of inhalation: Cough, pharyngitis, pneumonitis, pulmonary edema, dyspnea, cyanosis and respiratory depression.

In case of skin contamination: Skin irritation, burning, tingling, redness, swelling and blistering.

In case of eye exposure: Burning sensation, blurred vision, conjunctivitis and keratitis.

In case of ingestion: Headache, dizziness, weakness, fever, vomiting, diarrhea, hypoglycemia, metabolic acidosis, jaundice, ventricular fibrillation, shock, oliguria, anuria, seizures and coma.

Death due to this agent is either due to hepatic failure or respiratory depression.

Management

No specific antidote is available.

Supportive treatment is given.

Administer oxygen. Provide ventilation if required.

Give milk or water.

Activated charcoal is recommended.

Diazepam is given to treat convulsions. Following diazepam, either Phenytoin or Phenobarbitone needs to be given.

ETHYLENE GLYCOL

Ethylene glycol is main ingredient (upto 95%) in antifreeze. It is sometimes consumed as an alcohol substitute by alcoholics and children like its sweet taste.

Toxic dose: The approximate lethal oral dose of 95% ethylene glycol (e.g. antifreeze) is 1.5 mL/kg

Specific levels: Serious intoxication occurs when serum levels are >50 mg/dL. However, poisoning is not ruled out with lower levels as the parent compound may have already been metabolized. This is indicated by marked elevation in anion gap.

In case, facilities for measuring ethylene glycol levels are not available, it may be estimated by calculating the **OSMOLAR GAP:** To obtain serum ethylene glycol levels (in mg/dL), multiply osmolar gap by 6.2, which can be calculated by the following manner:

Osmolar gap = Measured - Calculated osmolality.

Calculated osmolality = 2[Na] + [Glucose]/18 + [BUN]/2.8.

Na (serum sodium) in meq/L.

Glucose and BUN (urea nitrogen) in mg/dL.

Signs and Symptoms

Seen in first 3-4 hours:

Inebriated state resembling ethanol ingestion.
Increase osmolar gap but not initial acidosis.
Gastritis with diffused abdominal pain and vomiting.

After 4-12 hours:

Severe intoxication:
Convulsions, Coma.
Cardiac arrhythmias.

Reversible renal failure.
Hyperventilation.
Anion gap acidosis.
Pulmonary and cerebral edema may occur.
Hypocalcemia occurs resulting in muscle spasm.

E

Management

Prevent aspiration of fluid. Assisted ventilation, if necessary, should be provided.

Ipecac induced emesis may be helpful if instituted within few minutes after ingestion of ethylene glycol (e.g. children at home).

Gastric lavage should be performed.

Activated charcoal is not helpful as it does not efficiently absorb glycols.

Administer glucose.

Adults: 50%, dextrose, 50 ml (25 gm) IV.

Children: 25% dextrose, 2 ml/kg IV.

For treatment of convulsions:

Diazepam followed by either Phenytoin or Phenobarbitone is recommended.

Administer sodium bicarbonate for correction of acidosis. Adjust dose according to requirement.

Dose: 500-800 ml IV (7.5/v/v). Maintain blood pH at 7.5 or higher.

Treat hypocalcemia with intravenous calcium gluconate or calcium chloride.

Calcium gluconate dose:

Adults: 10-20 ml of 10% solution.

Children: 0.2-0.3 ml/kg of 10% solution.

Calcium chloride dose:

Adults: 5-10 ml of 10% solution.

Children: 0.1-0.2 ml/kg of 10% solution.

To avoid cardiac effects intravenous calcium should be given very slowly.

Specific Therapy

Ethanol is the specific antidote for ethylene glycol poisoning and its use is warranted if:

1. Serum ethylene glycol levels are > 20 mg/dl or
2. There is positive history of ethylene glycol ingestion accompanied by osmolar gap > 5 mosm/L or

3. Anion gap acidosis is accompanied by glycol ingestion or presence of oxalate crystalluria.

Ethanol Therapy

Ethanol can be given orally or intravenously and the desired serum concentration of ethanol is 100 mg/dl (20 mmol/L). The intravenous loading dose should be given for a period of 20-30 minutes or longer.

Ethanol Dosing (Adults and Children)

Dose	*Intravenous*		*Oral*	
	5%	10%	50%	95%
Loading	**10 ml/kg**	**7-5 ml/kg**	**1.5 ml/kg**	**0.8-1.0 ml/kg over 30 minutes**
Maintenance in (non-drinker)	**2-4 ml/kg/h**	**1-2 ml/kg/h**	**0.2-0.4 ml/kg/h**	**0.07 ml/kg/h**
Maintenance during hemodialysis	**4-7 ml/kg/h**	**2-3.5 ml/kg/h**	**0.4-0.7 ml/kg/h**	**0.25 ml/kg/h**
Maintenance dose in chronic drinker		**1.96 mg/kg/h**	**0.46 ml/kg/h**	**0.32 ml/kg/h**

Hemodialysis efficiently removes ethylene glycol and its toxic metabolites. It is indicated:

a. In suspected cases of ethylene glycol poisoning with osmolar gap of over 10 mosm/L not accounted for by ethanol or other alcohols or if ethylene glycol concentration is above 20-50 mg/dl.
b. If renal failure is present.
   Dialysis should be continued until osmolar and anion gaps are normalized. **Ethanol infusion must be increased during dialysis. Patients should continue to receive ethanol atleast 24 hours after the last dialysis to avoid rebound increase in levels of ethylene glycol.**

Folic acid: It enhances the conversion of glyoxylic acid to non-toxic products.

Dose: 50 mg IV every 4 hours.

Pyridoxine: It enhances metabolic conversion of the glyoxylic acid to the non toxic product—glycine.

Dose: 50 mg IV or IM every 6 hours untill intoxication resolves.

Thiamine: It is given in ethylene glycol poisoning as it acts as a cofactor in the metabolism of glyoxylic acid.

Dose: Adults: 100 mg slow IV (over 5 minutes) or IM repeat every 6 hours.

Children: 50 mg slow IV (over 5 minutes) or IM repeat every 6 hours.

ETHYLENE GLYCOL MONO BUTYL ETHER (EGMBE), MONOETHYL AND MONOMETHYL ETHER

All belong to the group of chemicals called as glycols and are used extensively in industry and other areas and show common clinical picture during toxicity. **Their symptoms and management is common.**

Ethylene glycomonobutyl ether	*Ethylene glycolmonoethylether*	*Ethylenglycolmono methylether*
LD_{50}-(oral) Mouse a. 1230 mg/kg	LD_{50}-(Intraperitoneal) Mouse a. 1710 mg/kg	LD_{50}-(Intraperitoneal) Mouse a. 2147 mg/kg
LD_{50}-(Inhalation) Rat a. 2900 mg/kg —	LD_{50}-(oral) Mouse a. 4310 mg/kg LD_{50}-(oral) Rat a. 3000 mg/kg b. 3460 mg/kg	LD_{50}-(oral) Mouse a. 2560 mg/kg LD_{50}-(Intraperitoneal) Rat a. 2500 mg/kg
LD_{50}-(oral) Rat a. 1480 mg/kg b. 470 mg/kg	LD_{50}-(Subcutaneous) Rat a. 3160 mg/kg	LD_{50}-(oral) Rat a. 2370 mg/kg b. 2460 mg/kg (inhalation) Rat 25 ppm TcLO-(inhalation) human a. 25 ppm = CNS

Signs and Symptoms

Levels of 432 μg/ml have been associated with coma, hypotension and acidosis without an osmolar gap, oxalate crystals or renal dysfunction.

Management

Same as with other **Ethylene glycol** *(Refer page 122)*.

ETRIMFOS (Organophosphorus compound)

E

It belongs to organophosphorus group of widely used pesticides that may cause acute or chronic poisoning. It is a relatively less toxic organophosphorus compound with LD_{50} of 1800 mg/kg.

Signs, Symptoms and Management

Same as with other **Organophosphorus compounds** *(Refer page 219)*.

F

FENFLURAMINE

It is used to suppress appetite.

Symptoms of Toxicity

Euphoria, talkativeness, restlessness, tachycardia, peripheral vasoconstriction, tachypnea, tremors and dilated pupils may occur. Nausea, vomiting, facial flushing and sweating are other symptoms.

Confusion, delirium, hallucinations, paranoia are prominent symptoms.

Serious vascular, cardiac and neurological complications sumilar to cocaine and related products are also seen with this drug.

It can precipitate complications such as dissection of the aorta, myocarditis, myocardial infarction, dilated cardiomyopathy, cerebral infarction, transient cerebral ischaemic attacks, hyperpyrexia, convulsions, metabolic acidosis, impaired consciousness, impaired respiration, and paranoid psychosis.

Clinical Presentation: Nausea and vomiting frequently occur within 30-60 minutes after ingestion. Other symptoms are muscle weakness, tetanic contractions, respiratory muscle weakness and respiratory arrest. Cardiac arrhythmias may be associated with hypocalcemia, hypomagnesemia and hyperkalemia.

Management

There is no specific antidote available. Treatment is mainly symptomatic.

Activated charcoal to be administered

Maintain proper airway. Adequate ventilation is imperative if consciousness is impaired.

Arterial blood gas tension should be measured.

Hypoxia and metabolic acidosis corrected as required.

Convulsions and agitation: Should be managed in the usual way **(Diazepam** I.V. followed by either phenytoin or phenobarbitone).

Hypertension is controlled with **labetol** I.V. at a rate of 2 mg/min and escalated according to response, maximum dose should not exceed 200 mg/day.

Propranolol should be avoided because it can cause paradoxical increase in blood pressure so the use of any B-adrenoceptor blocker is contraindicated in control of hypertension due to feafluramine.

Arrhythmias: Extreme tachycardia due to this drug responds to beta adrenoreceptor blockers but extreme caution is necessary.

While other cardiac arrhythmias should not be treated unless life threatening.

Forced diuresis should not be produced because it can lead to serious trouble in case patient has hypertension and dysarrhythmias.

FENITROTHION (Organophosphorns Compound)

It is an organophosphorus compound.

Clinical Picture and Treatment

Same as of other **Organophosphorus drugs** *(Refer page 219).*

FENSULFOTHION (Organophosphorus Compound)

It belongs to organophosphorus group of widely used pesticides that may cause acute or chronic poisoning. It is a highly toxic organophosphorus compound with an LD_{50} of 2 mg/kg.

Clinical picture is same as with other organophosphorus compounds and the toxicity due to this agent is managed as of other organophosphates.

FENTANYL (Opioid Synthetic)

It is an opioid and is used for its analgesic activity and also in combination with droperidol to produce neuroleptanalgesia.

Clinical Features and Management

Same as of other **Opioids** *(Refer page 215).*

FENTHION (Organophosphorus compound)

It belongs to organophosphorus group of widely used pesticides that may cause acute or chronic poisoning. It is a moderately toxic organophosphorus compound with **LD_{50} of 250 mg/kg.**

Signs Symptoms and Management

Same as with other **Organophosphorus compounds** *(Refer page 219).*

FERRIC AMMONIUM CITRATE, FERROUS SULPHATE, FERROUS FUMARATE (Haematinics)

These are commonly used hematinics available over the counter. These are most common cause of childood accidental ingestions and the leading cause of fatal poisonings in children.

Toxicity depends on the amount of elemental iron present in the preparation.

Ferrous sulphate (hydrate)–20% elemental iron.

Ferrous sulphate (dried)–37% elemental iron.

Ferrous fumarate–33% elemental iron.

It is advisable to calculate the amount of iron ingested.

To get the amount of elemental iron ingested multiply the total mg of iron compound ingested by the % iron in the preparation.

Toxic dose: Toxicity is likely following ingestion of over 20 mg/kg elemental iron.

Most pediatric iron formulations contain 12-18 mg of elemental iron per dose while most adult preparations contain 60-80 mg of elemental iron per dose. The fatal amount of elemental iron is estimated to be between 180 and 300 mg/kg body weight. **Serious toxicity** occurs when 60 mg or more elemental iron/kg bodyweight has been ingested.

Toxic serum iron levels:

Mild toxicity >450-500 μg/dl.

Severe toxicity >800-1000 μg/dl.

Total iron-binding capacity is unreliable in iron overdose.

Symptoms of Toxicity

Most of the toxic effects are due to hemorrhagic necrosis in the GIT often leading to perforation. Absorbed iron causes cellular dysfunction resulting in lactic acidosis and necrosis. Clinical course runs in 4 phases.

Clinical Toxicity and Management

For details see **Iron** *(Refer page 160).*

F

FLOCOUMAFAN (Anticoagulant)

Symptoms

With ingestion of long acting preparation of this drug: bruising haematuria and menorrhagia, other symptoms can include backache, bleeding lips, mucus membranes hemorrhages, abdominal pain, vomiting and petechial rash. Later paralysis due to cerebral hemorrhage shock and death may occur.

Management

Cholestyramine orally enhances the elimination. Cholestyramine 4 gms orally in fruit juice every 6 hours before meals.

Parenteral vitamin K_1 60 mg/day with infusion of fresh frozen plasma.

FLUORIDE

It is used in petroleum industry, glass etching industry, aluminium production, vitamins or dietary supplements and tooth pastes to prevent dental caries.

Uses

Sodium fluoride, sodium duosilicate and crayolite are used as insecticides and rodenticides.

Sodium or stannous fluoride is used in tooth pastes. Fluoride promotes resistance of tooth decay in children.

Fluoride can increase the density and calcification of bone. It is recommended for individuals with osteoporosis.

It is commonly added to community drinking water in the west in India chronic toxicity is common as subsoil water in certain regions has high flouride content. It is also found in hydrofluoric acid. One cup of tea contains 1-4 mg fluoride. Acute toxicity is not common in India.

Management

Maintain patent airway and assist ventilation if necessary. Induce emesis or perform gastric lavage.

Activated charcoal does not absorb fluoride and is not likely to be beneficial.

Monitor ECG and serum calcium for at least 4-6 hours and admit symptomatic patients to intensive care setting.

Specific drugs and antidotes: When clinically significant hypocalcemia is present administer intravenous calcium (10-20 ml). Correct hypomagnesemia with intravenous magnesium sulfate (1-2 g).

Administer calcium salts e.g. calcium carbonate (TUMS), calcium lactate to form insoluble complexes with fluoride, thereby, minimizing absorption. For initial treatment of children at home who have ingested more than 5-10 mg/kg elemental fluoride, ipecac induced emesis may be useful.

Although fluoride is a small ion with minimal protein binding, it rapidly binds to free calcium and bone therefore **hemodialysis and hemoperfusion are unlikely to be beneficial.**

FLUORINATED HYDROCARBONS

Most fluorinated hydrocarbons are gases in their natural state. Dibromotetrafluoroethane is a liquid. Fluorinated compounds (e.g. enflurane, isoflurane) are used as anesthetic drugs. Flourinated hydrocarbons are used as refrigerants, industrial solvents, fire extinguishers, local anaesthetics, glass chillers, propellant in aerosols.

Uses of these compounds has been reduced due to its effects on ozone layer of the atmosphere.

Symptoms

Systemic effects of moderate exposure include headache, nausea and vomiting, mental confusion and appearance of drunkenness.

Management

Patient be evacuated from toxic environment, clothes removed and skin washed. No specific treatment is available. Management is symptomatic.

Maintain airway and assist ventilation if necessary.

Treat coma and arrhythmias if they occur. Avoid epinephrine or other sympathomimetic amines that may precipitate ventricular arrhythmias. Monitor ECG for 4-6 hours.

Inhalation: Remove victim from exposure and give supplemental oxygen if available.

On ingestion: Administer activated charcoal if available. Do not induce emesis because of rapid absorption and the risk of abrupt onset of central nervous system depression. Cathartic to be administered with charcoal.

There is no evidence for efficacy of diuresis, hemodialysis, hemoperfusion or repeat dose charcoal.

F

FLUOROACETATE (SMFA)

It is also known as compound Moso sodium monofluoroacetate (SMFA) and **sodium fluoroacetate is one of the most toxic substances known.** It is a tasteless, odorless, water soluble white crystalline powder.

Management

There is no specific antidote therefore symptomatic treatment is recommended.

Maintain the airway and assist ventilation if necessary. Administer supplemental oxygen.

Replace fluid losses due to gastroenteritis with intravenous saline or other suitable crystalloids.

Treat shock, seizures (diazepam followed by phenytoin or phenobarbitone) and coma if they occur. Monitor the ECG for at least 4-6 hours.

Activated charcoal: Administer activated charcoal and a purgative.

Skin exposure: Remove contaminated clothing and wash exposed skin thoroughly.

There is no role for forced diuresis and dialysis.

FLUOXETINE (Anti Depressant)

It is a selective serotonin reuptake inhibitor and is commonly used as an antidepressant.

Experience of overdosage with this drug is limited.

Therapeutic dose: Differs from patient to patient, but lies in the range of 20 to 60 mg/day.

Toxicity: Ingestion of 40 to 800 mg have produced minimal toxicity.

Seizures have been reported in adults after ingestion of 900 mg or more.

LD_{50}–(oral) mouse: 248 mg/kg.

LD_{50}–(oral) rat: 452 mg/kg.

Symptoms

a. **With therapeutic dose:** Adverse effects that may appear are: seizures, suicidal ideation, mania and paranoia, EPS, cardiac arrhythmia, hyponatremia and SIADH like symptoms. Serotonin syndrome also occurs.

b. **With poisoning:**
   i. Doses of 40 to 800 mg produce minimal, if any symptoms.
   ii. Effects in overdose include–blurred vision, vomiting, lethargy, dizziness, insomnia, diarrhoea, tremors, abdominal pain and rarely seizures.
   iii. Significant CVS toxicity is unusual but mild hypertension, tachycardia, bigeminy junctional rhythm and QTc prolongation have been reported.

Management

Supportive and symptomatic measures are required. **Repeated administration of activated charcoal is also beneficial.**

F

FLURAZEPAM (Benzodrazepine)

It is one of the benzodiazepines used for short term management of insomnia.

Symptoms

Mild: Drowsiness, ataxia, weakness.

Moderate to severe: Apathy, dizziness, lethargy, slurred speech, partial ptosis, nystagmus but **response to verbal stimuli may remain intact.** Hypotension respiratory depression are responsible for fatal outcome.

Management

Specific: Flumazenil. Adult - 0.2 mg I/V given over 30 sec. Repeat at 20 minutes interval. Maximum dose should not exceed 3 mg in an hour except in profound coma.

Supportive:

Gastric lavage:

Activated charcoal (if available) is helpful.

Adequate oxygenation, provide ventilatory support if required.

IV fluids.

Administer Dopamine at the rate of:

4-6 μg/kg/min intravenously.

F

FONOFOS (Organophosphorus Compound)

It belongs to organophosphorus group of widely used pesticides that may cause acute or chronic poisoning. It is a highly toxic organophosphorus compound with an LD_{50} of 8-17.5 mg/kg.

Clinical Picture

Same as with other **Organophosphorus compounds.**

The toxicity due to this agent is managed as other **Organophosphates** *(Refer page 219).*

FOOD POISONING: BACTERIAL

Food borne illness remains the most common cause of epidemic gastroenteritis.

Systemic infection in India can result from Salmonella, Shigella or Listeria.

Symptoms

Nausea, vomiting, abdominal cramps and diarrhoea. Fluid and electrolyte abnormalities may occur, especially in young children or elderly patients.

Fever, bloody stools and leukocytosis are common with invasive bacterial infections.

The presence of many white blood cells in a stool smear suggests invasive bacterial infection.

Management

Emergency and supportive measures: Replace fluid and electrolyte losses with intravenous saline or other crystalloid solutions. Patients with hypotension should be given large volumes of intravenous fluid. Resuscitation may be necessary.

Strong antidiarrhoeal agents such as lomotil should not be used because it may prolong the course of the infection.

Specific drugs and antidotes: There are no specific antidotes—except anti-microbial agents and these may be used once the stool culture reveals specific bacteria.

Pregnant women who have eaten Listeria contaminated food should be treated empirically even if only mildly symptomatic to prevent serious intrauterine infection. The antibiotic of choice is **ampicillin with gentamicin** added for treatment of severe infection.

FORMALDEHYDE (37% Formalin)

Often used as preservative in pathology.

Industrial/Household uses: It is used in fertilizers, insecticides, germicides, fungicides, herbicides, sewage treatment, paper making, preservative, dye fasteners, explosives, plywood, air freshners, cosmetics, wet tingement hardners and polishes, in hair shampoos, conditioners, water based paints.

It is present in building materials, insulations and items such as glues, preservatives, permanent press fabrics and other household products.

In smoking tobacco or marijuana that has been soaked in HCHO.

Symptoms of Poisoning due to ingestion:

Local effects: Burns on lips, oral mucosa, upper airway and oesophagus.

GIT: Drooling stridor, vomiting and gastrointestinal bleeding.

On Inhalation

Oedema of upper airway, dyspnea, wheezing, pulmonary oedema, pneumonitis, respiratory failure.

Exposure of eyes: Conjunctival irritation, corneal perforation, distortion of cellular membranes, loss of epithelium of cornea, conjuctiva and lens.

Skin exposure: Pain, redness, irritation, full thickness burns on skin.

Management

In case of ingestion:

Avoid inducing vomiting as well as gastric lavage.

Administer water or milk so that acid can be diluted. Irrigate mouth frequently in patients who are cooperative and conscious.

In case of inhalation: Patient should be removed from site of exposure and shifted to fresh air.

In case of eye exposure: Depending upon severity, irrigate with large volumes of 0.9% normal saline or water for 15 minutes or more.

Eyes should not be washed with soap solution. Remove contact lenses.

Wash affected skin with copious amounts of water or mild soap solution for atleast 6-8 hours.

In case of airway compromise undertake endotracheal intubation.

F

Administer 100% humidified oxygen for inhalation. Use respirator if available and if deemed necessary. Suction should be done using soft nasogastric tube.

IV fluids—the volume should be determined according to the condition of the patient. Vasopressors (dopamine) can be used if necessary.

Endoscopy should be performed within first 24 hours to detect absence or presence of perforation.

Chest X-ray for detecting mediastinitis or GI perforation.

Administer antibiotics if there is perforation.

Laparotomy should be done in case endoscopy reveals necrosis of oesophagus or stomach or when signs and symptoms of GI perforation are evident at the time of initial presentation and surgical treatment given.

FORMIC ACID (Organic Acid)

In Industry: It is used as a component of descaling and stain removing agents.

In Agriculture: It is used as an animal feed additive, food preservative, flavor enhancer and antiseptic.

In Therapeutics: It is used for removal of tattoos in skin.

As a food additive in small amounts (0.1 to 6 ppm) in icecreams, ices, candy and baked goods.

Symptoms of Toxicity

In case of ingestion: Severe burning pain in the mouth, throat, abdomen, dysphagia, gastritis, vomiting, diarrhoea (bloody, mucoid) hypotension with cold clammy skin and rapid pulse. Metabolic acidosis, hemolysis, massive fluid and electrolyte shifts (hyperkalemia, hyperphosphatemia, hypocalcemia and hyperchloremia) can occur.

In case of inhalation: Cough, dyspnea, pleuritic chest pain, pulmonary oedema, frothy sputum, hemoptysis, bronchospasm, hypoxia, pain in eyes and lacrimation.

In case of eye exposure: Irritation, pain, lacrimation, swelling, chemosis, photophobia, corneal erosion and perforation, necrosis of conjunctiva and cornea.

In case of dermal exposure: Burning pain, irritation, redness and blistering ulceration.

Management

In case of inhalation: Patient should be shifted to fresh air.

In case of eye exposure: Irrigate with large volumes of 0.9% normal saline or water for 15 minutes or more depending upon severity.

Eyes should not be washed with soap solution.

Wash affected skin with copious amounts of water or mild soap solution.

In case of Ingestion:

Do not induce vomiting.

Administer water or milk with a view to dilute poison and reduce irritation.

Do not give gastric lavage.

Endotracheal intubation to be done in case of airway obstruction.

Administer 100% humidified oxygen with assisted ventilation.

Suction should be done by soft nasogastric tube.

Irrigate mouth with water in cooperative patients or intubate unconscious patients.

Administer IV fluids, according to the need of the patient (saline or dopamine).

Vasopressors to be given if there is hypovolumea/ hypotension.

Antibiotics to prevent development of infections.

Exploratory endoscopy done within first 24 hours to detect perforation and chest X-ray for detection of mediastinitis or GI perforation.

Perform laparotomy in case endoscopy reveals grade B burns with thickness, necrosis of oesophagus or stomach or when signs and symptoms of GI perforation are evident at the time of initial presentation.

Precautions

Do not give excessive amount of milk or water as it provokes vomiting.

Do not give carbonated beverages or bicarbonate for neutralization.

FURNITURE POLISHES

Symptoms

Vomiting is common while diarrhoea is uncommon.

F

There may be initially some excitement, but in severe poisoning drowsiness is seen which may lead to coma.

The most common complication of this poisoning is pulmonary troubles which occur in about 60% of the cases and results from aspiration of the poison into the bronchial tree. This results into cough, choking, wheezing and breathlessness.

Clinical evidence of respiratory involvement is usually evident within few months after poisoning but in some cases it may be delayed for hours but not more than a day. Severe poisoning can cause hemorrhagic pulmonary oedema which is fatal. Pneumonities in most of the cases involves two or more lobes and is peripheral in distribution. Fever and polymorph leukocytes are common.

Rare complications include pneumatocele formation, intravascular hemolysis and renal failure.

Diagnosis of hydrocarbon ingestion may be confirmed by finding a double gastric level on the X-ray of the abdomen taken in the erect position.

Management

Gastric emptying is favoured if sufficiently large amount of the poison has been ingested, provided patient is sufficiently alert so that he can cough effectively and second the airway should be protected by cuffed entotracheal tube.

Indications for gastric emptying:

If the amount of ingested amount is more than 1 ml/kg of body weight.

Or

The solution contains another toxin (such as pesticide)

Or

Signs of serious poisoning are evident.

Antibiotics should be given in only those patients who develop secondary bacterial infection.

If cyanosis is present, oxygen may be necessary. Intermittant positive pressure is indicated for patients with pulmonary oedema.

Pulmonery oedema is treated with frusemide IV and morphine.